MANAGEMENT OF THE BURNED PATIENT

Edited by

Bruce M. Achauer, M.D.

Associate Adjunct Professor of Surgery
Director, Burn Center
University of California, Irvine Medical Center
Orange, California

Appleton & Lange

Norwalk, Connecticut/Los Altos, California

0-8385-6116-0

Notice: Our knowledge in clinical sciences is constantly changing. As new information becomes available, changes in treatment and in the use of drugs become necessary. The author(s) and the publisher of this volume have taken care to make certain that the doses of drugs and schedules of treatment are correct and compatible with the standards generally accepted at the time of publication. The reader is advised to consult carefully the instruction and information material included in the package insert of each drug or therapeutic agent before administration. This advice is especially important when using new or infrequently used drugs.

Copyright © 1987 by Appleton & Lange
A Publishing Division of Prentice-Hall

All rights reserved. This book, or any parts thereof, may not be used or reproduced in any manner without written permission. For information, address Appleton & Lange, 25 Van Zant Street, East Norwalk, Connecticut 06855.

87 88 89 90 91 / 10 9 8 7 6 5 4 3 2 1

Prentice-Hall of Australia, Pty. Ltd., Sydney
Prentice-Hall Canada, Inc.
Prentice-Hall Hispanoamericana, S.A., Mexico
Prentice-Hall of India Private Limited, New Delhi
Prentice-Hall International (UK) Limited, London
Prentice-Hall of Japan, Inc., Tokyo
Prentice-Hall of Southeast Asia (Pte.) Ltd., Singapore
Whitehall Books Ltd., Wellington, New Zealand
Editora Prentice-Hall do Brasil Ltda., Rio de Janeiro

Library of Congress Cataloging-in-Publication Data

Management of the burned patient.

   Includes index.
   1. Burns and scalds—Treatment.   I. *Achauer*, Bruce M.
[*DNLM:* 1. Burns—complications.   2. Burns—therapy.
WO 704 M2661]
RD96.4.M345 1987   617'.1106   86-28691
ISBN 0-8385-6116-0

Design: Kathleen E. Peters

PRINTED IN THE UNITED STATES OF AMERICA

TO THE BURN TEAM

This work was prepared by members of several U.S. burn teams. The concept of individuals working as a unit to achieve a goal otherwise unobtainable is crucial to modern burn care. As with any team effort, each member must compromise and keep the overall goals uppermost, constantly modifying personal priorities. Because of these selfless attitudes, tremendous gains have been made in burn care and rehabilitation. Not only are more patients surviving their injury, they are recovering more rapidly with less pain and complications and being returned to enjoyable and productive lives. Along with these advances, it is becoming more acceptable in the medical world to be involved in burn care. Long a step-child in the hierarchy of medicine, the immense personal rewards of burn care are starting to be realized by more and more people. This is team work! A lot of work remains to be done and effective teams are the key to success. This book is dedicated to these wonderful people.

ACKNOWLEDGMENTS

The majority of manuscript preparation was done by the secretaries of the Division of Plastic Surgery at the University of California, Irvine. Initially, Kathleen Mitchell-Welch had the project, then the very capable Lillian Richmond. Final drafts and correspondance was handled by the Administrative Assistant, Janet Inkster. Their efforts are greatly appreciated. John Brown of Orange, California did the excellent illustrations in chapters 6 and 8.

Contributors

Bruce M. Achauer, M.D.
Assoc. Adjunct Professor of Surgery, Director, Burn Center, University of California Irvine Medical Center, Orange, California

Louis A. Bonaldi, M.D.
Chief Resident, Division of Plastic and Reconstructive Surgery, University of California San Diego, La Jolla, California

Linda Chilstrom Giel, R.D.
Clinical Dietician, University of California Irvine Medical Center, Orange, California

William T. Choctaw, M.D.
Medical Director Burn Team, Queen of the Valley Hospital, West Covina, California; Assistant Clinical Professor of Surgery, Charles Drew Postgraduate School of Medicine, Los Angeles, California

Philip A. Edelman, M.D.
Chief Toxicology Service and Regional Poison Center, Consultant Burn Center, University of California Irvine Medical Center, Orange, California

Martin E. Eisner, M.D.
Assistant Clinical Professor of Surgery, University of California Irvine Medical Center, Orange, California; Surgical Director Intensive Care Unit, Western Medical Center, Santa Ana, California

David H. Frank, M.D.
Associate Professor of Surgery, Division of Plastic and Reconstructive Surgery, University of California San Diego, La Jolla, California

Joyce K. Friedmann, Ph.D.
Associate Clinical Professor of Psychiatry, Surgery, and Family Medicine, Chief of Mental Health Services Burn Center, University of California Irvine Medical Center, Orange, California

John German, M.D.
Assistant Clinical Professor of Surgery, University of Irvine Medical Center, Orange, California

Suzanne E. Martinez, R.N., M.S.N.
Nursing Manager, Burn Center, University of California Medical Center, Orange, California

Anthony A. Meyer, Ph.D., M.D.
Medical Director of Critical Care, Director, Surgical Intensive Care Unit, Assistant Director, North Carolina Jaycee Burn Center, Department of Surgery, North Carolina Memorial Hospital/University of North Carolina, Chapel Hill, North Carolina

Lawrence Plon, Pharm.D.
Associate Clinical Professor Psychiatry, Pharmacist Specialist, University of California Irvine Medical Center, Orange, California; Assistant Clinical Professor of Pharmacy, University of California, San Francisco, California

Robert M. Schneider, O.T.R.
Senior Occupational Therapist, Burn Center, University of California Irvine Medical Center, Orange, California

Johanna Shapiro, Ph.D.
Associate Professor, Director of Behavioral Science Program, Department of Family Medicine, University of California Irvine Medical Center, Orange, California

Shirley Simonton-Thorne, O.T.R., United Kingdom Diploma of Occupational Therapy
Senior Occupational Therapist, University of California Irvine Medical Center, Orange, California

James W. Thornton, M.D.
University of Michigan Medical Center, Instructor of Surgery, Section of Plastic and Reconstructive Surgery, University of Michigan, Ann Arbor, Michigan

Donald D. Trunkey, M.D.
Chairman, Department of Surgery, University of Oregon, Portland, Oregon

Naomi Uchiyama, M.D.
Assistant Clinical Professor, Department of Pediatrics, University of California Irvine Medical Center, Orange, California; Family Health Programs, Fountain Valley, California

Thomas L. Wachtel, M.D., F.A.C.S.
Director, Trauma Service and Burn Service, Good Samaritan Medical Center, Phoenix, Arizona; Clinical Associate Professor of Surgery, University of Arizona College of Medicine, Tucson, Arizona; Associate Clinical Professor of Surgery, University of California, San Diego School of Medicine, San Diego, California; Adjunct Professor, Chemical and Bio-Engineering, Arizona State University, Tempe, Arizona

Glenn D. Warden, M.D.
Chief of Staff, Shriners Burns Institute, Cincinnati Unit, Shrine Professor of Surgery, University of Cincinnati College of Medicine, Cincinnati, Ohio

Kenneth Waxman, M.D.
Associate Professor, Department of Surgery, University of California Irvine, Orange, California

Contents

Foreword xi
Introduction xiii

I. THE BURN PROBLEM 1

1. Causes, Prevention, Prehospital Care, Evaluation, Emergency Treatment, and Prognosis 3
   William T. Choctaw, Martin E. Eisner, and Thomas L. Wachtel

2. Pathophysiology of the Burn Wound 21
   Louis A. Bonaldi and David H. Frank

3. Immunology 49
   Glenn D. Warden

II. INITIAL THERAPY 65

4. Resuscitation 67
   James W. Thornton

5. Monitoring 79
   Kenneth Waxman

III. CARE OF THE BURN WOUND 91

6. Treating the Burn Wound 93
   Bruce M. Achauer

7. Outpatient Burns 109
   Suzanne E. Martinez

8. Extremities 121
   Bruce M. Achauer

IV.	SYSTEMIC EFFECTS	133
9.	Nutrition *Linda Chilstrom Giel*	135
10.	Pulmonary Management *Kenneth Waxman*	149
11.	Preventing and Treating Complications *Anthony A. Meyer and Donald D. Trunkey*	161
V.	SPECIAL CONSIDERATIONS	181
12.	Chemical and Electrical Burns *Philip A. Edelman*	183
13.	Pediatric Considerations *Naomi Uchiyama and John German*	203
VI.	RECOVERY AND REHABILITATION	211
14.	Nursing and the Burn Team *Suzanne E. Martinez*	213
15.	Treament of Joints and Scars *Robert M. Schneider and Shirley Simonton-Thorne*	223
16.	Psychosocial Treatment and Pain Control *Joyce K. Friedmann, Johanna Shapiro, and Lawrence Plon*	243
Index		263

Foreword

Burns can be a devastating form of trauma. Large segments of our society experience lesser burns, but it is the serious burn injury that is such a catastrophic event. These large and complicated injuries may be life threatening as a result of the complex pathophysiologic and metabolic processes involved—shock, infection, and the resultant multiple organ failure. Those burn victims who survive the sequelae often face prolonged hospitalizations associated with painful treatments, frequent operations, multiple complications and very expensive care that may leave unsightly physical and deep emotional scars. For the burned patients who succumb, their course may be every bit as difficult only to end in death days or weeks later despite a valiant effort on the part of both the patient and the burn team. In either category the personnel and resource cost and emotional drain is enormous.

During the past half century and particularly in the last decade great progress has been made in caring for burned patients, reducing morbidity and mortality and increasing the effectiveness of treatment. These improvements have been due to advances in two major areas. The first of these is the rapid growth in cognitive information related primarily to a better understanding of the pathophysiologic effects of burns. The second area of advancement has been through the use of high technology coupled with improved surgical techniques and wide spread utilization of the burn team concept.

The BURN TEAM of coordinated skilled specialists lending expert care to important segments of the burned patient's therapy using a systems approach under the leadership of a Burn Director has revolutionized burn care. Moreover, the development of burn facilities that specialize in the comprehensive care of these complex trauma victims has allowed rapid evaluation and broad application of new skills and knowledge. These developments have led to improved care at every level, from the first responder, to those who transport to the initial hospital caretakers, so that there is exemplary care of the burned patient during each step and phase of their treatment course.

Thus, it has become important for physicians, nurses, emergency services personnel, acute care hospitals, and intensive care providers to have competence in the initial and emergency treatment of the acutely burned patient, so that appropriate therapy as well as comfort, reassurance and confidence can be provided promptly. A review of this book will do much to assure that competent, state-of-the-art burn treatment is rendered.

Dr. Achauer's textbook on burns is comprehensive yet concise. It encompasses the philosophy and techniques of modern burn care. The text is divided into functional segments that identify the problems associated with burns, supply a clear basic understanding of the principles of burn wound care and serve as a springboard for logical therapy of the burned patient, including limiting or even reversing the burn injury.

In areas where controversy exists opposing views are presented but the author selects a course of treatment that is representative of accepted current methodology. The therapy is supported by reasonable theories of the pathophysiology and is directed by both general principles and precise methods and skills of care.

Capturing the voluminous amount of information on burns and burn care and tailoring it into a readable and usable textbook is a monumental task. The authors of each of these chapters have done a remarkable job in accomplishing this goal. There is a wealth of new ideas and new information presented in this treatis. The text is nicely illustrated with figures, photographs and tables to illuminate the more difficult concepts and highlight some of the simple but very important ones. The book should serve as a ready and useful reference for physicians, nurses, emergency department and intensive care unit personnel and technicians responsible for patients with burn injuries.

Thomas L. Wachtel, M.D., F.A.C.S.

Introduction

Our primary goal is a practical guide for the various disciplines caring for the burn patient. Because of the ubiquitous nature of burn injuries, many burn patients are not treated in burn centers. For those who do not see burn patients on a daily basis, this book should serve as a useful guide. Most medical personnel will at some time be involved in burn care. Many surgeons, internists, surgical house officers, medical students, occupational and physical therapists, nurses, nursing students, and psychologists will spend part of their training in a burn center. It is hoped that this book will help them understand the overall plan and purpose of burn care.

Beyond the necessary practical detail of burn treatment lies an understanding of the problems faced by the burn patient. An introduction to these issues is presented. Caring for the thermally traumatized patient presents one of the most challenging, frustrating and rewarding professional experiences encountered in all of the disciplines that converge on the burn patient. We hope that by presenting ideas, bibliographies and a thorough discussion of the pathophysiology we might stimulate the reader to further investigation.

Another major goal was to help each discipline involved in burn care to understand the others' role. Hopefully the discussions are succinct enough to sustain the interest of other members of the burn team. Successful care of the severely burned patient requires the mobilization of a great number of people, equipment and time. Unless all the elements of good burn care are available for every patient at the precise time that they are needed, a less than optimum result occurs. The social worker, psychologist and therapist are just as important in the first few days of injury as the intensive physiologic care. Conversely, successful rehabilitation involves the understanding of intensive care personnel as much as the other disciplines.

PART I
The Burn Problem

CHAPTER 1
Causes, Prevention, Prehospital Care, Evaluation, Emergency Treatment, and Prognosis

William T. Choctaw, Martin E. Eisner, and Thomas L. Wachtel

HISTORY

It took many years for physicians to appreciate the significance of depth of burn injury. This concept evolved over many years. In 1607, Wilheim Fabrey of Hildon presented the first classification of burn in his book, *De Combustionibus*.[1] It was a classification of intensity of surface burns as evaluated by external appearance. During the 18th century, Heister, Dupuytren, Hunter, and Kentish modified Fabrey's original classification of burns by trying to delineate various depths of injury from the external appearance of the burn. During the 19th century, Boyer developed three degrees—first, second, and third—of burn injury. The first authoritative description of burn injury occurred in the 20th century by Sonnenburg and Tachmarke, who distinguished between burns that healed from the edges and those that heal from remaining dermal elements. In 1942, the National Research Council of Canada introduced the terms "partial" and "full thickness" to burn injury. Partial thickness skin loss was characterized by partial loss of the entire epidermis and part of the dermis with remaining growth of tissue from the sweat glands and hair follicles.[2] Full thickness skin loss was characterized by complete destruction of the epidermal and dermal elements causing healing to occur by migration from the wound edge (Fig. 1–1).

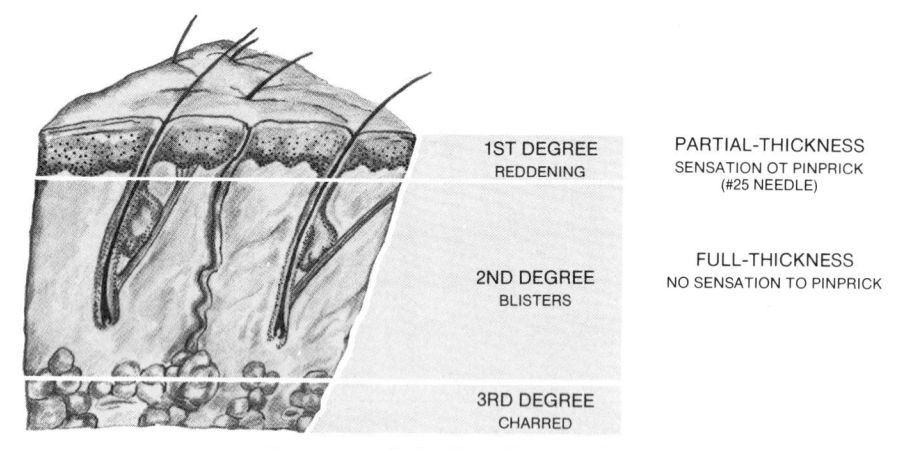

Figure 1-1. Estimation of burn depth.

THE SIZE OF THE BURN PROBLEM

It has been estimated that 1 percent of the population of the United States, i.e., over 2 million people, is burned each year.[3,4] One-half of these injuries are severe enough to cause restriction to daily activities (school, work, housework) or require medical attention (Fig. 1-2). One-fourth of these injuries

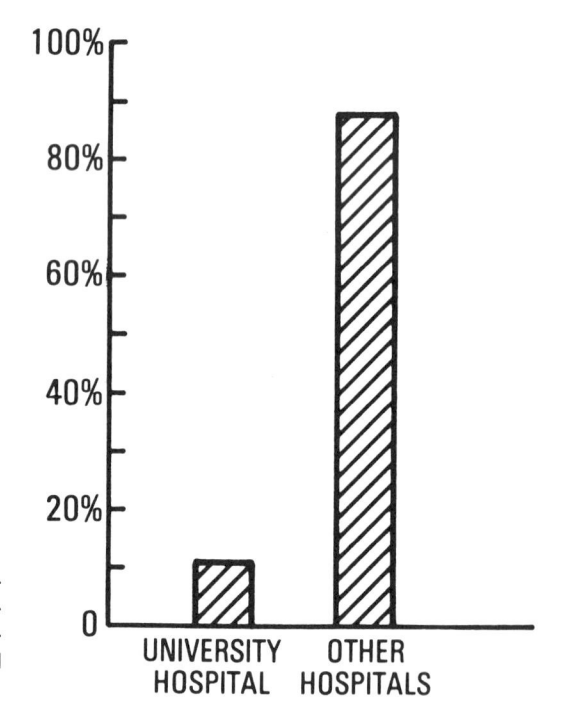

Figure 1-2. Burned patient emergency room visits from the Regional Burn Care System Demonstration Project: San Diego and Imperial Counties, California.

require confinement to bed.[4] Hospital admissions are estimated to be between 70,000 and 108,000. Burn deaths per year are between 6,500 and 12,000 depending on the source of information.[3-5] Property loss from fire and smoke in 1977 was estimated at $3.4 billion excluding automobile fire injuries and deaths.[5]

Burns are distributed unevenly, geographically in this country (Fig. 1–3). People living in the southeastern areas of the United States face a much greater risk of sustaining thermal injuries than do those living in other parts of the country. In Mississippi and South Carolina, death from fire exceeds that from falls.[4] Despite the high standard of health in America, our death rate (4 per 100,000) exceeds that of other civilized nations such as Denmark (1 per 100,000) and England (1.6 per 100,000), even though our survival rates are better than those of England or Denmark.[4] In other parts of the world, particularly in developing nations, the toll from burns is much higher than ours.[6]

SITES OF INJURY

The majority of significant burns occur in the home (68 percent), some in industry (24 percent), and in other places (8 percent).[3,7,8] Moreover, about 75 percent of all deaths from fire occur in the home.[4] Most burns in the home

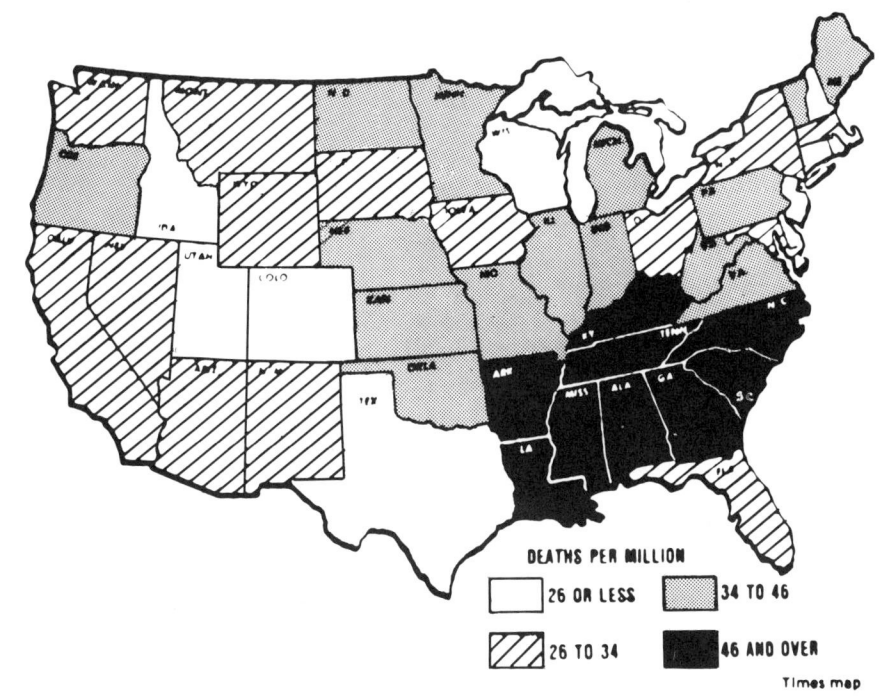

Figure 1–3. State fire death rates. *(Copyright 1980, Los Angeles Times, reprinted with permission.)*

occur in the kitchen followed closely by the bathroom. Most lethal burns, however, occur in the bedroom.[3] Many of these are related to smoke and toxic gases produced by the fire rather than the victims actually being burned.[3] These figures vary with the socioeconomic status of the victims, the type of home, household energy sources, and the frequency of light or heavy industry in the area.

The burns often involve the upper extremity (71 percent) or the head and neck (52 percent) regions of the body (Fig. 1–4) The upright nature of the human being and the attempts to extinguish the fire or remove scalding clothing may explain the predilection for these smaller anatomic areas sustaining the majority of the burns. The causes of burns are shown in Figures 1–5 and 1–6.

FIRE PREVENTION

Prevention is the most effective and least expensive form of burn treatment. There are two types of preventive programs—educational and environmental change. The first involves changing human behavior and the second usually involves regulations or new technology.

Fire and smoke detectors are relatively inexpensive and provide an early warning necessary to allow all to exit safely. Inherent in this concept is a plan

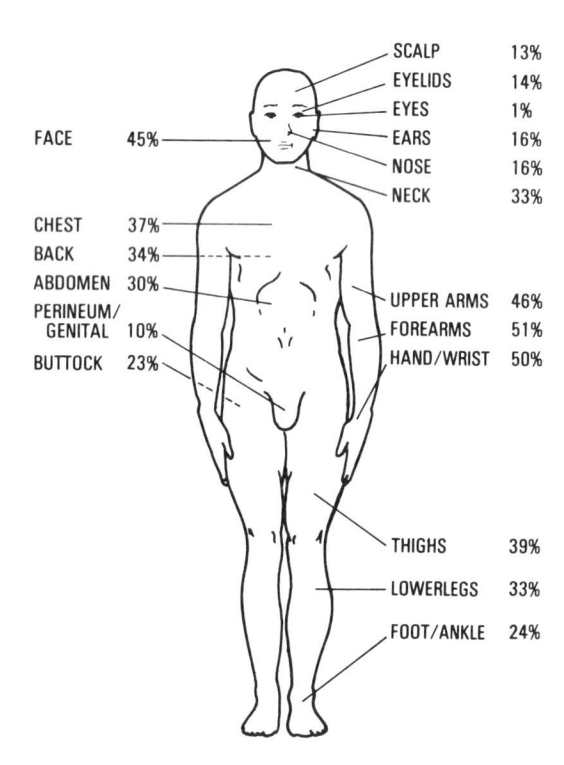

Figure 1–4. Frequency of anatomical regions burned in 939 patients admitted to the Regional Burn Center, UCSD. *(From Wachtel TL, Frank DH, Frank HA: Management of burns of the head and neck. Head Neck Surg 3:458, 1981, reprinted with permission.)*

Region	%
FACE	45%
SCALP	13%
EYELIDS	14%
EYES	1%
EARS	16%
NOSE	16%
NECK	33%
CHEST	37%
BACK	34%
ABDOMEN	30%
PERINEUM/GENITAL	10%
BUTTOCK	23%
UPPER ARMS	46%
FOREARMS	51%
HAND/WRIST	50%
THIGHS	39%
LOWERLEGS	33%
FOOT/ANKLE	24%

1. CAUSES, PREVENTION, CARE, AND PROGNOSIS   7

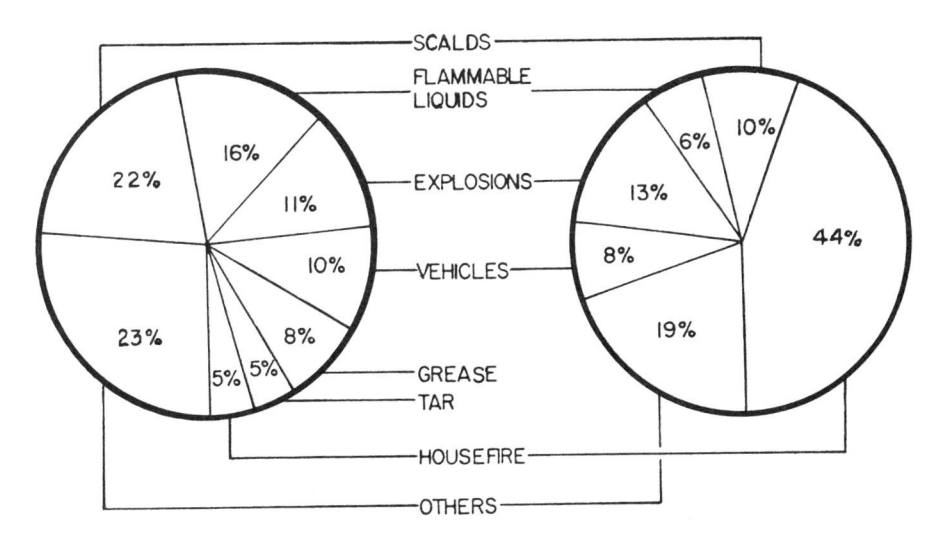

Figure 1-5. Burn injury: Adults. *(From Jay KM, Bartlett RJ, Danet R, Allyn PA: Burn epidemiology: A basis for burn prevention. J Trauma 17:945, 1977, reprinted with permission.)*

for exiting the home (or school, work place, hospital, hotel, or building). Fire survival skills must be learned; they are not instinctive.[3]

Automatic fire suppression systems are thought to be too expensive for the home, but some areas are starting to require them. Their use has shown a dramatic decrease in burns and fire deaths in public buildings. Appropriate

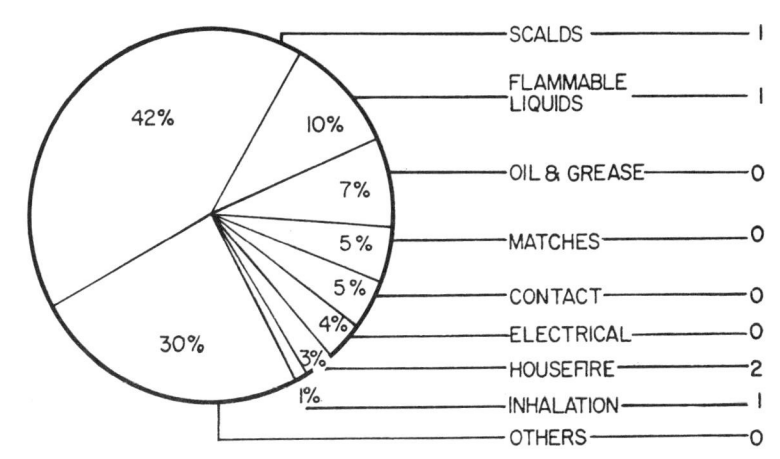

Figure 1-6. Burn injury: Children. *(From Jay KM, Bartlett RJ, Danet R, Allyn PA: Burn epidemiology: A basis for burn prevention. J Trauma 17:946, 1977, reprinted with permission.)*

storage and use of fuel, flammable aerosol products, and chemicals is easy to recite, but much more difficult to put into practice.[3] Home storage of gasoline was particularly disastrous during the gasoline shortage.

Decreasing the hot water temperature at the outlets to 120°F (49°C) by reducing the hot water heater temperature appropriately would eliminate most household scalds and save energy (and dollars).[3,9]

Kitchen safety improvements could result in dramatic decreases in burn injury. Some of these measures are turning the handles of vessels on the stove inward, using pot holders or mitts, using only rear burners whenever possible, not allowing the cords of appliances to hang over the counter top, using only low profile designed vessels and safety tea kettles on the stove, and keeping children away when hot liquids are being prepared and transported. Keeping matches out of reach of children is also very important.

Many burn injuries and nearly one-half the burn deaths result from lit cigarettes and other smoking materials.[9] Many involve secondary ignition of fabric or upholstery. Thus, another area of potentially high public benefit is in the development and widespread use of "fire safe cigarettes." Chemicals added to the cigarettes and cigarette design prevent the cigarette from self-extinguishing when it is unattended and not being smoked.[9] As a result, cigarettes continue to burn for up to 45 minutes instead of self-extinguishing in 4 to 5 minutes if unattended. We have the technology to make a safer cigarette that would have a lesser potential for fires and burn injuries.[9]

Fire retardant fabrics are available and required for new children's sleepwear (Flammable Fabrics Act of 1967 with 1974 extension). Fire safety standards for hospital sleepwear, carpets, and mattresses have eliminated many burns among the elderly and those with hindrance of self-care. The one major area not covered is the fabric used for most clothing, especially the daytime clothing worn by children.[3] Except where the law requires immediate replacement, old, flammable fabrics, sleepwear, mattresses, and tents will be eliminated gradually from our society because it is unlikely that usable goods will be thrown away. In fact, by giving these items to charitable organizations, this practice may continue to be reflected in a higher incidence of burns among the lower socioeconomic groups discussed before. Cotton, cotton-polyester, rayon, and linen are at the high end of the scale and burn most rapidly, whereas fiberglass, asbestos, and metallic fabrics are almost flameproof.[3] People in high thermal environments (e.g., firemen, race drivers, aviators) have already realized the benefits of state of the art fire retardant fabrics for reducing burn injuries.[3] The design, fit, weave, weight, texture, and composition of the fabric determine the specific hazard in any given situation. A tightly woven, close fitting, heavy fabric that has a smooth texture presents a much lower risk of ignition than a loose fitting, loosely woven, lightweight fabric with a fuzzy finish.[3]

Crash-worthy fuel systems in automobiles and general aviation would prevent many burn injuries and decrease the number of multimillion dollar settlements for unsafe fuel systems.[9] Electronic pilot lights would decrease accidental ignitions and perhaps lower the incidence of asphyxia from gas leaks as well. Banning fireworks except for well-controlled public displays and public "fire" acts by rock groups would prevent additional burn injuries.[9]

BURN PREVENTION

When clothing ignition occurs, serious burns can be avoided by immediately applying a sequence of *STOP, DROP,* and *ROLL* (or *ROCK*). This will extinguish the flames and limit the extent of the burn. The sequence should be practiced to condition oneself to respond immediately and correctly in the event of clothing ignition.

Learning how to use and maintain fire extinguishers that are easily accessible but slightly away from potential fires (e.g., kitchen, garage, car, workroom) is a valuable adjunct to fire safety training.

EVALUATION

Basic care of the patient who has sustained a burn begins with the basics of all injured patients. Evaluation of the ABCs of care (airway, breathing, and circulation) starts the process of reducing morbidity and mortality from serious burns, which may occur concomitantly with other injuries. The nature of the accident may give the prehospital care personnel (e.g., emergency medical technicians, paramedics) an insight into the possibility of related injuries sustained by the patient, e.g., a closed space fire associated with carbon monoxide inhalation.

The evaluation of what to do first starts with an evaluation of the scene of the accident. The first objective at the scene is the prevention of injury to those who are rescuing the victims. Authorities must also secure the scene to prevent injury to those who have come to watch the disaster. In treating a patient with an electrical burn, those in charge must insure that electrical lines are marked and electricity turned off so the people working with the patient do not come in contact with live wires. When treating patients with chemical burns, one must take care to avoid contact with the chemicals on the patient that could possibly cause the same type of injury to the rescuer. In case of flaming clothing, flames must be extinguished. This is accomplished by using a blanket or by rolling the patient on the ground.

The evaluation of the scene may give a clue to the type of any associated injury or to the best treatment plan. A flame burn sustained in a closed area may be associated with carbon monoxide poisoning, or a glove-like hand burn in a small child may be indicative of child abuse. Chemical burns need to have the type of chemical identified, and the best source of this information available at the scene is the container or label, which should be transported with the patient. The electrical burn's voltage and amperage are important if one is to calculate the depth and extent of the burn.

Immediate evaluation of the patient's extent of injury, after the scene is secured, is accomplished by ABCs, control of hemorrhage, and a quick secondary survey. This must include inspection of the nares and mouth for burns and carbon particles, indicating possible inhalation injury and the need for immediate supplemental oxygen. At this early stage in patient care, a basic history must be taken while the patient is most alert. This should include allergy, medications, serious medical problems, such as cardiovascular, pulmonary, diabetes, seizure disorder, or immunologic deficiency. If there is too long of a delay in obtaining this information, it may become unavailable from the delirious or unconscious patient. Evaluation of burn size and determination of major or minor burns is essential. The "Rule of Nines" (Fig. 1–7A) is very useful. Major and moderate injuries (Fig. 1–8) require admission and should be taken to the nearest burn facility. Burn injuries to the face, hands, and perineum are considered major burns, even though they may cover a smaller percentage of body area.

TREATMENT ON THE SCENE

Initial care of the patient by paramedical personnel includes the application of fluids to the burned area taking care, particularly in cold climates, to avoid hypothermia. Lactated Ringer's is the fluid most available to paramedic personnel. Its local use should be confined to burns of less than 20 percent body surface. In burns greater than 20 percent, the only local care necessary is to keep the burn clean. The patient should not be tightly wrapped, but should be loosely covered to avoid contamination. The intravenous (IV) line, if ordered by the base station physician, should not be placed through the burned area, if at all possible.

Intravenous line placement is generally not necessary for most burn victims within the first 30 minutes postburn, but may be indicated as a lifeline. This is especially true for older individuals who have suffered severe burns and have concomitant cardiovascular or pulmonary disease. Cardiac monitoring, with transmission to the base station, is indicated in these patients. The addition of carbon monoxide poisoning and inhalation burn to a compromised pulmonary or cardiovascular system may predispose the victim to cardiac arrhythmias. These patients need immediate treatment using the lifeline.

The transport time and patient's condition, as determined by the base station physician, will dictate the treatment rendered enroute to the hospital, as this physician will be the medical authority directing the field care of the burn victim. In cases of multiple victims, it is extremely important for the prehospital personnel (paramedics, EMTs) to be able to evaluate the extent of the burn and other injuries to provide information to the physician for proper triage.

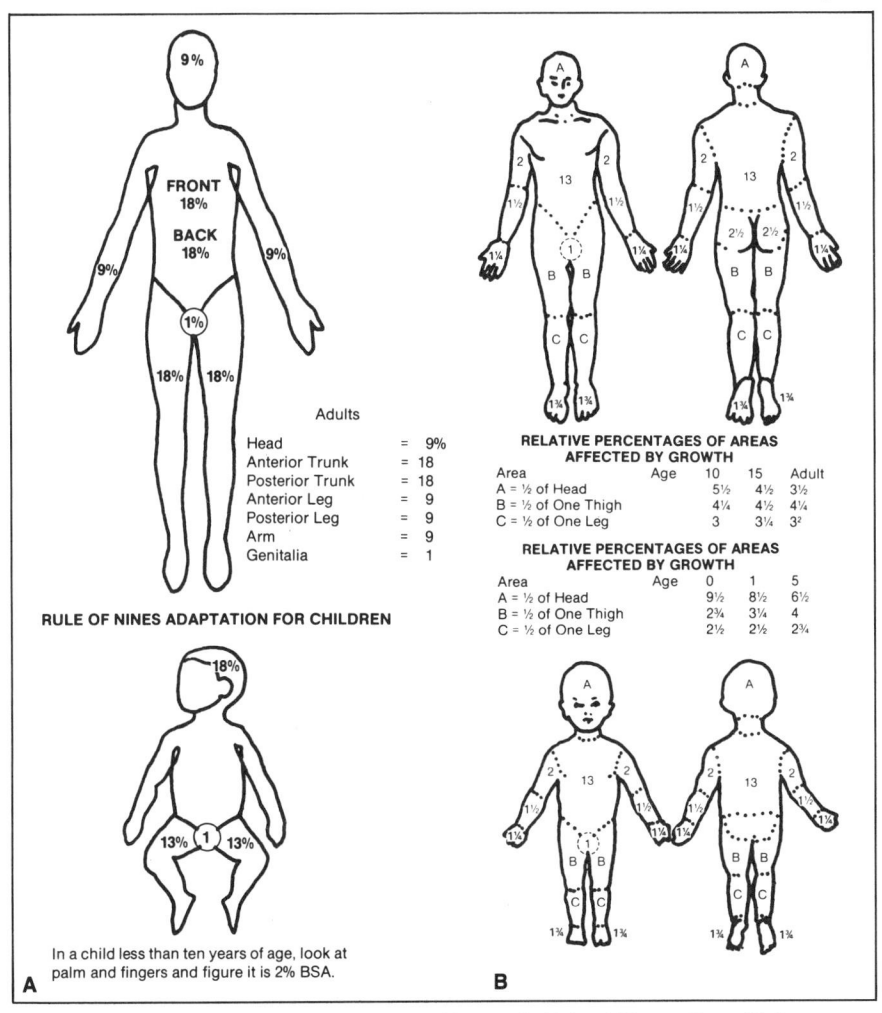

Figure 1-7. Evaluation of the extent of burns. **A.** Rule of Nines. *(From Wallace AB: The exposure treatment of burns. Lancet 1:501, 1951.)* **B.** Lund and Browder Chart. *(From Lund CC, Browder NC: The estimation of areas of burns. Surg Gyn Obstet 79:352, 1944.)*

Chemical Burns

Chemical burns differ from other types of burns in that the chemical agent will continue to burn as long as it remains in contact with the skin. The use of copious irrigation is the mainstay of prehospital treatment. Since many chemical burns are industrial in origin, it is suggested that the local burn center provide preaccident information to personnel so they can begin lavage, thus reducing the burn injury. Most industrial plants have lavage systems and stressing the importance of starting lavage in the first few moments after

Type of Burn	Admission Factors	Facility
Minor	0	Emergency Department (any hospital)
Moderate	0	Burn Unit/Center
Major	0	Burn Unit/Center
Any severity	+	Burn Unit/Center

Figure 1-8. Appropriate disposition of burn injury patients.

injury will reduce burn morbidity. In cases where the chemical is not water soluble, as in phenol burns, extensive lavage may be necessary if appropriate solvents are not available. The length of time of lavage is of primary importance. It could take longer than 30 minutes for thorough lavage of acid burns and perhaps longer for alkali burns. If the patient is otherwise stable, transport of the patient to a medical facility is of secondary importance to thorough lavage of the burn at the scene. Lavage of eye burns is particularly important. A good ocular lavage setup can be made of lactated Ringer's and IV tubing and should be continued until arrival at the hospital. In the prehospital setting, lavage is adequate for most burns (see Chap. 12).

Electrical Burns

The prehospital care of electrical burns is threefold: (1) stopping the source of electrical contact to the injured patient while avoiding electrical burns to the rescuers; (2) monitoring and correction of possible ventricular arrhythmias (defibrillation, lidocaine) and establishment of an IV lifeline; and (3) immediate fluid resuscitation to decrease renal injury and hyperkalemia associated with the severe tissue destruction of electrical injuries. The patient should then be transported to the burn center while being monitored to reduce the possibility of cardiac arrhythmias not recognized during transport.

TRANSPORT OF THE PATIENT

The patient may have only a short distance from the scene to the vehicle, or it may be a complicated journey from the top of a high rise apartment building. In cases where there is a burn injury alone, care must be taken to avoid further injury to the burned areas. If possible, straps that hold the patient on the stretcher should not be placed over the burned areas. In transporting the burn patient, time is usually not a major factor unless additional traumatic injuries that cause the patient to be hypotensive are present. In cases of hypotension secondary to other major trauma, the Military Anti-Shock Trousers (MAST) suit may be indicated if the blood pressure cannot be maintained by infusion of crystalloid solution. IV infusion will be beneficial in patients with burns of over 25 percent and transport time greater than 30 minutes. The rate for infusion can be easily calculated by the physician using the information transmitted by the paramedics. Infusion rates may have to be greater to keep blood pressure at near normal levels, if a great deal of time has elapsed from time of burn to initial treatment or if the patient was exposed to high environmental temperatures.

In most cases, burns greater than 20 percent in adults will indicate that the patient should be transported to a burn center, although this will vary from one area of the country to another. If the patient also has other associated injuries, such as intra-abdominal hemorrhage from liver, spleen, aorta, or other injuries, it is imperative that the patient be taken to the nearest trauma center for the care of these immediate life-threatening injuries. This is simplified if the burn and trauma centers are at the same hospital. If they are not, however, then transport to the trauma center would be appropriate. It is unwise to triage a patient to a burn center that is greater than 30 minutes away if there are injuries, other than the burn, causing shock. Burns do not produce hypotension in the first 1 to 2 hours. These life-threatening injuries need to be treated before transport to the burn center. The stabilized, postoperative patient may then be transferred.

Evacuation of the injured is a consideration that needs early attention. This can be accomplished by ambulance or helicopter, depending upon need and availability. One should consider transporting to a facility with a hyperbaric chamber in cases of severe carbon monoxide poisoning that is nonresponsive to 100 percent oxygen therapy. In cases of multiple patients, evacuation to several hospitals better able to care for patients with less than 25 percent burn area, as opposed to the triage of a great number of patients to the burn center at the same time, is recommended. Interhospital transfer could be accomplished after initial stabilization and resuscitation at a facility without a burn center.

The transmission of significant associated diagnostic features by the paramedic personnel will aid the base station physician in assuring consideration of all possible diagnoses. In assessing the patient, one must include a thorough secondary survey, checking for carbon particles on the tongue or in the sputum, burned hairs in the nares, hoarse voice, or any signs of respiratory distress which may include stidor, wheezing, or dyspnea. The evaluation of lung sounds may also disclose evidence of pulmonary injury or insufficiency. The unburned areas may reveal the cyanosis of respiratory insufficiency or the red color of carbon monoxide poisoning. The use of oxygen in the field is generally recommended. Patients with chronic obstructive pulmonary disease (COPD) and who have sustained inhalation injuries need oxygen supplementation even more than other patients. A decreased respiratory effort that may occur in these patients can be alleviated by bag or valve mask use of oxygen.

MULTIPLE DISASTER BURN VICTIMS

The current technologic advancements of our society also bring the attendant risk of mass casualty problems. The logistics of caring for hundreds of patients who may have sustained burns, as well as multiple trauma, present a major medical and administrative problem. The organization of available medical resources united with the paramedical, police rescue, and other manpower needs a united effort for optimal patient care and outcome. In trying to care for these large numbers of patients, triage is the mainstay for appropriate therapy. The patients with hypotension, respiratory difficulties, and obvious severe head trauma or facial injuries must be transported to a medical facility for definitive care with the least possible delay. The burn patients should be grouped by severity at the scene so that burns of greater than 50 percent are transported first, followed by 25 to 50 percent, and, finally, the group with less than 25 percent burns. The victims must be kept in an area that will not cause them to lose excessive fluid. In one disaster exercise, the burn patients were placed in direct sunlight on a hot day with resulting excessive fluid losses. The opposite situation may also be true in a cold climate where body heat loss (secondary to skin and thermoregulatory mechanism injury) increases the risk of hypothermia and, therefore, ventricular fibrillation. In these circumstances, blankets become a basic necessity.

The availability of beds may also be a severe problem. The burn patient without the additional problems of trauma, airway, or head injury could have IV placement and treatment while being transported to facilities which may be out of the region for his or her care. The need for multiple IV therapy sets (lactated Ringer's solution and IV administration sets) necessitates a mass casualty disaster box containing the IV sets and appropriate tape, bandages, blankets, and basic first aid equipment in a large enough quantity to care for the needs of 200 or more patients. The rotation of this stock with participating hospitals is necessary to keep the medications from becoming out of date.

The disaster drill with the participation of the hospitals in the area provides the necessary rehearsal for disaster. This allows the staff of each hospital to interact and help to establish communication before such an event. Communication is particularly important to establish the available bed and medical manpower in these cases where medical resources are pushed to the limit.

ASSESSMENT IN THE EMERGENCY DEPARTMENT

Extent of Burn Injury

An estimation of the extent of burn injury is best expressed as the percent of body surface area (BSA) injured in relation to the total body area. In adults, the "Rule of Nines" (see Fig. 1–7A) is a very convenient and clinically practical method to determine the extent of burn injury by dividing the body into multiples of nine. This method must be modified for infants and small children less than 10 years of age since the head has a larger percentage and legs a smaller percentage of the total BSA. For greater accuracy, the Lund and Browder Table (see Fig. 1–7B) is best to define the extent of burn injury by the burn center. These tables are difficult to memorize, however, and frequently are not available in emergency departments and hospitals that do not have a burn care facility. The "Rule of Nines" method is very practical for the emergency department.

Depth of Burns

In spite of all the increased attention in research done to more accurately determine depth of burn injury, probably the most reliable and practical method still used is "pinprick sensation." Patients with a partial thickness burn will usually have nerve endings that are intact because the endings are at the dermal–epidermal junction and these patients will have pinprick sensation. Those with full thickness burn injury where the burn has extended through the entire dermis and epidermis will have destruction of these nerve endings and will consequently have no sensation to pinprick.

TREATMENT IN THE EMERGENCY DEPARTMENT

When respiratory compromise is present due to circumferential burn injury, an escharotomy of the chest should be done immediately; bleeding is minimal if the diagnosis is correct. The Doppler and wick catheter are adjuncts to clinical evaluation of vascular compromise in an extremity due to circumferential full thickness burn (see Chap. 8). Prior to transfer to a burn facility, a nasogastric tube should be inserted in all patients with a greater than 30 percent burn, intoxicated patients, intubated patients, and those being transferred by air. Heavy sedation should be avoided for this may impair adequate respiration and compromise the burn facility's ability to re-evaluate the patient. A burn transfer checklist (Fig. 1–9) should be present in each emergency room that treats burn patients. Completion of this form greatly expedites the care of the burn patient within the first few hours of injury.

Disposition

After initial stabilizing procedures have been performed in the emergency room and the injuries evaluated, the next most critical decision is where the patient can best be treated. This decision should be made with a knowledge of the available burn care facilities in the area and their levels of expertise (Fig. 1–10).

There are three levels of burn care: (1) basic emergency department burn care (outpatient), (2) general hospital, and (3) burn center. The presence of any of the admitting factors shown in Table 1–1 should strongly suggest admission to a burn unit (see Fig. 1–8). Specific admitting criteria of the American Burn Association and the American College of Surgeons are listed in Table 1–2.

A burn unit is a facility with a trained burn team that provides specialized, high quality care to patients with burn injury. With the team approach, all areas of concern—hands, burn wound, nutrition, and psychological problems—are met immediately and in a coordinated effort. Appropriate isolation and equipment are also readily available.

DATE _____	TIME OF CALL _____	AM PM

REFERRING DOCTOR _____
REFERRING HOSPITAL _____
PHONE # _____

CLOSED SPACE	YES NO
ENDOTRACHEAL TUBE	YES NO
VENTILATOR	YES NO
IV LINES	YES NO

(size & site _____

CONSCIOUS NOW	YES NO
DIABETES	YES NO
HEART DISEASE	YES NO

Type _____
ALLERGIES?   YES NO
To What? _____

ASSOCIATED INJURIES: (Fracture, abdominal or chest injury, head trauma, etc.) _____

THERAPY GIVEN THUS FAR
IV's _____ cc Normal Saline
     _____ cc Ringer's
     _____ cc D$_5$W
Foley _____ cc Urine total
     _____ cc urine last hour

IF PATIENT IS ACCEPTED SUGGEST:

1. Avoid heavy sedation
2. NG tube for burns over 30% or if drunk or intubated - if transported by air.
3. IV fluids - Ringer's fast enough to produce urine output.
4. NO topical cream, antibiotics IM meds of any kind.
5. Eshcarotomy if needed
6. Inform family of transfer

PATIENT NAME _____
DATE & _____ TIME OF BURN _____

TYPE OF BURN: FLAME   SCALD
ELECTRICAL   CHEMICAL   RADIATION

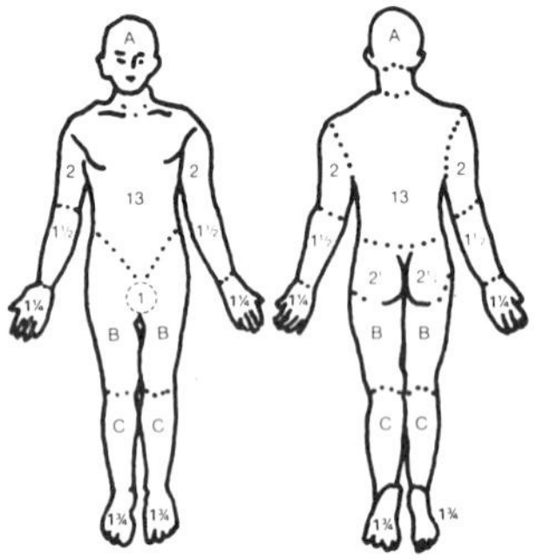

RELATIVE PERCENTAGE OF AREAS
AFFECTED BY GROWTH
(Age in Years)

A:	½ of head	9½	8½	6½	5½	4½	3½
B:	½ of thigh	2¾	3¼	4	4¼	4½	4¾
C:	½ of leg	2½	2½	2¾	3	3¼	3½

Total Percent burned _____ 2+ _____ 3= _____

INSURANCE DATA:
Type: _____
Policy # _____
Workmen's Compensation!   YES   NO
Resident making report _____
Senior resident notified _____
Attending notified _____
Accept patient _____
Refer to _____

Figure 1-9. Burn transfer checklist.

TABLE 1-1. ADMITTING FACTORS

1. All electrical burns greater than 1000 volts because there is a high incidence (30%) of delayed arrhythmias.
2. Patients with complicating medical conditions such as diabetes and COPD.
3. Very young (younger than 3), very old (over 60).
4. Moderate or major burn.
5. Patients whose environment prevents adequate care at home.
6. Burns of hands, feet, eyes, ears, face, and perineum.
7. Inhalation or electrical injury.
8. Fracture of other major trauma.
9. Poor risk (intercurrent disease).

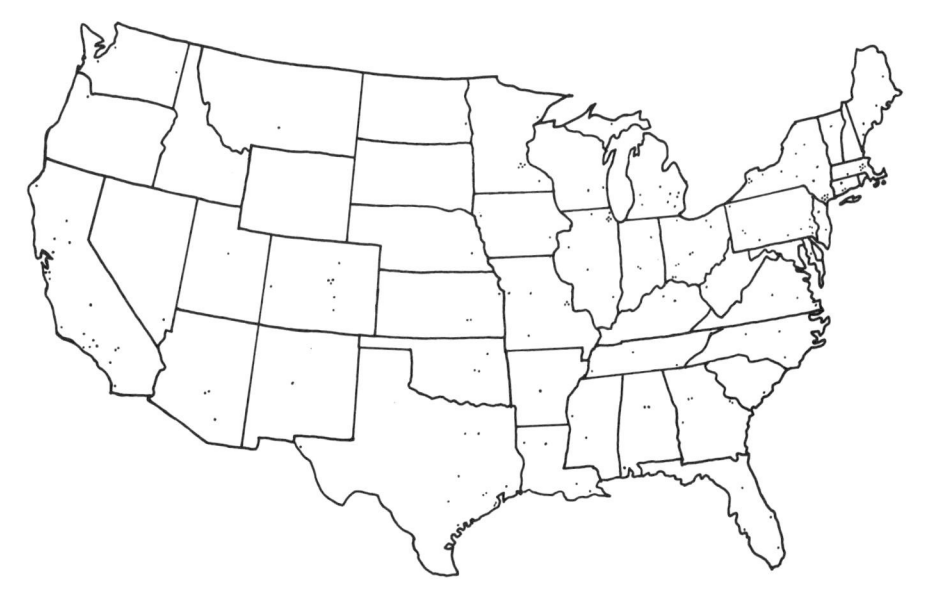

Figure 1–10. Burn care facilities in the United States.

Prognosis

Two-thirds of the fire fatalities are male.[3,5] The death rate is higher among children and the elderly[10] with more than half the deaths reported in some series involving children under the age of 14 years or the elderly.[3,4] Often individuals sustain lethal burns because of "hinderance to self-help" (e.g., bedridden, intoxicated, too young to act, physical handicaps, asleep, mentally ill or senile, suicide).[4] The death rate among all American nonwhites is about three times that of all whites.[4,5,7] This disadvantage for nonwhite children under 10 years is four to six times greater than for all white children.[4]

Our ability to care for the burn patient has significantly improved in the last decade. This improvement has been most noticeable in major burn injury patients (Fig. 1–11). Much of this improved care can be attributed to an increase in the number of burn care teams within hospitals that not only have special skills, but lack the fatalistic attitude regarding burn survival that was previously so prominent. This fatalistic attitude was encouraged by inadequate assessment of burn severity and poor therapy, usually due to limited experience of the health care team. Other factors contributing to improved survival of the major burn patients are advances in critical care medicine, improved infection control, better nutrition, and improved prehospital trauma care.

With consistent data from various burn care facilities available, information can be compiled to accurately determine the probability of fatal outcome in burn patients. Bull[10] in 1971 used the age of the patient and percentage of BSA burn to predict probability of mortality. His work and others have allowed burn units to evaluate their individual performance with a statistically valid model. These data not only give overall survival but can identify those

TABLE 1-2. CRITERIA OF BURN INJURY SEVERITY

	American Burn Association		American College of Surgeons	
	Adults Degree %	Children Degree %	Adults Degree %	Children Degree %
Minor	2nd — < 15 3rd — < 2	2nd 3rd } < 10	2nd 3rd } < 15	2nd 3rd } < 10
Moderate	2nd — > 15–25 3rd — < 10	2nd — > 10–20 3rd — < 10	2nd 3rd } 15–25	2nd 3rd } 10–20
Major	2nd — > 25 3rd — > 10	2nd — > 20 3rd — > 10	2nd — > 25 3rd — > 10	2nd — > 20 3rd — > 10

patients at greatest risk for high mortality. Our ability to accurately predict patient survival has not come without a price. With it has come the realization that there are some patients who have a 100 percent mortality and for whom there is no precedent for survival. Some suggest these patients should be queried on admission as to whether they want an all-out effort made to save their life or just "ordinary care."[11] They relate that it is imperative that these patients have autotomy. Others suggest that patients are not rational after just sustaining an immediate, severe burn injury, and for the physician to suggest anything less than an all-out effort to save the patient's life is immoral.[12,13] This controversy will continue because, for obvious reasons, one cannot do a randomized prospective double-blind study to resolve this issue. Generally, the burn patient should be treated as any trauma patient and have all efforts made to assure survival.

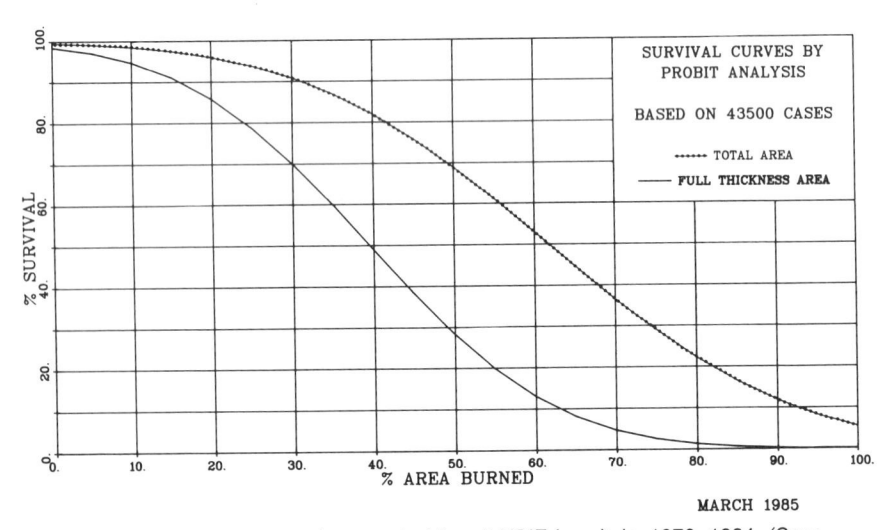

Figure 1-11. Burned patient survival for all NBIE hospitals, 1976–1984. *(Courtesy of National Burn Information Service, Ann Arbor, Michigan. I. Feller, M.D., Director.)*

REFERENCES

1. Jackson DM: A historical review of the use of local physical signs in burns. B J Plast Surg 23:211, 1970
2. Choctaw WT: Emergency Management of Burns. Los Angeles, Alicia Ann Rusch Burn Foundation, 1981
3. Maley MP: Burn education and prevention. In Hummel RP, Wright J (eds): Clinical Burn Therapy. Boston, PSG, Inc., 1982, pp. 509–540
4. Monafo WW: Socio-economic factors of importance in the treatment and prevention of burns. In Monafo WW (ed): The Treatment of Burns. St. Louis, Warren H. Green, 1971
5. Feck G, Baptiste M, Greenwald P: The incidence of hospitalized burn injury in upstate New York. Am J Public Health 67:566, 1977
6. Somaya PM: A survey of burn accidents in the city of Bombay. Vocational Rehabilitation Administrating U.S. Government Research Project on Rehabilitation of Burns, 1968
7. Edlich RF, Glasheen W, Attinger EO, et al.: Epidemiology of serious burn injuries. Surg Gynec Ostet 154:505, 1982
8. Frank HA, Wachtel, TL, Berry CC, Johnson RW: Demonstration of a regional burn care system: Sub-task C-1: Development of a burn injury severity grading system. Final Report to Department of Health and Human Services, Health Services Administration, Bureau of Medical Services, Division of Emergency Medical Services, Washington, D.C., September 1980
9. McGuire A: Prevention of burns. Crit Care Quart 1(3):1, 1978
10. Bull JP: Revised analysis of mortality due to burns. Lancet 2:1133, 1971
11. Imbus SH, Zawacki BE: Autonomy for burned patients when survival is unprecedented. N Engl J Med 297:308, 1977
12. Bailey J: Moral and ethical aspects of fluid resuscitation. Proc NIH Consensus Devel Conf on Supportive Therapy in Burn Care. J Trauma 19:870, 1979
13. Pruitt BA: Fluid resuscitation for extensively burned patients. Proc Second Conf on Supportive Therapy in Burn Care. J Trauma 21:690, 1981

CHAPTER 2
Pathophysiology of the Burn Wound
Louis A. Bonaldi and David H. Frank

LOCAL EFFECTS OF THERMAL INJURY

The burn wound is made up of varying degrees of cellular impairment following exposure to thermal energy. The mechanisms involve denaturation of cellular protein, inhibition of cellular metabolism, and secondary interference of local vascular supply. The factors that determine the extent of injury are: (1) the heat intensity to which the cells are exposed, (2) the duration of the exposure, and (3) the conductance of the tissue involved.

Intensity and Duration
There is an inverse relation between the intensity of heat and the duration of exposure that is required to produce a given degree of tissue injury. This relationship is nonlinear. Moritz and Henriques[1] were able to show that at surface temperatures of 44°C, local tissue damage does not occur unless exposure time exceeds 6 hours. At temperatures between 44 and 51°C, the rate of epidermal necrosis nearly doubles with each degree rise in temperature. At 70°C and greater, the exposure time required to cause transepidermal necrosis is less than 1 second. Figure 2–1 graphically illustrates the time–intensity curve for burn injury.

Although pressure may increase the rate of heat transfer to the skin by improving interface contact, there is no evidence to suggest that compressive occlusion of dermal blood vessels has any effect on the susceptibility of the epidermis to thermal injury. When hot water is applied to the surface of the

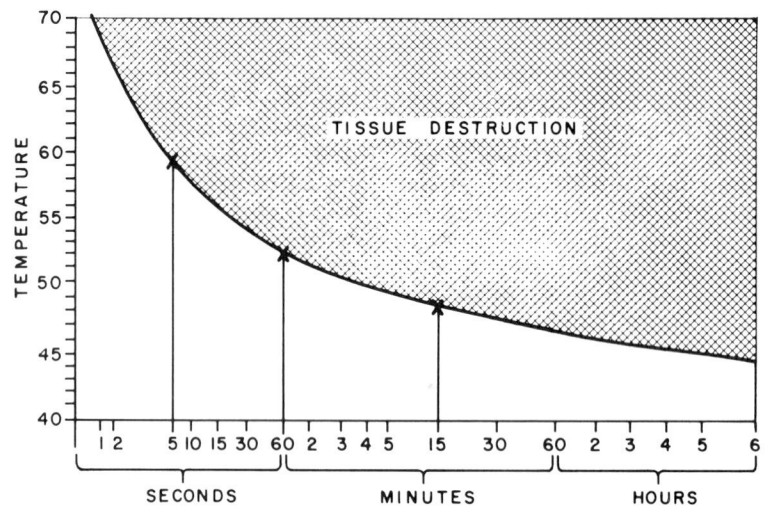

Figure 2–1. Temperature duration curve. Tissue destruction proceeds logarithmically with increasing temperatures as a function of time exposure. *(From Robson MC, et al., 1979, reprinted with permission.[3])*

skin at different pressures, compressive ischemia is observed, but does not alter the rate at which burning occurs.[1]

The type of energy source which is supplying the thermal energy does influence the degree of tissue injury. Radiant heat of 4.8 cal/cm of 0.54 sec exposure time has been shown to cause a full thickness burn to human skin.[2] This is approximately equivalent to holding your hand 2 cm away from a 100 watt light bulb for 15 seconds. Exposure to 85°C water for 10 seconds results in a similar injury. Part of this variability is caused by the specific heat content of the transferring medium, and part is influenced by the ability of the skin to conduct heat away from the surface and thus limit the temperature increase and potential damages.

Conductance

The human body has substantial ability to regulate skin temperature. Both internal heat from metabolism and external heat from the environment can be dissipated by evaporative losses, inherent thermal conductivity, and systemic blood supply (at the rate of 0.04 cal/sec/cm^2). This ability is needed because we constantly live within 6° of our thermal death. Core temperatures above 43°C for any length of time will lead to tissue damage. Since flash exposure may deliver nearly 30 cal/sec/cm^2, it is clear that our inadequate ability to dissipate heat at that rate will result in thermal injury.[3,4]

The physical principal of conductance, involving transfer of heat from an object of higher temperature to one of lower temperature, becomes important when discussing the depth of burn injury. Conduction, or the rate of absorption of dissipation of heat, determines the final temperature of the tissues involved and is dependent on several factors. These include peripheral circulation, water content of the tissue, thickness and pigmentation of the skin, and the presence or absence of insulating substances such as skin oils or hair. Of these factors, the most significant seems to be the peripheral circulation. Altering the rate of blood flow through tissue exposed to excess heat rapidly alters the local net accumulation of heat and is of major importance in determining the amount of cellular destruction.

Classification of Burns

One of the first classifications of burns was proposed by Fabry[5] in 1614 and contained no reference to the depth of burn injury. His classification was based on the intensity of surface burning, judged purely by external appearance. This type of classification stood with only minor modification for nearly 200 years. As understanding of the functional physiology of the skin and its layers increased, particularly with regard to its ability to withstand bacterial invasion and to regenerate itself, the depth of the burn became the basis for classification. It is the functional capacity of the residual skin that determines the ultimate prognosis of the burn wound.

Traditionally, burns have been differentiated into first, second, third, and fourth degree injuries. Diagnosis at the time of injury or for several days after is not always possible with any degree of assurance. This classification is in many respects retrospective. If the skin healed by peeling, without blistering, it is said to have been a first degree injury. If blisters formed and the wound healed by re-epithelialization, it is labeled a second degree injury. A wound which fails to heal by regeneration of epithelium from within the wound margins is assumed to be a full thickness skin loss and is called third degree. Fourth degree wounds are those which are discovered to involve muscle or other tissue deep to the skin after the skin has been removed. This morphologic classification served well for many years while burn shock and gross wound infection were the principal concerns of burn physicians and researchers. While this traditional classification is still present in our literature, it is being rapidly abandoned for a functional and descriptive classification that allows a more precise description of the burn wound.

Burn wounds are now classified into superficial, partial thickness, or full thickness wounds. The partial thickness wounds are frequently separated into superficial and deep subgroups. The spectrum of both eventual outcome and treatment varies greatly from the superficial burns to those of full thickness. It is thus important to choose a grading system that will allow the most complete understanding of the pathophysiologic process taking place in the burn wound.

The Superficial Burn Wound. These wounds are frequently the result of either prolonged exposure to low intensity heat, e.g., sunburn, or to a short duration flash exposure to a high intensity heat source. Erythema of the skin with edema confined to the basal layers is the result. Irritation of naked nerve endings occurs but swelling is not consistently present. In some cases, cell death at the level of the stratum granulosum does occur. This results in desquamation for 2 or 3 days following the burn and is recognized as the typical peeling following a sunburn. There is no significant, early clinical consequence to burns at this level. The wounds heal rapidly without leaving a trace of scar. Late changes, such as an increased rate of neoplastic degeneration, are well recognized following solar and ionic radiation, but have not been documented for flash explosion burns.

The Partial Thickness Burn Wound. A *superficial partial thickness* burn is equivalent to the classic second degree blister burn. These injuries are the result of either increased exposure time or higher intensity flash exposure, and implies further cellular destruction than is present in a simple superficial burn. The basal layer of the skin provides the line of demarcation between the deep and superficial partial thickness injury. In the superficial (second degree) burn, the basal layer is not totally destroyed. As in the first degree burn, erythema is a prominent feature; however, blistering is the hallmark of this level of burn. Cellular destruction of the stratum granulosum and stratum corneum occurs forming the covering of these blisters. The vascular response of the subpapillary plexus within the dermis results in edema formation at the dermal–epidermal junction. As fluid accumulates, the junction separates forming the blister. The epidermis itself may become swollen and edematous. Again, nerve endings are irritated and these can be extremely painful injuries.

It is clear that the blister membrane, in its intact condition, forms a sterile environment preventing excessive water loss from the wound. Fallon and Moyer[6] were able to show that merely stripping the stratum corneum resulted in accelerated insensible water loss 10 to 20 times that of normal skin. The "dry" burn eschar transmits water 75 times faster than that of normal skin, thus its dry appearance. Since the basal layer is, for the most part, left intact, the superficial partial thickness burn heals without scarring between 10 and 14 days after injury. In some cases, a significant number of melanocytes are lost which results in a minor and sometimes permanent color change. Secondary infection of the superficial wound is rare, but may occur. This can be explained by plasma inhibition of the antistreptococcal properties of sebum.[3]

The *deep partial thickness* burn consists of a wound with complete disruption of the epidermis and destruction of most of the basal layer. Sparing of dermal appendages such as hair follicles and sweat glands allows the wound to potentially regenerate and is thus partial thickness. The events that occur in the subpapillary plexus characterize the major histologic changes in this injury. Edema fluid infiltrates the dermal–epidermal junction. Ischemic (coagulation) necrosis of the epidermis occurs, followed by an inflammatory cellular response incited at the basilar level resulting in further tissue destruction. Blistering may occur; however, this is not an essential component. The wound is more often characterized by eschar formation. Microhygrometer readings of deep partial thickness burn eschar demonstrates massive fluid loss.[7] Of major clinical importance and a significant difference from the superficial burn is the loss of the cellular barrier which protects against bacterial invasion and wound sepsis.

Sensation in this type of burn is diminished because of actual destruction of nerve endings in the basal layer of the skin. And, with disruption of the deeper skin layers, wound healing takes longer and more scar is formed.

The Full Thickness Burn. Based on the work of Order and Moncrief,[8] the differences between deep partial thickness and full thickness burns can be broken down into five characteristics (Table 2–1).

It is evident from the above that in the full thickness injury the epidermis is destroyed along with dermal appendages and supporting structures. The wound is characterized by coagulation necrosis of cells, and only at the edges of the wound do edema and cellular infiltrates occur. As with the deep partial thickness wound, a thick, leathery eschar forms that allows copious fluid losses and fails to prevent bacterial invasion and wound sepsis. Granulation tissue consisting of new fibroblasts and endothelial tissue develops as the result of an inflammatory response at the margin of the wound (both the edges and the undersurface of the coagulated eschar). The eschar becomes loosened and will eventually slough. Because of the lack of skin appendages, the wound will heal by contraction and epithelial growth from the edges. For most wounds of any size, the result of such natural wound healing is a contracture deformity and unstable scar. In clinical practice, skin grafts are applied to seal the wound and speed the healing process.

The Fourth Degree Burn. Severe incineration injuries represent the extreme full thickness wound in which the level of injury extends well beyond the skin. The terminology from the traditional classification is retained. In these injuries, subcutaneous tissue, muscle, fascia, periosteum, and even bone can

TABLE 2–1. CHARACTERISTICS OF DEEP PARTIAL AND FULL THICKNESS BURN WOUNDS

Characteristic	Deep Partial	Full Thickness
Vascularity	Never totally ischemic	Arterial occlusion and devitalization
Dermal cellular inflammation	Present	Absent
Revascularization	Arterial patency re-established 1 week postburn	Neovascular granulation tissue 3 weeks postburn
Granulation tissue	In the dermis	In the fascia
Healing by	Epithelial growth	Eschar separation No epithelial growth Requires autograft

be destroyed. Coagulation necrosis of the tissues occurs and cellular inflammation is absent except at the periphery. Because of massive muscle destruction, myoglobinuria can become a significant clinical problem and may lead to renal failure in the poorly hydrated patient.

Tissue Response to Burn Injury

Thermal injury is the result of denaturation of cellular protein and disruption of cellular metabolic process which lead to cellular necrosis. Some cells are instantly destroyed, others are irreversibly injured, and others are injured but are capable of survival under appropriate conditions. In 1953, Jackson[9] described three concentric zones of thermal injury (Fig. 2–2). The innermost "zone of coagulation" appears as white coagulated skin and on microscopy is characterized by obliteration of vessel lumina. The outermost "zone of hyperemia" is the area least affected. Biopsies show complete loss of epidermis without apparent structural damage to the dermis. The subpapillary plexus and capillary loops are patent. This zone is typically healed by the seventh day. Between these two zones lies the intermediate "zone of stasis." This zone initially resembles the zone of hyperemia in that it is erythematous and blanches with pressure. But, at 24 to 48 hours following injury, petechial hemorrhages may be visible without magnification, and on microscopic examination the superficial capillaries are dilated and packed with red blood cells. Complete stasis has occurred and progresses to cell death.

The zone of stasis has been the subject of much recent research which suggests that stasis is a reversible phenomenon and not inevitable. Environmental and pharmacologic manipulation of the burn wound may prevent progression to cell death. This is discussed further in the section on modification of the burn wound.

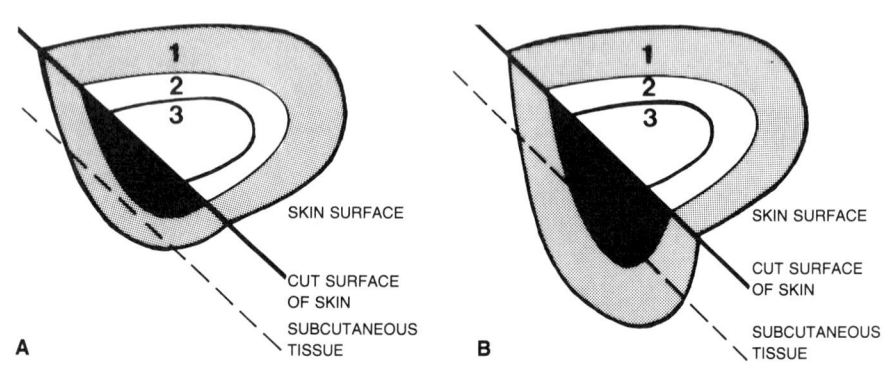

Figure 2–2.A. Shows the three zones of intensity: (1) the zone of hyperemia (peripheral); (2) the zone of stasis (intermediate); (3) the zone of coagulation (central). The two inner zones of necrosis (*shaded black*) do not penetrate the skin. **B.** Shows the same surface appearance associated with complete skin destruction, the zones of necrosis (*shaded black*) penetrating the full thickness of the skin. *(From Jackson DM, 40, 1953; reprinted with permission[9].)*

Whether or not the zone of stasis progresses, the eventual zone of coagulation can be related to our classification of the burn wound in the previous section. If the zone of coagulation lies above the level of the dermal appendages, the wound will be partial thickness and have the potential for spontaneous healing. If the zone of coagulation extends below this level, a full thickness wound is produced.

Vascular Response to Burn Injury

The microcirculation of the skin is composed of three separate capillary plexuses: the subpapillary plexus, the dermal plexus, and the subdermal plexus within the subcutaneous tissue (Fig. 2–3). The vascular dynamics of the burn wound have been studied by many techniques. Microangiography has been used to demonstrate the destruction of the vascular bed following burn injury. Immediately after burning, there is cessation of flow through arterial and venous channels within the zone of coagulation. This is due primarily to thrombosis. Using the scald burn model described by Zawacki[10] for measurement of dermal ischemia, Robson et al.[11] studied the intermediate zone of stasis. A uniform thickness, 10 percent body surface area (BSA) scald burn was created in albino guinea pigs. At timed intervals, the guinea pigs were killed and the aortas cannulated. Sixty milliliters of India ink were injected at a constant pressure of 400 mm Hg using a pneumatic injection device. This calculated volume and pressure insured maximal filling of the microcirculation. The burn wounds were then biopsied and fixed for microscopic examination. The level at which vessels were filled with India ink was noted and compared to levels of the capillary plexuses within the dermis. In normal, unburned skin, 95 percent of the dermal thickness was perfused, as was the case immediately postburn. By 2 hours postburn, the India ink was limited to 80 percent of the dermal thickness, and at 8 hours only to the lower 40 percent. At 24 hours, the ink was not seen above the subdermal plexus. This suggests that there is progressive loss of dermal perfusion with time. With extensive thrombosis of the initial wound, circulation cannot be re-established and progression to a zone of coagulation has occurred.

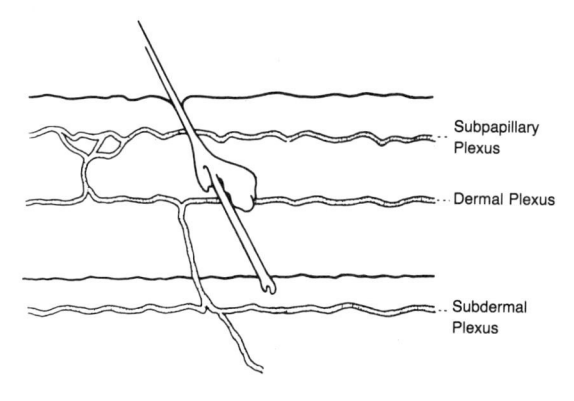

Figure 2–3. Lack of circulation of the skin is composed of three separate capillary plexuses: the subpapillary plexus, dermal plexus, and subdermal plexus. *(From Robson MD, et al.: 1978, reprinted with permission.[31])*

Massiha and Monafo,[12] using both venographic and arteriographic techniques, were able to demonstrate that the venous circulation is initially compromised with the zone of stasis to a greater degree than that of the arterial side. Their data suggest that it is the progressive venous thrombosis which causes the arterial abnormalities. These data are supported by the work of Robb[13] using cinephotomicrography. He demonstrated venous platelet aggregation and embolization while pulsatile arteriolar conditions continued. The cause of platelet thromboembolism is not clear, but appears to be related to several factors including endothelial damage, injury to the platelets themselves, and release of tissue or red cell adenosine diphosphate (ADP).

Recently, a new group of compounds, the thromboxanes and prostaglandin precursors (endoperoxides), have been implicated in this process.[11,14-16] These compounds produce platelet aggregation and contraction of vascular and airway smooth muscle. Thromboxane B2 (TXB2), a metabolite of the biologically active but short-lived thromboxane A2 (TXA2), has been identified and quantified in human blister fluid.[14] New but indirect evidence for the role of these compounds in burn wound pathophysiology is derived from studies using nonsteroidal prostaglandin synthetase inhibitors. In some situations, these compounds will inhibit progression of the burn injury. This topic will be discussed further in the section on modifying the burn wound.

The effect of bacterial toxins on the microcirculation is well established, but appears to vary with the organism. Platelet aggregation and embolization was demonstrated following injection of *Escherichia coli* into the vascular system of rabbit bowel mesentery.[13] The topical application of staphylococcal endotoxin causes immediate precipitation of platelets. Thus, infection resulting in stasis, anoxia, and subsequent cellular necrosis can greatly extend the depth of the partial thickness burn wound.

Edema Formation Following Burn Injury

Thermal injury to skin will cause all of the physical findings of inflammation including heat, redness, pain, swelling, and loss of function. The progressive onset of swelling is the most dramatic. The rapid formation of edema is due mainly to increased microvascular permeability and marked vasodilation. Netsky and Leitek[17] in 1943 first demonstrated the increased microvascular permeability of plasma proteins following thermal injury. They measured the extravasation of horse serum across the capillary endothelium of a dog. These results were subsequently confirmed by others using radioactive and vital dyes as test substances.[18-20]

Using a plethysmograph technique to measure tissue swelling, Arturson et al.[18] applied thermal trauma to a cat's hind paw (Fig. 2–4). The highest rate of edema formation (20 to 40 ml/min/mm Hg/100 g of tissue) occurred in the early phase a few minutes after injury. In less than 20 minutes, the tissue had doubled its original weight due to fluid transfer. With time, there was a gradual decline in the rate of extravasation. The capillary filtration coefficient (CFC) increased rapidly from 0.04 to 0.10 ml/min/mm Hg 100 g of tissue; this,

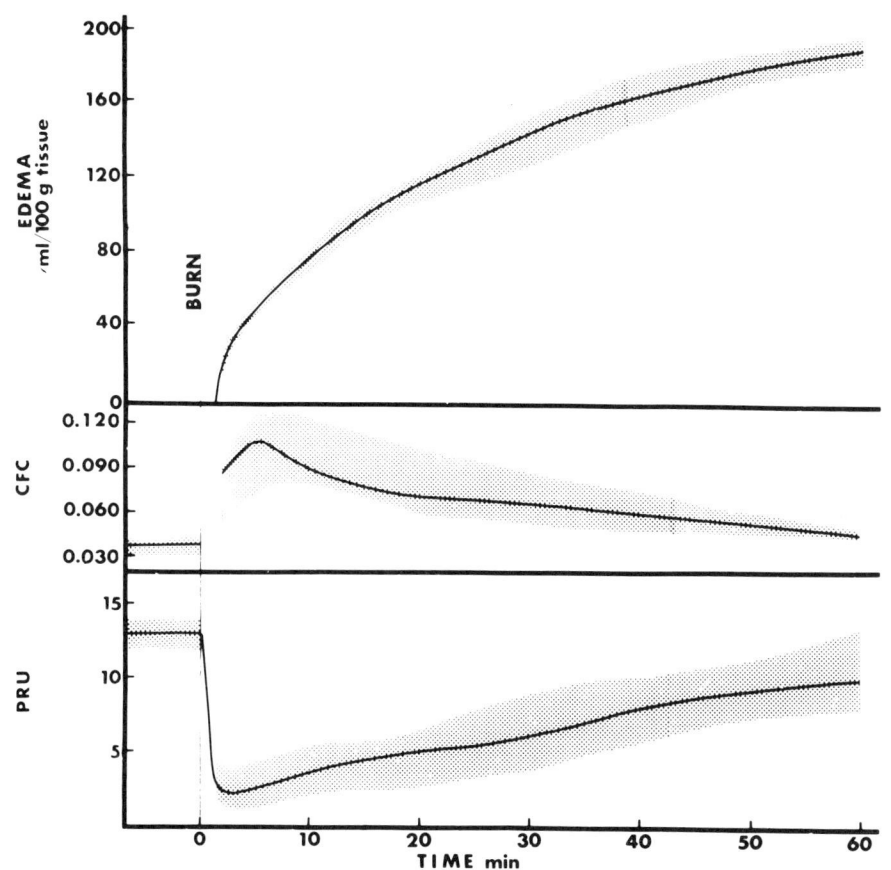

Figure 2-4. Effects on dermal burns on net transcapillary fluid movement (edema), on capillary filtration coefficient (CFC), and on resistance of vessels (PRU) in the cat hind paw. Solid lines represent means of five experiments, shaded areas the range of individual experiments. *(From Arturson G, 1980, reprinted with permission.[22])*

up to 300 percent increase, occurs within 5 to 10 minutes of injury directly reflecting an increase in microvascular permeability. The rate of lymph flow was also noted to increase and showed its highest values at the same time that the wound edema was maximal.

It is a well-known clinical observation that when the primary area of thermal damage is large enough (greater than 25 to 30 percent in humans), it will exert an influence on the systemic circulation resulting in generalized edema. Arturson et al.[18] investigated this phenomenon and found increased microvascular permeability in the nonburned areas simultaneous with an increased infiltration rate across the blood–lymph barrier. Using fluorescein-labeled dextran, the leakage sites were found to occur mostly at the postcapillary venules (Fig. 2–5).

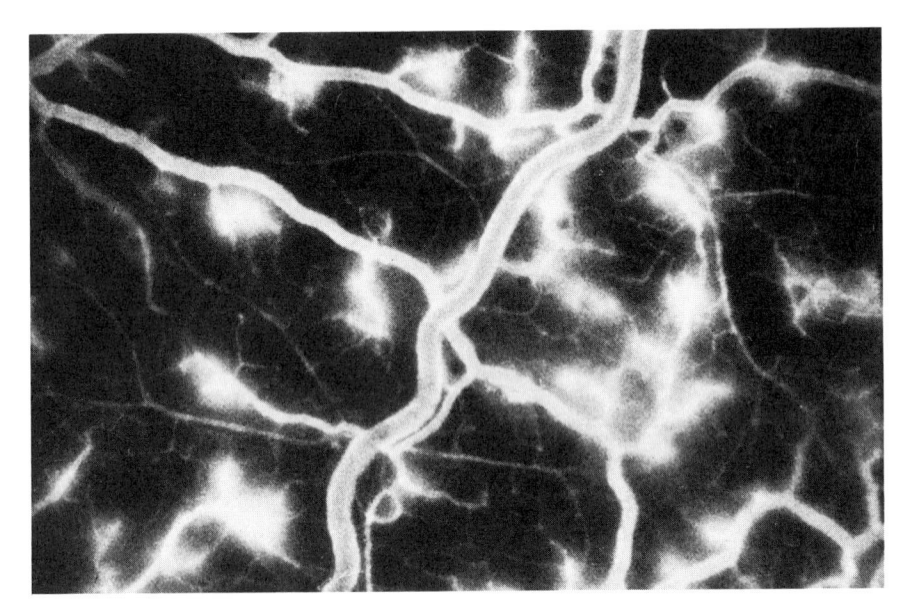

Figure 2-5. Fluorescein extravasation postburn injury. Photograph in fluorescent light showing extravasation of fluorescein-labeled dextran M_W = 145.000 from postcapillary venules 10 minutes after a mild thermal injury of a hamster cheek pouch preparation. ×34 magnification, 100 μm is indicated. *(From Arturson G, 1980, reprinted with permission.[22])*

In an attempt to explain the mechanism behind this edema formation, Eriksson and Robson[21] observed the mesenteric microcirculation of rats following a major (20 percent) cutaneous burn. Arteriolar constriction of up to 25 percent occurred with a smaller percent dilation of venules. Adherence of white blood cells appeared to obstruct venular flow. They were able to quantitate the number of white cells that stuck and also to demonstrate and calculate an increase in postcapillary resistance. This would tend to increase hydrostatic capillary pressure and result in increased transcapillary filtration pressure.

Additionally, a systemic transcapillary osmotic pressure gradient is immediately created following thermal injury by mechanisms that are not understood, but probably relate to release of intracellular molecules from the thermally injured cell. Finally, the increased permeability of the endothelium to passage of macromolecules causes an effective decrease in plasma oncotic pressure. This also promotes the accumulation of tissue edema.

The loss of protein to the extravascular space is tremendous. Twice the normal plasma pool of albumin is lost from the vascular space within the first 4 days following a moderate-sized burn injury.[4] Half of this is lost through the wound surface and the other half remains within the interstitial space.

Inflammatory mediators also play an ill-defined role in edema formation. Histamine is thought to be the first vasoactive substance released following burn injury, and elevated levels have been measured in lymph drained from a thermally injured area. The early transient stage of vasodilation and increased venular permeability is probably due to this substance. Prostaglandins of the E and F series, along with their precursors, have been isolated from human blister fluid in amounts three to seven times above levels known to have vasodilatory effects.[14–16,22] High concentrations of these substances have been documented beginning immediately postburn and continuing until epithelialization of the wound is completed. PGE1 is recovered during the first few hours and is later replaced in higher concentration by PGE2 and PGF2 (alpha).[16]

Following thermal injury, coagulated protein located outside of blood vessels is thought to activate the complement cascade which then acts as a trigger stimulus for the acute inflammatory process. Once the complement system is activated, a host of permeability factors are liberated at the site of injury (mainly histamine and prostaglandins). The coagulation system is also activated causing release of 5-hydroxytryptamine from platelets and formation of the vasoactive kinins.

The formation of edema following thermal injury is a complex balance between many systems which regulate microvascular permeability. The major pathways which we now are aware of are schematically summarized in Figure 2–6.

Thermal injury

↓

Modified protein

Activation complement system → $C_{3,5}$ → Histamine ; C_9 → Prostaglandins

Activation clotting system → Platelets → 5 HT ; Hageman factor → Kinins

→ Increased microvascular permeability

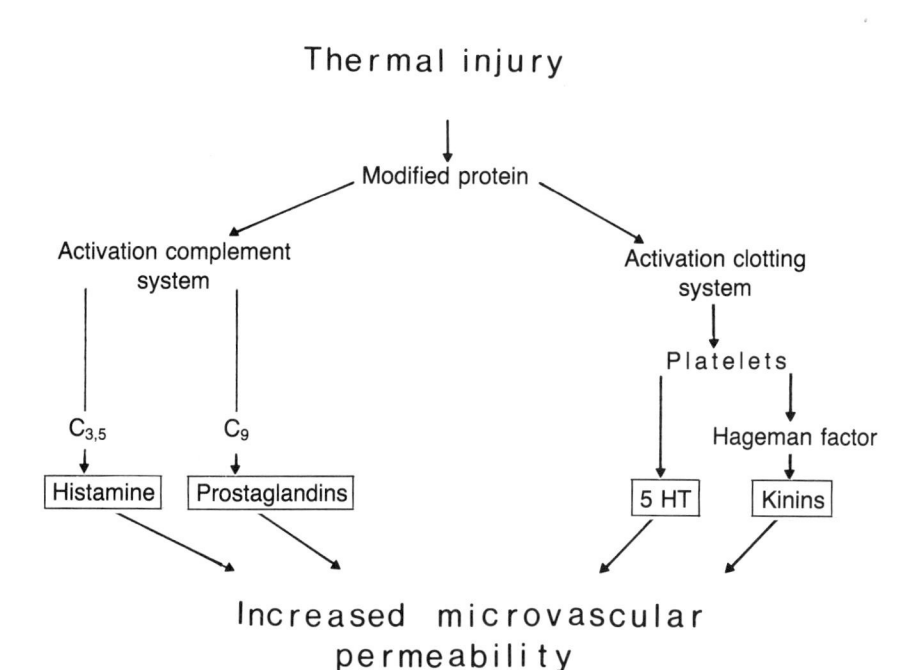

Figure 2–6. A scheme showing some of the inflammatory factors involved in the "acute phase" of the burn syndrome. *(From Arturson G, 1980, reprinted with permission.[22])*

Evaporative Water Loss

In addition to the extravascular fluid sequestration of edematous tissue, fluid loss through the surface of the burn wound contributes significantly to the hypovolemia following thermal injury. Normal intact skin limits the amount of water loss in addition to being a physical barrier to the outside environment. Using extraction techniques, Jelenko et al.[23,24] isolated a hexane-soluble lipid (ethyl linoleate) from normal skin. This lipid was found to be absent from burned skin and is thought to explain why water vapor transmission is at least four times more rapid than through normal skin.

Vapor pressure of normal skin is 4 to 5 mm Hg as compared to 30 to 35 mm Hg observed 4 days following a full thickness burn. In partial thickness burns, the evaporative loss of water is greatest on the day of injury, while in the full thickness burn, the peak evaporative loss is reached gradually by the fourth day. The average fluid loss has been calculated to be about 150 milliliters per square meter of body surface per hour. A 70 kilogram man with 1.85 M^2 surface area, sustaining a 40 percent burn, would lose over 2500 milliliters of fluid from evaporation alone.

As previously described, partial thickness wounds will convert to full thickness wounds in the presence of sepsis or dehydration. Intact blisters not only form a barrier to infection, but also to wound dehydration. Wheeler and Miller[25] have shown that the evaporative water loss from the surface of a burn blister is essentially the same as that for normal skin. When the blister is removed, water loss is initially more than 100 times normal and remains 20 to 50 times normal throughout the first week (Fig. 2–7). The high rate of water loss is associated with an increased depth of wound destruction and a thickening of the overlying crust. Microscopic sections show previously viable dermis incorporated into the crust. However, the dermal loss is negligible when the blister is left intact.

Oxygen Free Radicals in Thermal Injury

It has recently been suggested that oxygen free radicals are likely to be involved in thermal injury. When reduction of oxygen occurs by the monovalent pathway, superoxide radical (O_2) and hydrogen peroxide (H_2O_2) are formed. Under normal conditions, these will be scavenged by superoxide dimutases (SOD) and peroxidases (PO) respectively. Should this not occur, hydroxyl radical ($=OH$) and possibly singlet oxygen ($=O$) will result; neither of which are well tolerated by the living cell. Arturson[22] noted that NADPH-oxidases in the phagosome wall of the polymorphonuclear neutrophil leukocyte (PMN) undergo a burst of oxidative metabolism during the ingestion of particulate matter—the so–called oxygen burst. Incomplete reduction of oxygen to the superoxide radical and H_2O_2 occurs which kills bacteria and other related phagocytized material. The scavenger enzymes (SOD and PO) convert these radicals to water and oxygen (Fig. 2–8). Measured levels of these enzymes are known to be very low and insufficient to destroy the free radicals released from injured tissue.

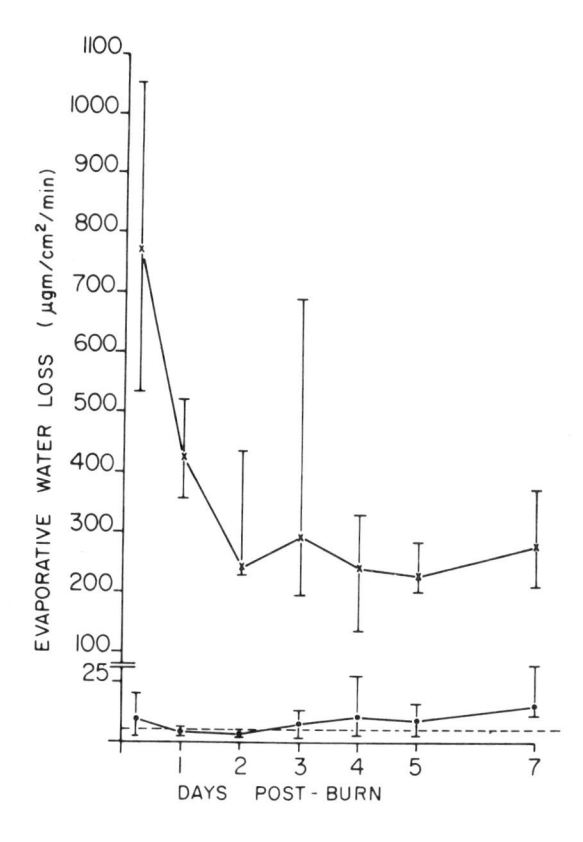

Figure 2-7. Evaporative water loss from the wound surface. Brackets represent the range of the highest and lowest recordings. – – –, mean value for normal skin; X, exposed wounds; •, blister-covered wounds. All values are significant (p 0.001). *(From Wheeler ES, Miller TA, 1976, reprinted with permission.[25])*

In the burn wound, release of oxygen free radicals from PMNs occurs without benefit of enzymatic degradation. Hydroxyl radicals may be formed. This results in enhanced membrane phospholipase activity and release of arachidonic acid. Regeneration of prostaglandins (PGE2), endoperoxidases, and other prostaglandin precursors takes place. These substances are thought to cause endothelial contraction resulting in leakage of macromolecules from the intravascular space. Bjork et al.[26] used the rat-foot burn model to test this hypothesis by measuring edema formation following pretreatment with SOD and catalase. They found that if the plasma concentration of these enzymes could be kept sufficiently elevated using an exogenous supply, i.e., polyethylene glycol coupled SOD and an activated form of catalase reversibly bound to plasma proteins, a significant reduction in postburn edema could be achieved.[22,26] This suggests that at least part of the increased vascular permeability observed after thermal injury may be related to oxygen free radical damage initiated by invading leukocytes.

Overview of Wound Physiology

From the foregoing discussion of burn wound pathophysiology, it is clear that many factors influence the final outcome of the burn wound with respect to

Figure 2-8. Scavengers in the monovalent pathway of oxygen reduction. The monovalent pathway for the reduction of molecular oxygen to superoxide anion radical, hydrogen peroxide, hydroxyl radical, and water. The enzymatic defense mechanisms to bypass and prevent the accumulation of reactive intermediates namely the functions of the scavenger superoxide dismutases and catalases are also indicated. *(From Arturson G, 1980, reprinted with permission.[22])*

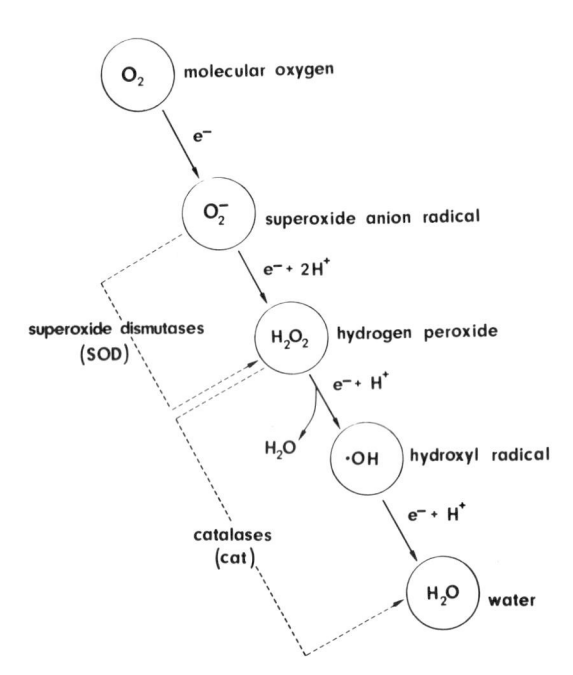

severity, depth, and probability of developing wound sepsis. These factors include the intensity and duration of heat exposure, amount of edema formation, and the degree of wound dehydration. The role of vasoactive mediators and of cellular adherence within the wound microvasculature was discussed in light of their importance to the natural progression of the burn wound.

With this in mind, it seems evident that there exists great potential for influencing the final severity of the burn wound. The key to success lies in manipulation of the area described by Jackson[9] as the "zone of stasis." The potential for preventing progression of this zone to ultimate cell death and thus markedly limiting the final extent of the burn wound has been the subject of extensive and promising research in recent years. In the following section, we will discuss this research. It will become clear, however, that many avenues, especially in the area of pharmacologic manipulation, have yet to be explored.

Modifying the Depth of the Burn Wound

Now that we have reviewed the various pathophysiologic mechanisms involved in creating a burn wound, we should consider ways of modifying the eventual outcome of the burn. Our attention for this purpose will once again be focused on the intermediate zone of stasis.

Cooling the Wound. The benefits of immediately cooling a burn wound have long been appreciated as a matter of common sense and subjective pain relief. Recent experimental evidence has demonstrated objective benefits. Ofelgsson et al.[27] studied scald burns in rats. They found that cooling the wound with water at 25°C for 30 to 45 minutes, even if delayed, limited the extent of necrosis. Repair was established earlier and was usually complete in 30 days, at which time deep ulceration persisted in the control group.

De Camara, Raine, and Robson[28] studied the effects of cooling on the morphology of partial thickness scald burns in guinea pigs. They used ice water immersion at 10 minutes postburn. Comparing these wounds to those of untreated wounds, they found reduced loss of epidermis, reduced damage to the basement membrane, less damage to the dermal microvasculature, and less edema fluid (Figs. 2–9 and 2–10). At later stages, the cooled wounds demonstrated minimal dermal hemorrhage and PMN infiltration in contrast to the untreated wounds. They concluded that on a cellular level, cooling produced beneficial effects on the experimental burn wound.

Boykin and Crute[29] have suggested that several different mechanisms are involved in the beneficial effects of cold water treatment of burn wounds. These all involve the stabilization of membranes and the active compounds which interact with membranes (Fig. 2–11).

It is because of repeated similar experimental data and anecdotal clinical stories that cooling of burn wounds continues as one of the more important initial emergency treatment measures for small burns. The risk of inducing systemic hypothermia precludes its use in patients with large surface area burns.

Prevention of Dehydration. Using an India ink perfusion technique to study partial thickness scald burns, Zawacki[10] investigated the effects of dehydration on eventual burn depth. He found that reversal of capillary stasis was complete and necrosis absent when blisters were left intact or replaced by fresh split thickness porcine skin. Reversal of capillary stasis was least and progressed to full thickness necrosis in undressed wounds with blisters removed (Fig. 2–12). This suggests that capillary stasis can be reversed and wound necrosis avoided with proper measures to prevent dehydration.

Pharmacologic Manipulation. As one might guess, many agents have been used in an attempt to prevent progression of the burn wound. These have ranged from the Aloe vera plant of folk medicine to specific chemical substances produced in the laboratory. Noble et al.[30] found that pretreatment of rats with systemic doses of heparin preserved capillary integrity for up to 72 hours postburn. Animals given heparin postburn showed no change in the pathologic process. They concluded that there is ongoing insult to the rheologic properties of the microvasculature that could be modified. As we have seen, this probably relates to cellular sludging and white blood cell adherence.

Robson et al.,[31] using this premise was able to show that topical 1 percent methyprednisolone acetate improved dermal perfusion (India ink method), and preserved dermal appendage survival ninefold without potentiating wound sepsis. These effects were initially attributed to the steroid-mediated inhibition

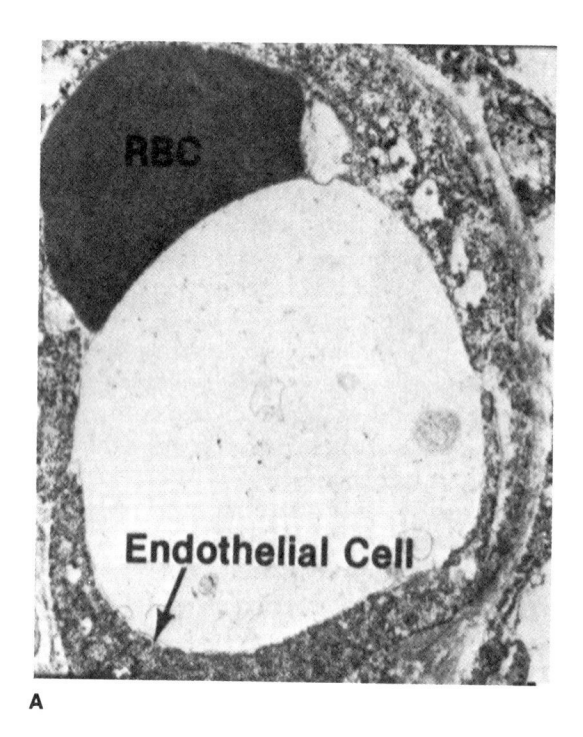

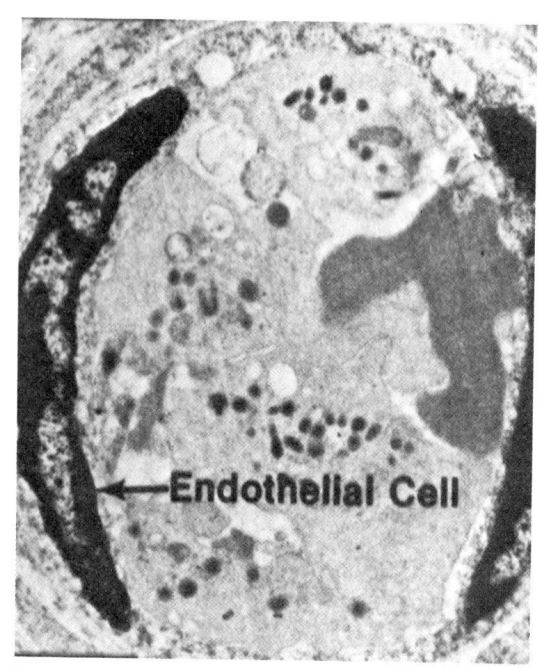

Figure 2–9.A. Capillary 2 hours postburn with swelling and vacuolization of endothelial cells: a red blood cell (RBC) is seen with the lumen. ×11,500. **B.** Cooled capillary 2 hours postburn with some vacuoles within endothelial cells but no disruption or cell gaps. Lumen is filled with platelets. ×11,500. *(From de Camara DL, Raine T, Robson MC, 1981, reprinted with permission.[28])*

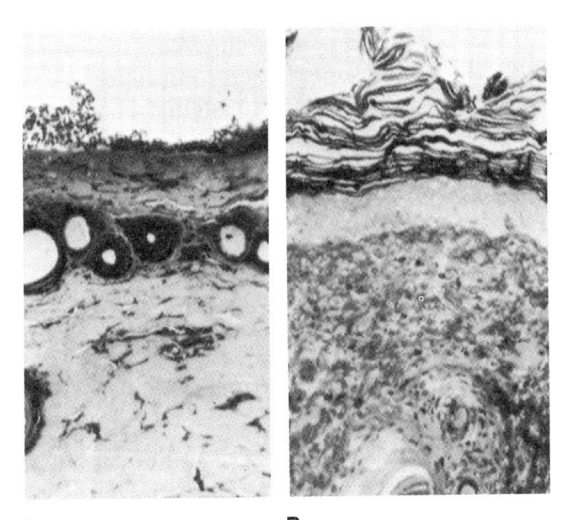

Figure 2–10.A. Ninety-six hours postburn skin from an untreated animal showing complete loss of epidermis. Red blood cells and cellular debris are noted on the burn wound surface with edema separating collagen in the dermis. ×500. **B.** Ninety-six hours postburn in the cooled skin showing near normal structure with adherence of the epidermis to dermis. Epidermis cell outlines are maintained with little dermal edema noted. ×500. *(From de Camara DL, Raine T, Robson MC, 1981, reprinted with permission.[28])*

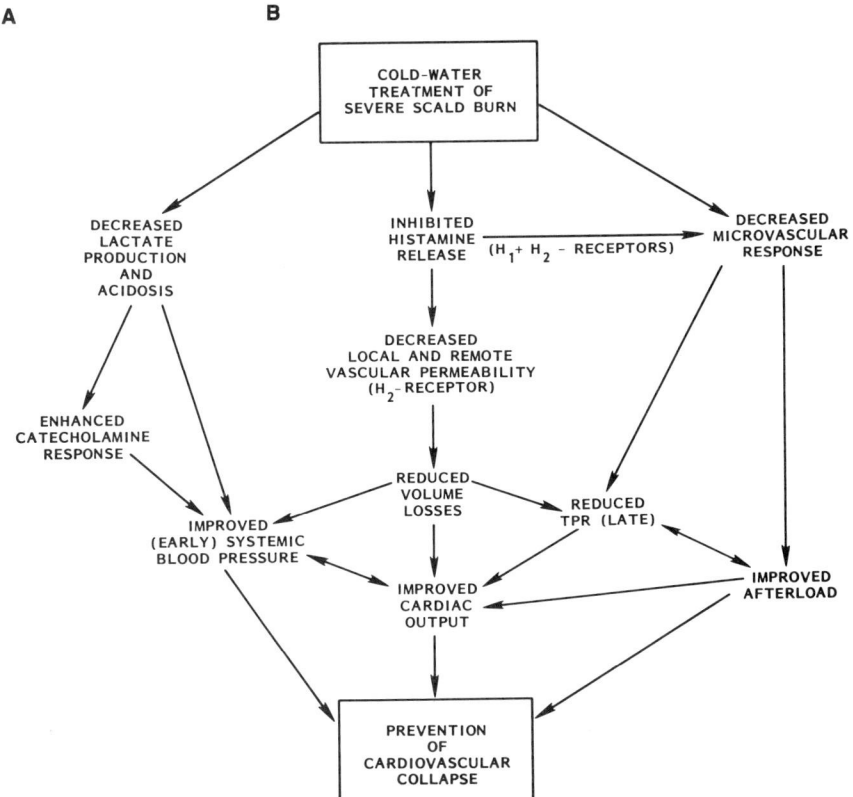

Figure 2–11. Cold-water treatment of severe scald burn. Schematic display of CWT-related factors contributing to burn shock aversion and prevention of cardiovascular collapse following unresuscitated, severe scald injury. *(From Boykin JV Jr, Crute SL, 1982, reprinted with permission.[29])*

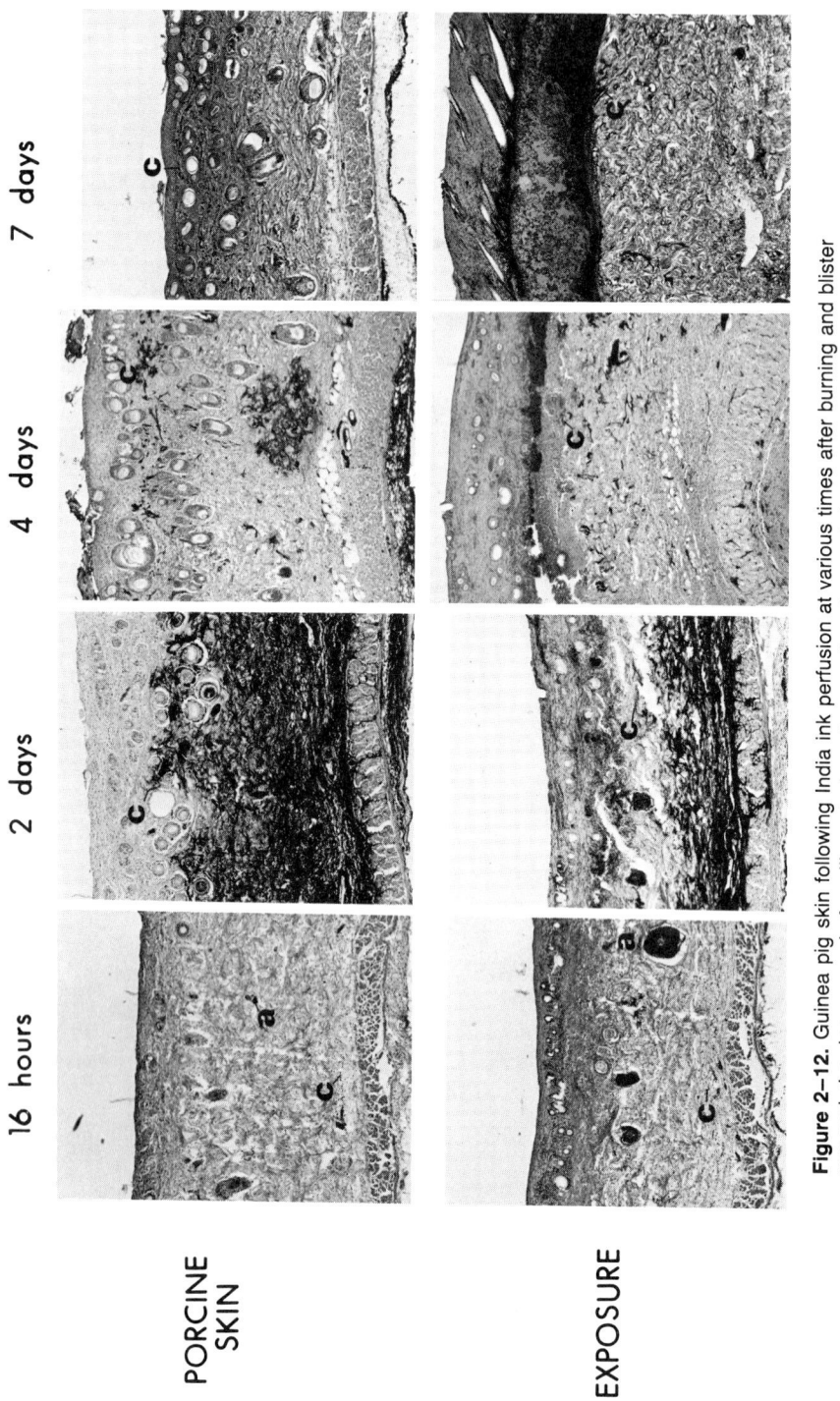

Figure 2–12. Guinea pig skin following India ink perfusion at various times after burning and blister removal showing reversal of capillary stasis and prevention of necrosis by application of porcine skin. (*From Zawacki B, 1974, reprinted with permission.*[10])

of leukocyte sticking in inflammatory conditions as described by MacGregor et al.[32] Robson and others have subsequently demonstrated the ability of steroids to interfere with prostaglandins as vasoactive mediators.[11,14–16] Steroid-mediated inhibition of bradykinin effects have also been described.[33]

Other agents have been used experimentally to influence the amount of edema and to some extent inhibit progressive ischemia in the burn wound. Nonsteroidal prostaglandin synthetase inhibitors, in particular indomethacin (Fig. 2–13)[18] and acetylsalicyclic acid (Fig. 2–14),[15] fall into this category. Extracts of the Aloe vera plant also contain significant levels of a salicylate-

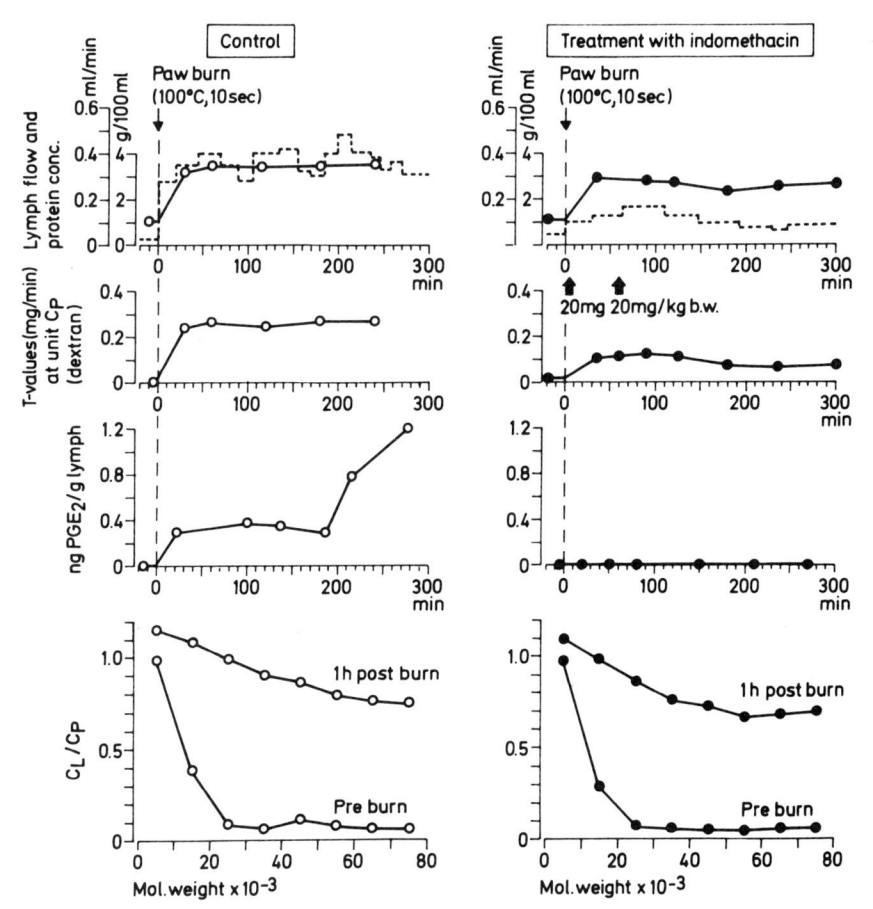

Figure 2-13. Lymph flow, total protein concentration of lymph, T-values (T = the net transport of dextran from blood to the lymph cannula at unit plasma concentration, ml/min), efflux of prostaglandins and C_l/C_p ratios for dextran in lymph from paws scalded for 10 seconds at 100°C in two dogs, one without treatment (A) and one treated with indomethacin 20 mg/kg body weight immediately and 1 hour after scalding (B)._ _ _ _, lymph flow, O_ _ _ _O, protein concentration. *(From Arturson G, Jonsson CE, 1979, reprinted with permission.[18])*

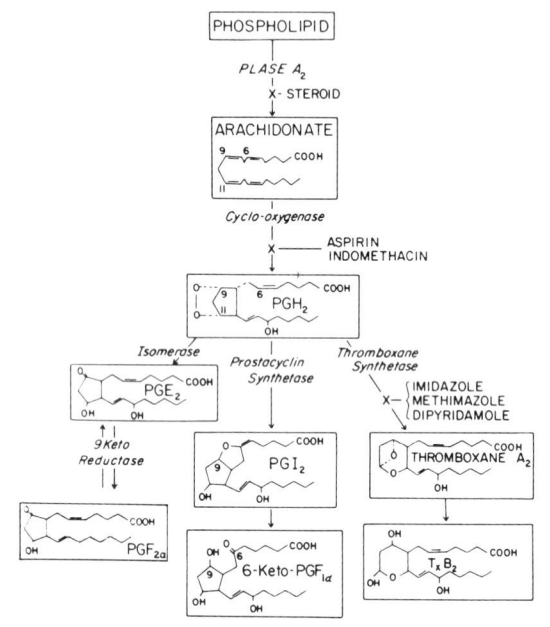

Figure 2-14. Schematic representation of arachidonic acid metabolism to prostaglandins and thromboxanes showing steps of inhibition by blocking agents. (From Robson M, et al., 1980, reprinted with permission.[15])

related substance which has prostaglandin inhibitory activity, and thus is a potential explanation for its reputed effectiveness on burn wounds.[34,35]

Histamine antagonists have also been evaluated in the prevention of burn wound edema. Yoshioka et al.[36] found that large doses of the H2 antagonist cimetidine significantly inhibited edema formation in thermally injured rat muscle. Tissue sodium influx and potassium efflux were sharply restricted. The minimal effective dose was found to be between 0.1 and 0.2 mg/g (Fig. 2-15). It should also be noted that cold water treatment has been shown to inhibit histamine-mediated burn edema.[29,37]

Over the next few years as the chemistry and physiology of prostaglandins and other vasoactive substances are explored, we should be better able to understand and perhaps clinically manipulate the zone of stasis within the partial thickness burn wound.

SYSTEMIC EFFECTS OF THERMAL INJURY

The high mortality rate suffered by patients who experience extensive thermal injury is not only a consequence of the burn wound and its potential for sepsis, but also to the extensive effect of thermal injury on virtually every organ system in the body. Alterations of many aspects of the immune system

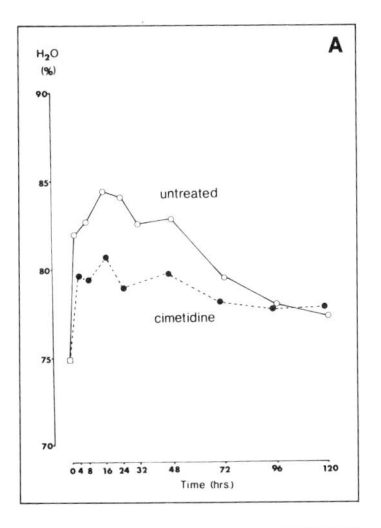

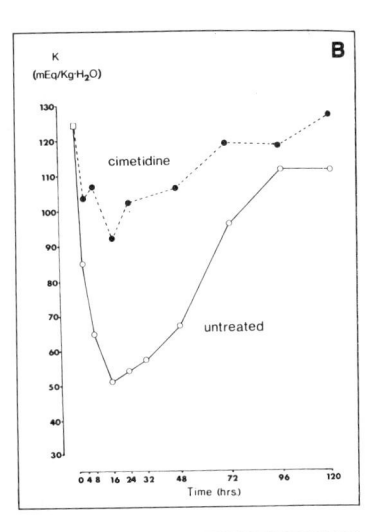

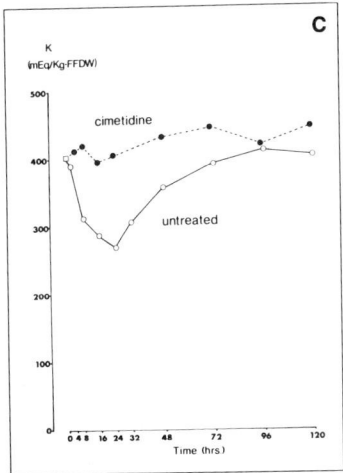

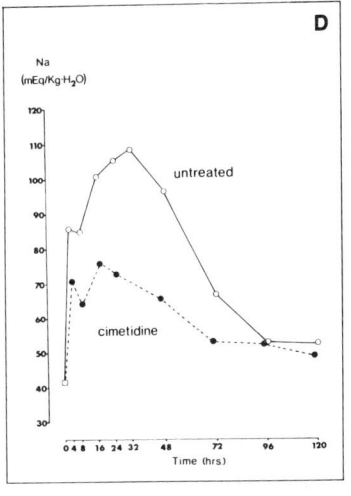

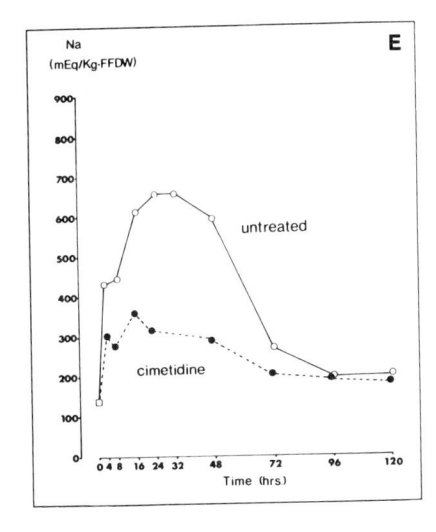

Figure 2–15. The changes in water, sodium, and potassium levels of muscle after injury: effects of pretreatment with cimetidine. The differences between the control and cimetidine-treated groups are relatively significant at all intervals between 8 and 72 hours (p 0.05). Normal values are shown as unshaded squares. FFDW, fat-free dry weight. *(From Yoshioka T, et al., 1978, reprinted with permission.[36])*

have long been known and studied, and impaired immune response remains one of the more difficult management problems in the burned patient. In addition, marked changes in the endocrine and metabolic milieu, as well as hemodynamic, hematologic, pulmonary, renal, and gastrointestinal functions occur. This section will focus on these alterations and new avenues for their investigation.

Hematologic Changes Following Thermal Trauma

A variety of hematologic changes occur following major thermal trauma.[38] These include thrombocytopenia, secondary thrombocytosis, increased platelet adhesiveness, decreased platelet survival, elevated fibrinogen levels, elevated levels of Factors V and VIII, along with increased fibrin split products. An increased erythrocyte destruction rate also occurs for several weeks after thermal injury. This results in a moderate to severe postburn anemia apart from any blood lost during excisional treatment of the burn wound.

Although hemoconcentration increased the hematocrit to 132 percent of normal at 6 hours postburn (untreated 50 percent scald burn model in dogs), Heideman[39] demonstrated hemolysis of 30 percent of the circulating erythrocytes. Erythrocyte destruction corresponded to simultaneous complement consumption. In 1955, Troell et al.[40] documented similar findings in humans. In addition to the initial direct thermal destruction of erythrocytes, it is postulated that C3-mediated red cell lysis occurs. It appears that a lytic process is initiated at a site (the burn wound) distant to normal cell membranes and makes them sensitive to an attack by C8 and C9 with subsequent lysis as a final result.

Endocrine and Metabolic Changes Following Thermal Injury

The increase in metabolic rate and heat production is greater following thermal injury than in any form of trauma. All of the principal metabolic fuel pathways are utilized. While it has long been presumed that this increase was under hormonal control, the details of the endocrine and metabolic pathophysiology of burns have only recently begun to be understood.

Following thermal trauma, metabolic heat production is substantially increased. This is partially balanced by a pronounced increase in evaporative heat loss and, to some extent, by convective and radiative heat loss. Were this not to happen, core temperatures would quickly reach lethal levels. Wilmore et al.[41] have shown that the average core temperature of burned patients is elevated and that the mean skin temperature is increased above normal.

The amount of heat and water lost following thermal injury is controlled by the temperature, humidity, and movement of the surrounding air, and the distribution of radiant energy over the body surface. Evaporative heat loss accounts for the greatest percentage of the heat transfer which takes place. Patients with extensive burns lose a tremendous amount of heat for several weeks following the burn injury, and they invariably have the subjective sensation of feeling cold even though their measured core temperature may be elevated. If the burned patient is exposed to a cool environment, such as the usual hospital room, the body is unable to respond appropriately and conserve heat by peripheral vasoconstriction. Instead, any drop in body temperature is countered with a costly increase in heat production. This places an additional metabolic load on the already high nutritional requirements which these patients have.

Associated with the transcutaneous loss of water and energy from the burn wound is an increase in resting oxygen consumption and excessive nitrogen wasting. A massive catabolic drive results and is manifested by early suppression of insulin secretion with associated increases in production of the catabolic hormones, i.e., catecholamines, glucagon, and probably cortisol. These in turn stimulate lipolysis, ketogenesis, proteolysis, gluconeogenesis, and substrate flow to the liver. Skeletal muscle is the substrate used for protein degradation and not only supplies fuel, but also carbohydrate intermediates.

Insulin release is inhibited by the alpha adrenergic response that dominates the early postburn state. In severe burns, the low plasma insulin is accompanied by a higher serum glucose than would be expected, suggesting both insulin resistance and impaired insulin secretion. It is speculated that the high serum glucose is the result of increased gluconeogenesis.[42] Additionally, insulin enhances amino acid uptake and protein synthesis.[43] The net effect is a decrease in amino acids released into the circulation. Arturson[42] describes these initial events as the ebb phase. With time, this is followed by a flow phase which is characterized by increased oxygen consumption and heat production, negative nitrogen balance, and weight loss (Fig. 2–16). This phase seems to be directed by catecholamines and glucagon. The ratio of insulin to glucagon is important in determining the flow of substrate to the liver. Glucagon is increased relative to insulin and leads to increased glycogenolysis, gluconeogenesis, and ureagenesis at the expense of protein synthesis.

Taking advantage of recent advances in radioimmune assay techniques, Dolecek et al.[44] studied the hormonal response to thermal injury in 82 patients. They concluded that the endocrine and metabolic systems have three main tasks following thermal trauma: (1) to supply enough fuel, (2) to repair damage, and (3) to protect the burned organism from infection. They characterized the endocrine response as one of markedly increasing catabolism, markedly decreasing anabolism, and a change in the endocrine priorities such that these demands can be met. Impaired glucose tolerance and insulin resistance were demonstrated, while human growth hormone (HGH) levels were normal or slightly increased. Renin and angiotensin II levels were high to very high in almost all burned patients. Adrenocorticotropin hormone (ACTH) levels were unpredictable and ranged from normal to very high with no correlation to the 17-OHCS levels. Serum follicle-stimulating hormone (FSH) and testosterone levels were low to very low, while luteinizing hormone (LH) levels were high in 25 percent, normal in 31 percent, and low in 44 percent. In some patients, LH serum levels had a tendency to increase during stress.

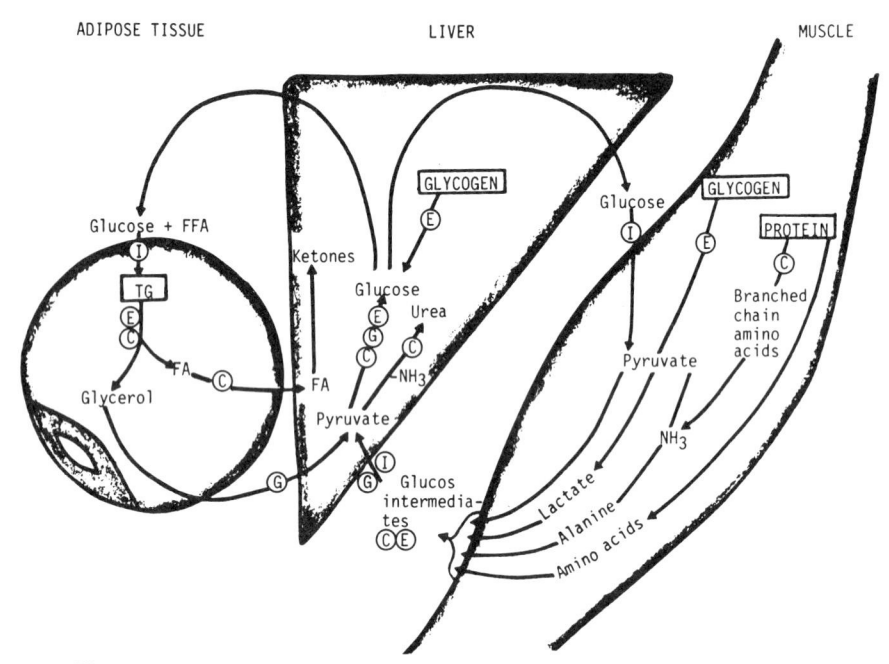

Figure 2–16. Interrelationship between hormones and substrates in the "flow phase" after thermal injury characterized by enhanced lipolysis, protein breakdown, and gluconeogenesis from three carbon glucose intermediates and glycerol. TG, triglyceride; FFA and FA, free or nonesterified fatty acids; C, cortisol; E, epinephrine; G, glucagon; I, insulin. *(From Arturson G, 1978, reprinted with permission.[42])*

Smeds et al.[45] followed thyroid function for 4 to 6 weeks in 12 thermally injured patients and found serum T3 to be low, while thyroxine and the free T4 index were within normal range. TSH was initially low, but gradually returned to normal. They concluded that the thyroid hormones are depleted at the cellular level after burn injury and are not responsible for postburn hypermetabolism.

While researchers agree that the sequence of metabolic events following thermal trauma is hormonally mediated, there is disagreement on the relationship between the specific hormones and the observed metabolic changes. Immediately after the burn injury, the adrenal cortex is stimulated to form glucocorticoids by ACTH release from the anterior pituitary. Elevated levels of free urinary cortisol reflect this increase in adrenocortical activity. Aldosterone secretion parallels that of cortisol probably as a result of sodium depletion and hypovolemia. Plasma cholesterol levels rise as a result of increased cortisol production. Batstone et al.[46] have demonstrated high plasma cortisol concentrations up to 5 days postburn and correlated it with increased protein catabolism. Others have suggested that adrenocortical hormones have only a permissive role in the metabolic response and do not control or alter metabolism.[47,48]

REFERENCES

1. Moritz AR, Henriques FC Jr: Studies of thermal injury. II. The relative importance of time and surface temperature in the causation of cutaneous burns. Am J Pathol 23:531, 1947
2. Yarbrough D III: Pathophysiology of the burn wound. In Wagner M (ed): Care of the Burn-Injured Patient. Littleton, Mass. PSG Publishing, 1981, p 21
3. Robson M, Krizek T, Wray R Jr: Care of the thermally injured patient. In Zuidema GD, Rutherford RB, Ballinger WF (eds): The Management of Trauma. Philadelphia, Saunders, 1979, pp 662–682
4. Moncrief J: The body's response to heat. In Artz C, Moncrief J, Pruitt B. (eds); Burns. A Team Approach. Philadelphia, Saunders, 1979
5. Sonnenburg E, Tschmarke P: Die Verbrenuungen und die Erfrierungen. Stuttgart, Enke, 1915, pp 6, 18
6. Fallon RH, Moyer CA: Rates of insensible perspiration through normal, burned, tape stripped, and epidermally denuded living human skin. Ann Surg 158:915, 1963
7. Cohen S: An investigation and fractional assessment of the evaporative water loss through normal skin and burn eschars using a microhygrometer. Plast Reconstr Surg 37:475, 1966
8. Order SE, Moncrief JA: The Burn Wound. Springfield, Ill., Chas. C Thomas, 1963
9. Jackson DM: The diagnosis of the depth of burning. Br J Surg 40:588, 1953
10. Zawacki B: Reversal of capillary stasis and prevention of necrosis in burns. Ann Surg 180:98, 1974
11. Robson MC, Del Beccaro J, Heggers JP: The effect of prostaglandins on the dermal microcirculation after burning, and the inhibition of the effect by specific pharmacological agents. Plast Reconstr Surg 6:781, 1979
12. Massiha H, Monafo WW: Dermal ischemia in thermal injury: The importance of venous occlusion. J Trauma 14:705, 1974
13. Robb HJ: Dynamics of the microcirculation during a burn. Arch Surg 94:776, 1967
14. Jonsson CE, Granström E, Hamberg M: Prostaglandins and thromboxanes in burn injury in man. Scand J Plast Reconstr Surg 13:45, 1979
15. Robson M, et al.: Increasing dermal perfusion after burning by decreasing thromboxine production. J Trauma 20:722, 1980
16. Harms BA, Bodai BI, Smith M, et al.: Prostaglandin release and altered microvascular integrity after burn injury. J Surg Res 31:274, 1981
17. Netsky MG, Leitek SS: Capillary permeability to horse proteins in burn shock. Am J Physiol 140:1, 1943
18. Arturson G, Jonsson CE: Transcapillary transport after thermal injury. Scand J Plast Reconstr Surg 13:29, 1979
19. Garlick DG, Renkin EM: Transport of large molecules from plasma to interstitial fluid and lymph in dog. Am J Physiol 219:1595, 1970
20. Ham KN, Hurley JV: An electron microscopic study of the vascular response to mild thermal injury in the rat. J Pathol Bact 95:175, 1968
21. Eriksson E, Robson M: New pathophysiological mechanism explaining post burn edema. Burns 4:153, 1977
22. Arturson G: Pathophysiology of the burn wound. Ann Chirig Gynaegol 69:178, 1980

23. Jelenko C, Wheeler ML, Scott TH Jr: Studies in burns X, ethyl linoleate: The water holding lipid of the skin. A. The evidence. J Trauma 12:968, 1972
24. Jelenko C, Wheeler ML, Scott TH Jr: Studies in burns X, ethyl linoleate: The water holding lipid of the skin. B. Effects on in vivo burn eschar. J Trauma 12:974, 1972
25. Wheeler ES, Miller TA: The blister and the second degree burn in guinea pigs: The effect of exposure. Plast Reconstr Surg 57:74, 1976
26. Bjork J, del Maestro RF, Arfor KE: Evidence for participation of hydroxyl radical in increased microvascular permeability. Agents Actions (Suppl) 7:208, 1980
27. Ofeigsson OJ, Mitchell R, Patrick RS: Observations on the cold water treatment of cutaneous burns. J Pathol 108:145, 1972.
28. De Camara D, Raine T, Robson M: Ultrastructural aspects of cooled thermal injury. J Trauma 21:911, 1981
29. Boykin JV Jr, Crute SL: Mechanisms of burn shock protection after severe scald injury by cold-water treatment. J Trauma 22:859, 1982
30. Noble HGS, Robson M, Krizek TJ: Dermal ischemia in the burn wound. J Surg Res 23:117, 1977
31. Robson M, Kucan JO, Paik KI, et al.: Prevention of dermal ischemia after thermal injury. Arch Surg 113:621, 1978
32. MacGregor RR, Spagnolo PJ, Lentner AL: Inhibition of granulocytic adherence by ethanol, prednisone, and aspirin measured with an assay system. N Engl J Med 291:642, 1974
33. Zweifach BW: Functional Behavior of the microcirculation. Springfield, Ill., Chas. C Thomas, 1961
34. Robson M, Heggers JP, Pineless GR: Myth, magic, witchcraft or fact? Aloe vera revisited. Abstr. 31, Am Burn Assoc, 11th Annual Meeting, March 15–17, 1979
35. Heck E, et al.: Aloe vera (gel) cream as a topical treatment for outpatient burns. Burns 7:291, 1981
36. Yoshioka T, Manafo WW, Ayvazian VH, et al.: Cimetidine inhibits burn edema formation. Am J Surg 136:681, 1978
37. Boykin JV, Eriksson E, Sholley MM, et al.: Histamine-mediated delayed permeability response after scald burn inhibited by cimetidine or cold-water treatment. Science 209:815, 1980
38. Gehrke CE, Penner JA, Niederhuber J, et al.: Coagulation defects in burned patients. Surg Gynec Obstet 133:613, 1971
39. Heideman M: The effect of thermal injury on hemodynamic, respiratory, and hematologic variables in relation to complement activation. J Trauma 19:239, 1979
40. Troell L, Norlander O, Johanson B: Red cell destruction in burns. Acta Chir Scand 109:158, 1955
41. Wilmore DW, Mason AD, Johnson DW, et al.: Effect of ambient temperature on heat production and heat loss in burn patients. J Appl Physiol 38:593, 1975
42. Arturson G: Metabolic changes following thermal injury. World J Surg 2:203, 1978
43. Fulks RM, Li JB, Goldberg AL: Effects of insulin, glucose, and amino acids on protein turnover in rat diaphragm. J Biol Chem 250:290, 1975
44. Dolecek R, Adámková M, Sotorníkova T, Závada M, Kračmar P: Endocrine response after burn. Scand J Plast Reconstr Surg 13:9, 1979

45. Smeds S, Kagedal B, Lieden G, et al.: Thyroid function after thermal trauma. Scand J Plast Reconstr Surg 15:141, 1981
46. Batstone GR, Alberti KGMM, Hinks L, et al.: Metabolic studies in subjects following thermal injury. Burns 2:207, 1976
47. Wilmore DW: Hormonal responses and their effect on metabolism. Surg Clin North Am 56:999, 1976
48. Johnston IDA: The endocrine response to trauma in parenteral nutrition. In Lee HA (ed.): Acute Metabolic Illness. London, Academic Press, 1974, p 211

CHAPTER 3
Immunology
Glenn D. Warden

Infection continues to be the leading cause of death in thermally injured patients, in spite of the many improvements in burn care which have been introduced during the past decades. Numerous conditions contribute to the increased susceptibility of burn patients to infection, including the presence of open wounds (inevitably contaminated with bacteria), increased metabolic requirements, decreased nutritional intake, loss of plasma protein from the burned area, and active suppression of immune defense mechanisms. Alteration of host immune defense following thermal injury has been studied since the early 1950s.

It is the purpose of this chapter to review the immune alterations following major thermal injury and to try to correlate these alterations within the complex totality of host defense.

COMPONENTS OF THE IMMUNE RESPONSE

Nonspecific Immunity
The skin functions as an aesthetic container for the human body, providing protection for internal organs, regulation of temperature, and a barrier to prevent protein and water loss. In addition, the skin is the most important defense mechanism against microbial invasion. Any injury which compromises skin integrity threatens the ability to coexist with surrounding microorganisms.

Any organism taking advantage of a wound to gain access to the human body must first survive local conditions at that portal of entry. The violation of organisms into the body results in a local inflammatory response. The inflammatory response is initiated by vasoactive amines, such as histamine and serotonin, kinin polypeptides, and other chemical mediators. These mediators act by constriction of venular sphincters and by dilation of the capillaries. In addition, the kallikrein–kinin system is responsible for increased vascular permeability and the adherent properties of the venular endothelial surfaces. The vascular changes result in fluid and fibrinogen leaving the dilated, permeable vessels, creating a fibrin and thrombin network which functions to localize invading bacteria. The adherent capillary endothelial walls marginate circulating phagocytic cells and allow migration out through the widened endothelial spaces. Leukotaxis has also been found to be aided by the kinin system. Nonspecific inflammation also places the microorganisms in contact with serum. Serum contains at least two classes of protein which function in nonspecific resistance. One, a heat-stable protein called beta-lysin is lethal to gram-positive organisms, and the other, a heat-labile group of proteins collectively known as complement is effective against gram-negative organisms. In addition, complement promotes effective phagocytosis by polymorphonuclear leukocytes.

If local mechanisms are not effective in containing the infection, the invading microorganisms are transported by the lymphatics to the regional lymph nodes where fixed macrophages phagocytize the organisms. These cells contain enzymes which may destroy the bacteria. In addition, specific immune responsiveness is initiated by lymphocytes at this location. Beyond the lymph nodes, the bacteria enter the general circulation. Specific immune mechanisms now become all important in the survival of the host. These defenses include the generation of specific, protective antibodies, and the generation of specific, cytotoxic lymphocytes that are effective against intracellular infection. The success of these specific immune mechanisms in containing the infection depends upon many factors including the previous exposure of the host to the invading microorganism, and the virulence, growth rate, and toxin production of the organism.

Specific Immune Response
The lymphocyte is the central cell in specific immune responsiveness. Lymphocytes form two response systems: the thymus-derived (T cell) system which is commonly associated with the concept of cell-mediated immunity, and the bone marrow-derived (B cell) system which is associated with humoral or antibody-mediated immunity (Fig. 3–1). The lymphoctye is not the most aggressive cell in the body (neutrophils, for example, are more efficient at disposing of antigens) but it is the only cell which is capable of specifically recognizing an antigen as foreign and of initiating specific mechanisms to dispose of the invader. Both B and T lymphocytes arise from a common bone marrow stem cell. Cells which mature under the influence of the thymus differentiate into mature T lymphocytes. A second population of cells, B lymphocytes, avoids thymic processing.

Upon reaching maturity, B and T lymphocytes seed the peripheral lym-

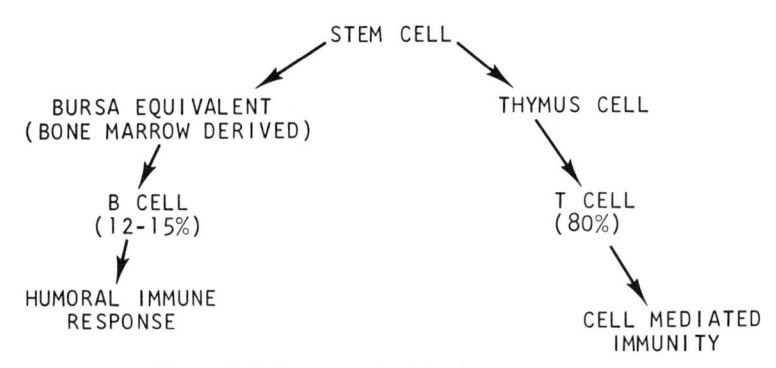

Figure 3-1. Components of the immune response.

phoid organs. There are approximately 80 percent T cells and 12 to 15 percent B cells in the normal human peripheral blood lymphocyte compartment. Varying proportions of each cell type are present in the lymphoid organs of the body. Despite the division of lymphocyte response into cell-mediated and humoral immunity, investigators have begun to uncover a complex array of interactions between these two aspects of immune reactivity that is blurring a once sharp distinction between cell types and cell functions. The discovery of additional subpopulations of lymphocytes has further complicated this once clear dichotomy. An interrelationship between lymphocyte types is a factor in most aspects of the immune response.

Cell-Mediated Immunity

The mechanisms involved in T cell function and cell-mediated immunity have been extensively studied. Briefly, when stimulated by antigen, T lymphocytes undergo blast transformation and then proliferate following a number of directions or pathways (Fig. 3-2). T lymphocytes can differentiate into memory cells which live as long as 20 years, and are capable of early and accelerated

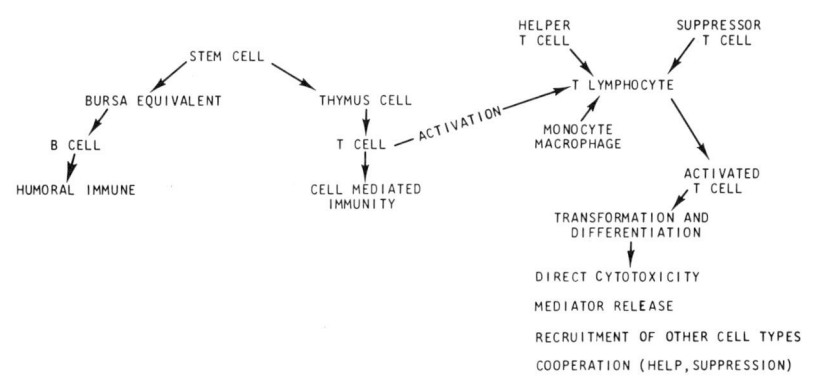

Figure 3-2. Cell-mediated immunity.

response when restimulated by the original or cross-reactive antigenic determinants. This memory characteristic is particularly relevant in continued immunity against reinfection with the same or closely related organisms following natural infection or immunization. A similar mechanism involving memory cells also occurs in antibody (B lymphocyte) response to infection. In addition, T cell cooperation is thought to be essential for most B cell responses to occur.

Another characteristic function of T lymphocytes is to elaborate and secrete a variety of soluble mediators of immune reactivity called lymphokines. These lymphokines are directly involved in the stimulatory as well as the inhibitory capacities of T lymphocytes. In addition to regulating specific immune response, the soluble products of T lymphocytes effectively amplify the nonspecific immune response. Both macrophage inhibitory factor (MIF) and lymphocyte-derived chemotactic factors recruit other uncommitted lymphoid cells as well as monocytes, neutrophils, and eosinophils. The recruited cells are then active in destroying invading microorganisms. Lymphokines derived from T cells also activate macrophages to greater microbicidal activity; an important factor in host defense against a variety of infections.

Helper and suppressor T cells and the products of these cells are also essential elements in host defense against microbial invasion. Both T cell responses and many B cell responses are dependent upon interactions with activated regulatory T cells. Adequate helper T cells are clearly required for antibody responses to at least some of the organisms that are primarily held in check by humoral immune defenses. Suppressor T cells are also important regulators of these immune responses. Elevated suppressor cell activity has been associated with impaired host defenses in many crucial situations involving intracellular parasites.

Altered cell-mediated immunity following thermal injury has been recognized since the 1950s with the demonstration of prolonged survival of skin allografts in patients with very extensive burns.[1] Further evidence of T cell abnormality was confirmed with the demonstration that the anamnestic response to tetanus toxoid was abrogated following thermal injury. A decline in the response of peripheral blood lymphocytes to the T cell mitogens phytohemagglutinin and *Candida* has also been demonstrated following thermal injury. Direct measurement of the number of peripheral blood lymphocytes has demonstrated a decrease in T cells while B cell number apparently remained normal. Extensive suppressor T cell activity has been found in thermally injured patients.[2,3] A serum-borne factor and a specific subset of B lymphocytes have been implicated in the generation of such suppressor cells.[4] In addition, the cytotoxic activity of lymphocytes from spleen, abdominal lymph nodes, and peripheral blood is decreased following thermal injury.

Humoral Immunity

The hallmark of humoral immunity in host defense against infection is the production by B lymphocytes and their plasma cell progeny of specific antibodies directed toward microorganisms and their products (Fig. 3–3). Five major classes of immunoglobulin have been identified which are antigenically and, in some ways, functionally distinct. The immunoglobulin types which are known to have functionally significant antibody activity against microorganisms are IgG, IgM, and IgA. Most immunoglobulins are the result of a complex series of events that begin with the activation of B lymphocytes through T lymphocyte cooperation.

All immunoglobulins are decreased in quantity during the first week postburn, but then returned to normal levels during the second week postinjury.[5] The initial decrease is proportional to the extent of the injury. The IgG decreases are far greater than either IgA or IgM, and the administration of gamma globulin or plasma does not influence serum protein concentrations. The initial depression of IgG and IgA levels are followed by higher than normal concentrations. Such elevations could be anticipated considering the antigenization to which burn patients are subjected during their clinical course. In addition, the serum IgM following burn injury is predictably elevated, particularly in patients with large injuries, and may well be due to widespread fungal infection in this group of patients. There is an initial depression in the level of alpha$_2$ macroglobulin. This protein has received considerable interest since it is a protease inhibitor and is thus active in limiting tissue damage by the release of proteolytic enzymes from neutrophils during the inflammatory response. In addition, alpha$_2$ macroglobulin has been associated with the development of functional lymphocytes.

It must be remembered, however, that the techniques used for measuring serum immunoproteins are generally limited to measuring classes of immunoglobulins rather than to specific immunoglobulins produced against specific antigens. Antibodies have multiple roles in host defense including toxin neutralization, bacteriolysis in the presence of complement, and opsonization of bacteria resulting in enhanced phagocytosis. Thus, any defect in antibody production would result in altered complement and white cell function since opsonization has an important role in leukocyte phagocytosis. Furthermore, these systems interact also with cell-mediated immunity since increased suppressor T cell activity results in altered B lymphocyte activation and subsequent changes in immunoglobulin production.

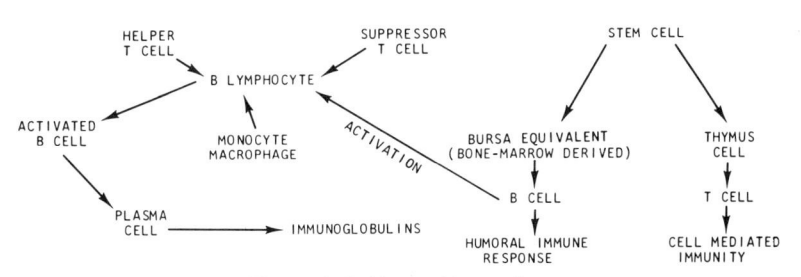

Figure 3–3. Humoral immunity.

The Complement System

The complement system is a highly complex integrated network of serum proteins which bridges both specific and nonspecific immunity. When activated, these serum proteins mediate inflammation, tissue damage, and facilitate ingestion of microorganisms by phagocytic cells.[6] The complement system plays a role in bacterial activity, neutralization of viruses, changes in vascular permeability, leukocyte chemotaxis, and opsonization leading to phagocytosis of microorganisms. Fresh human serum has bacterial activity that is dependent on an intact complement system (Fig. 3–4). Complement activation results in bacteriolysis, however, the functional properties of the cleavage products of complement activation may be more important in host defense against infection than are the actual bacteriolytic reactions themselves.

Both C5a and the molecular fragment C3a have glycoprotein components which have an affinity for cell membranes, resulting in increased vascular permeability, which is part of the inflammatory response associated with many host defense reactions. In addition, the components of C3a and C5a and C567 all have potent chemotactic properties for polymorphonuclear leukocytes. The complement system interacts with humoral immunity in that, with alterations of immunoglobulin or antibody production, there may not be activation of the complement system.

A decrease in the complement components C3a and C5a occurs in the circulation following thermal injury suggesting that thermal injury nonspecifically activates the complement system.[7] Activation of complement in the injured tissue results in an inflammatory response due to the release of histamine and serotonin by C3a and C5a. Thus, edema formation in the injured tissue may be complement dependent. In addition, a consumptive opsoninopathy of C3, properdin, and Factor B occurs following thermal injury.[8] Thus, if complement activity is suppressed, the response of chemotactic cells and subsequent phagocytosis is also depressed.

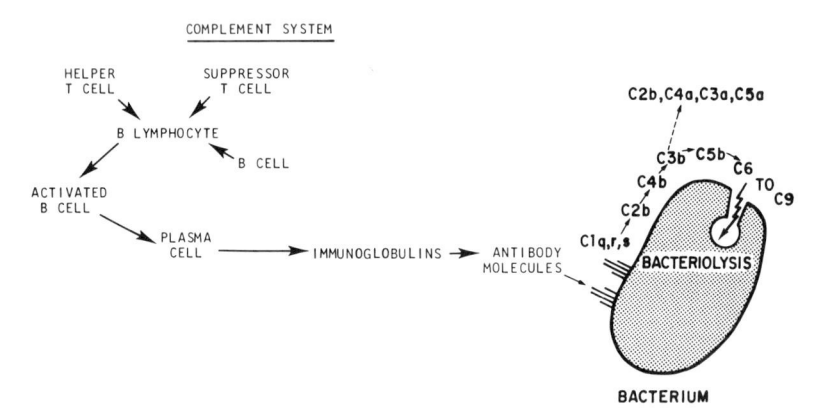

Figure 3–4. Complement system.

Phagocytic Cells

There are two major categories of phagocytic cells in man: the circulating phagocytes of the blood which include the granulocytes (neutrophils, eosinophils, and, to a much less extent, the basophils) and the monocytes; and the fixed phagocytes or macrophages of the tissue, known collectively as the reticuloendothelial system (RES).

The neutrophil is primarily a circulating cell involved in host defense against infectious agents. It is present in higher numbers and possesses much greater phagocytic capabilities than do other circulating leukocytes. The neutrophil becomes available to blood and tissues as a result of an intricately regulated kinetic pattern.[9] The neutrophil (PMN) function in response to stimulation is shown in Figure 3–5. In the marginal pool, leukocytes adhere to postcapillary venules but are in constant equilibrium with the circulating pool. The mechanisms involved in the normal emigration of neutrophils from the circulation are poorly understood. Within minutes of tissue damage or microbial invasion, however, neutrophils adhere to the endothelium of the blood vessels and subsequently migrate into the involved tissues. The migration of neutrophils outside the circulation to the tissues is considered an end stage activity since there is no substantial return to the blood.

In the peripheral tissues, neutrophils, eosinophils, and monocytes all demonstrate chemotaxis or directional migration in response to various stimuli. Chemotactic factors or chemoattractants are present in serum or plasma. The best described chemotactic factors are the products of complement activation, namely C3a, C5a, the trimolecular complex C567, and the fibrolytic and kinin-generating systems. In addition, leukocytes that participate in the inflammatory response elaborate products which can also function as chemoattractants.

Altered leukocyte chemotaxis has been demonstrated following thermal injury.[10] The interaction of polymorphonuclear chemotaxis and the other immune components is demonstrated in Figure 3–6. A depressed cell-mediated

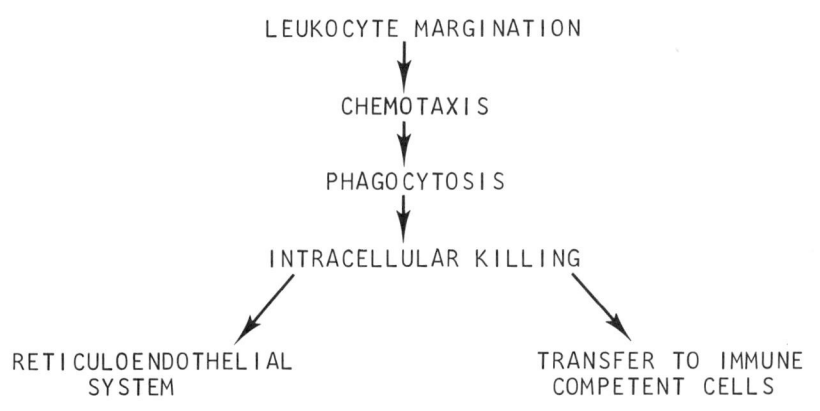

```
              LEUKOCYTE MARGINATION
                      ↓
                  CHEMOTAXIS
                      ↓
                 PHAGOCYTOSIS
                      ↓
              INTRACELLULAR KILLING
                 ↙            ↘
     RETICULOENDOTHELIAL      TRANSFER TO IMMUNE
          SYSTEM                COMPETENT CELLS
```

Figure 3–5. PMN function.

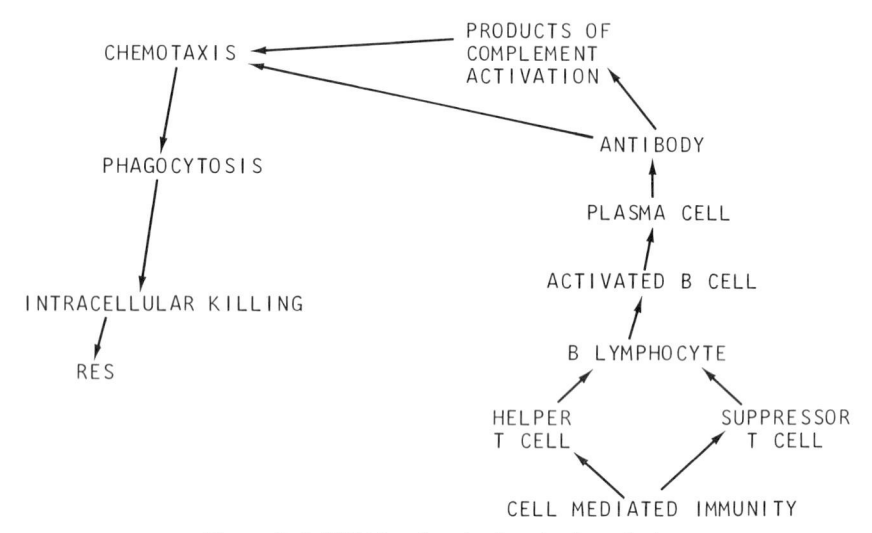

Figure 3-6. PMN function: Leukocyte chemotaxis.

immunity and activation of suppressor T cells resulting in an altered B cell activation and antibody formation can lead to abnormal complement system function, thus resulting in depressed leukocyte chemotaxis.[11]

Next in the sequence of leukocyte function is phagocytosis (Fig. 3-7). Phagocytosis can be greatly enhanced by various humoral factors which are collectively termed opsonins. These diversified substances act predominantly on the target particle itself, rendering it more susceptible to phagocytosis. The best described opsonins are antibodies which are heat stable and add specificity to the phagocytic process. Complement, however, is heat labile

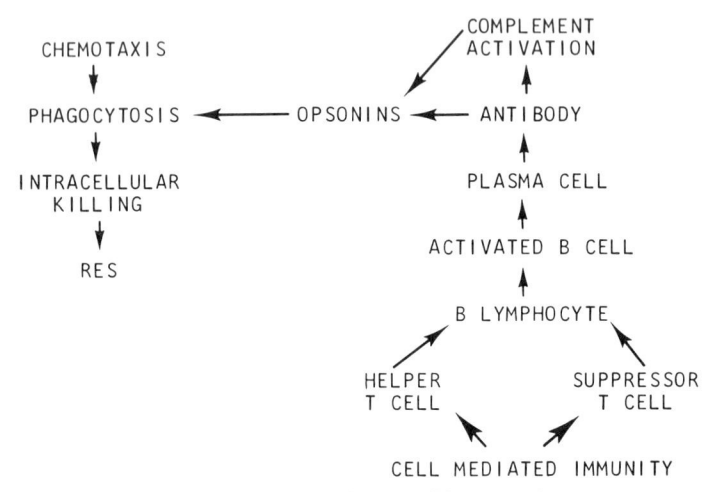

Figure 3-7. PMN function: Phagocytosis.

and nonspecific. In addition, other noncomplement thermolabile serum factors, as well as lysozyme, can serve as opsonins.

The fixed phagocytes or macrophages of the RES most likely arise from bone marrow monocyte precursors which pass through the blood as circulating monocytes and are ultimately deposited in various tissues. In man, the major organs in which tissue macrophages are found are in the spleen, liver (Kupffer cells), lung (alveolar macrophages), and bone marrow. These tissue macrophages are major participants in host defense. Not only are they extremely effective in clearing and killing microorganisms, they are also present in enormous numbers in the body. It has been estimated that there are approximately 200 billion macrophages in the human spleen, liver, and bone marrow.

The macrophage, once considered to be strictly phagocytic and only a peripheral component of the immune system is now emerging as a central cell in the immune response. It is capable of at least three immune-related activities. The first two, phagocytosis and chemotaxis, have already been discussed briefly. Like the lymphocyte, however, the macrophage must undergo a process of activation in order to become maximally efficient. One of the ways in which this can occur is through the release of stimulatory soluble substances by antigen-activated lymphocytes. Thus, macrophage phagocytosis is linked directly to the lymphocytic immune response.

The third and perhaps most important function of the macrophage is to express antigen on its surface. Antigen presented in this manner is immunogenic, and lymphocytes that interact with macrophage-bound antigen become immunologically activated. Antigen which escapes the macrophage will stimulate only a weak immune response, may fail to evoke any response at all, or may be instrumental in the generation of suppressor T cells. Macrophages which act to promote an effective immune response have recently been labeled facilitory macrophages to distinguish them from a recently discovered second population of suppressor macrophages which exert a negative influence upon specific immune reactivity.

INTERACTION OF SPECIFIC IMMUNE RESPONSES WITH NONSPECIFIC IMMUNITY FOLLOWING THERMAL INJURY

The combination of a neutrophil host defense system and a network of circulating and fixed monocytes or macrophages provides a highly diversified, adaptable, and effective phagocytic defense against microbial invasion.

Leukocyte phagocytosis is depressed following thermal injury, however, neutrophil function is not altered immediately following thermal injury. The neutrophil ingestive capacity is not decreased until more than 5 days following injury.[12] In addition, not all severely burned patients displayed these defects in phagocytic function.

Depressed RES functions occur following major burns. The RES defects are indirect consequences of thermal injury, and are due to the interface between specific immune responses and phagocytosis.[13]

The interactions of cell-mediated immunity, humoral immunity, and the complement system have a direct effect on opsonization (see Fig. 3–7). A decreased antibody production, activation of the complement system along with consumption of opsonins results in decreased phagocytosis. In the case of the macrophage, decreased phagocytosis means decreased antigen processing and a decreased specific immune response, as well as an increased likelihood that suppressor cells will be generated.

The opsonic activity of surface binding alpha-glycoprotein fibronectin is a key determinant of RES function. This protein appears to be greatly decreased in quantity immediately following trauma and major burns; a decrease which also contributes to RES phagocytic depression.[13]

Intracellular killing of microorganisms is the most important consequence of neutrophil phagocytosis and is associated with a complex series of metabolic events within minutes of phagocytosis of microorganisms.[14] The biology of the "respiratory burst" which is associated with intracellular killing capacity has been studied extensively[15] and is associated with a number of metabolic events including: (1) increase in glycolysis and lactate production; (2) fall in pH within the phagocytic vacuole; (3) increase in oxygen consumption; (4) increase in hexose monophosphate shunt activity; (5) increase in NADPH and NADH oxidation (metabolic reduction of the dye tetrazolium (NBT) to blue formazen by NADH oxidase measures this); (6) increase in H_2O_2 and superoxide formation; (7) increase in membrane lipid synthesis; and (8) oxidation of chloride and iodide ions via myeloperoxidase catalysis of H_2O_2 (Fig. 3–8). All of these metabolic events have been demonstrated to be decreased following major thermal injury resulting in decreased leukocyte intracellular killing capacity.[16]

ETIOLOGY OF IMMUNE DEFECTS FOLLOWING THERMAL INJURY

It is obvious that the altered immune response following thermal injuries is a complex interaction of the components of the immune response as well as interaction of the metabolic alterations and the burn environment (Fig. 3–9).

The immune defects have several possible contributing factors. Defects, for example, might be caused by either altered host environment or by an injury-triggered host deficiency state.

The internal environment in which immune function is carried out within the host is indeed altered following thermal injury. Normal lymphocyte function is suppressed in the presence of burn sera.[17,18] Normal leukocytes demonstrate depressed leukocyte chemotaxis and superoxide activity when incubated in burn serum.[10] In addition, burn serum contains an inhibitor of C3 conversion which would lead to decreased opsonization and PMN

PMN FUNCTIONS

1. INCREASE IN GLYSOLYSIS
2. FALL IN PH
3. INCREASE IN O_2 CONSUMPTION
4. INCREASE IN HEXOSE MONOPHOSPHATE SHUNT
5. INCREASE IN NADPH AND NADH OXIDATION
6. INCREASE IN H_2O_2 AND SUPEROXIDE FORMATION
7. INCREASE IN MEMBRANE LIPID SYNTHESIS
8. OXIDATION OF CHLORIDE AND IODIDE IONS VI MYELOPEROXIDASE CATALYSIS OF H_2O_2

CHEMOTAXIS → PHAGOCYTOSIS → INTERCELLULAR KILLING → RES

RESPIRATORY BURST

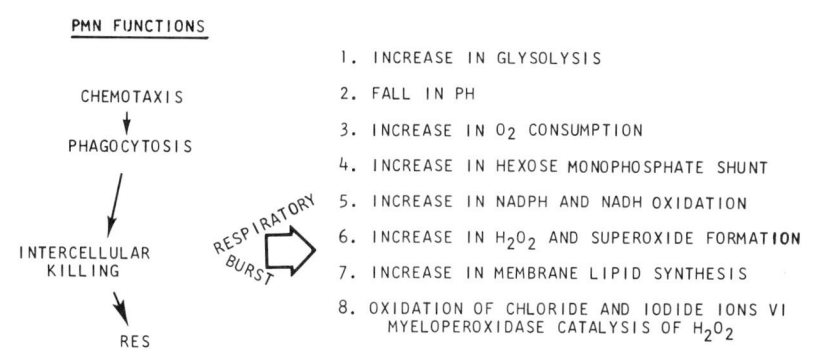

Figure 3-8. PMN function: Intracellular killing.

function.[8] Also, burn generated toxins may play a role in the immunosuppression following thermal injury.[19] The many hormonal changes that occur following thermal injury can also produce changes in the metabolic functions of the various cells of the immune system.[20] In addition, other exogenous inhibitors, such as endotoxin, and endogenous regulators, such as prostaglandins, have been demonstrated in the serum of burn patients. These substances, when incubated with normal cells, result in suppressed function.[21]

The other etiologic category of the immune defect is host deficiency. A complex interaction between nutrition, hormonal balance, and immunologic deficiency exists following thermal injury, major trauma, and in seriously ill patients. When burn cells are incubated with normal plasma or fresh frozen plasma, the depressed function returns toward normal. The phenomenon has been demonstrated in leukocyte chemotaxis, in reference to function and various intracellular metabolic functions of leukocyte intracellular killing.[10]

Whether or not the alteration in immune function following thermal injury is a deficiency disease, or is due to circulating toxins and factors, or a combination of the two, it is now obvious that the final result is an overstimulation of some immune system components (suppressor T cell stimulation, complement activation) and a depression of other components (T helper cell and T killer cell activity, PMN function).

HUMORAL IMMUNE RESPONSE (B CELL) ← HELPER T CELL / SUPPRESSOR T CELL / MONOCYTE → CELL MEDIATED IMMUNITY (T CELL)

ANTIBODY → COMPLEMENT ACTIVATION → PMN FUNCTION

CHEMOTAXIS → PHAGOCYTOSIS → INTERCELLULAR KILLING

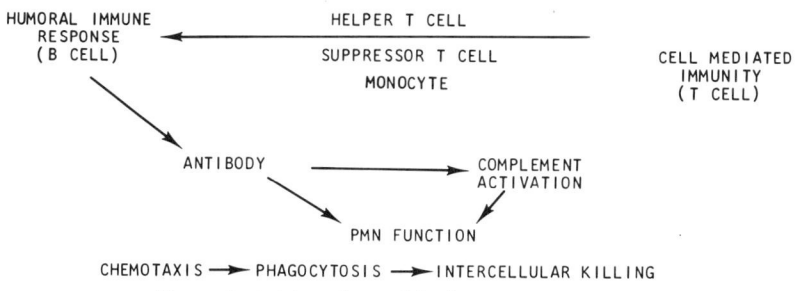

Figure 3-9. Interactions of the immune responses.

FUTURE MANAGEMENT OF THE IMMUNOLOGIC ALTERATIONS FOLLOWING THERMAL INJURY

Only recently has major trauma, including thermal injury, joined transplantation, cancer, and the congenital immunodeficiency syndromes as area of immunologic interest. During the past few years, new developments in immunologic monitoring and modulation have been described. It is exciting to anticipate what the future holds for the problem of reversing the immunologic effects of injury. The following are possible therapeutic approaches that have been suggested, some of which are current and already reported while others are only theoretical.[22]

The ideal immunomodulator should have the following characteristics: (1) rapid action, (2) broad spectrum, (3) inactivity on the suppressor cell population, and (4) minimal side effects. Four areas of approach to immunorestoration have been suggested, including biologic, pharmacologic, immunologic, and physical.

In the area of biologic approaches are the nonspecific immunomodulatory agents such as *Corynebacterium parvum*, Calmette–Guerin bacillus, and levamisole. The agents act by triggering the target cell to a state of accelerated metabolic activity, increased DNA synthesis, and a more rapid and efficient performance of its biologic function. The target cells in this category are macrophages and T lymphocytes and to some extent the B lymphocytes. The major problem with these agents is the inability to differentiate between lymphocytes or macrophages of different biologic function; thus suppressor cells are activated. In addition, these agents clearly require pretreatment before injury and infection to be effective. The future potential of these agents will be the development of precise dose response curves so that enhancement of helper function is maximized, and suppressor function is minimized. More promising will be the development of biologic agents that are specific activators of helper T cells and macrophages at needed times postinjury and with a wide variety of dose ranges.

In the pharmacologic category, stimulation of an immunologic active cell by influencing an intracellular enzyme system or messenger system is attempted. The semisynthetic polynucleotides, such as poly (IC), and poly (AC) and adenylcyclase activators accelerate protein synthesis in the cell. These agents have the same basic disadvantages as the biologic modulators in that they are unable to distinguish between helper and suppressor cells. In addition, these agents are quite toxic. Muramyl dipeptide may be an exception, and initial studies suggest that this agent is fairly specific for helper stimulation. The future is unlimited for development of more double-stranded, semisynthetic polynucleotides that have specific actions upon helper cell, macrophage, and T cell functions.

Other biologic approaches that may be listed in the same category are interleukin 1 and 2, other lymphokines, and the immunologically active thymic hormones. Acceleration of the maturation process of T cells by the use of thymosin or thymopoietin is currently being evaluated, but is plagued by the risk of maturing suppressor cells along with the helper cells. Recent work with the use of very small doses of polymyxin B to block the attachment of endotoxin to the receptor sites of suppressor T cells is another immunologic approach.

In the area of immunologic approaches are classic vaccines, synthetic vaccines, and hybridomas. One of the earliest attempts at immunomodulating the thermally injured patient was the *Pseudomonas* active and passive vaccine studies of the 1960s and 1970s. The development of regional burn units, improved nursing techniques, nutrition, and modern surgical management of the burn patient have decreased the seriousness of *Pseudomonas* infections and the human source for the passive immunoglobulin program. In underdeveloped countries, where well-isolated burn or trauma units are not available and mortality from contact-transmitted organisms even in small burns is still high, benefits can still be derived from this treatment modality.

The recent development of synthetic vaccines such as hepatitis B and influenza have demonstrated that the antigenic components of gram-negative bacteria can be coded and replicated, and synthetic vaccines may be possible. The potential for the development of antibacterial hybridomas with production of monoclonal bacterial antibodies is only theoretical but may be developed in the future.

Mechanical and physical approaches to immunomodulation would either remove serum-mediated inhibitors of immunocyte function or replace deficiency factors which have been demonstrated in thermally injured patients. Evidence for the relevant role of serum inhibitory factors is quite overwhelming. Plasmapheresis with replacement of fresh frozen plasma has already been used in burn patients with correction of normal lymphocyte suppression by burn serum and for burn shock resuscitation.[23] Exchange transfusion therapy has also been used in pediatric burns. With the development of improved filters, dialysis of specific immunosuppressive factors offer potential for the future. Granulocyte and specific lymphocyte or macrophage therapy may offer temporary support of the immunologic system. With the evidence that granulocytes and lymphocytes function normally when removed from the burn environment, however, the wide use of immunocyte therapy in burn patients without the addition of other adjuvant measures will not become a practical therapeutic approach.

It is apparent that the future holds new and exciting approaches to immunomodulation in thermally injured patients. Moreover, a single panacea does not appear to be the answer. Routine laboratory immunologic monitoring will become a daily automated event. Depending on the trend, appropriate immunomodulation techniques will be initiated. The future will undoubtedly see the transfer of diagnostic measures from the research laboratory to the clinical laboratory, with an increase in accuracy and speed, the frequent monitoring of the parameters of failure in host defense, and specific therapies aimed at appropriate defects.

REFERENCES

1. Ninnemann JL, Fisher JC, Frank HA: Prolonged survival of human skin allografts following thermal injury. Transplantation 25:69, 1978
2. Baker CC, Miller CL, Trunkey DD, Lin RC: Identity of mononuclear cells which compromise the resistance of trauma patients. J Surg Res 26:478, 1979
3. Miller CL, Baker CC: Changes in lymphocyte activity after thermal injury: The role of suppressor cells. J Clin Invest 63:202, 1979
4. Ninnemann JL: Suppression of lymphocyte response following thermal injury. In Ninnemann JL (ed): The Immune Consequences of Thermal Injury. Baltimore, Williams & Wilkins, 1981
5. Ninnemann JL, Fisher JC, Wachtel TL: Effect of thermal injury and subsequent therapy on serum protein concentrations. Burns 6:165, 1980
6. Raddy S, Gigli I, Austen KF: The complement system of man. N Engl J Med 287:489, 545, 592, 695, 1975
7. Heideman J: The effect of thermal injury on hemodynamic, respiratory, and hematologic variables in relation to complement. J Trauma 19:239, 1979
8. Bjornson AB, Altemeier WA, Bjornson HS: Changes in humoral components of host defense following burn trauma. Ann Surg 186:88, 1977
9. Klebanoff SJ: Antimicrobial mechanisms of neutrophilic polymorphonuclear leukocytes. Semin Hematol 12:117, 1975
10. Warden GD, Mason AD, Pruitt BA Jr: Evaluation of leukocyte chemotaxis in vitro in thermally injured patients. J Clin Invest 54:1001, 1974
11. Waldmann TA, Border S: Suppressor cells in the regulation of the immune response. In Schwartz RS (ed): Progress in Clinical Immunology, vol 13. New York, Grune & Stratton, 1977
12. Alexander JW, Wixon D: Neutrophil dysfunction of polymorphonuclear leukocytes in patients with burns and other trauma. Surg Gynecol Obstet 130:431, 1970
13. Saba TM, Blumenstock FA, Scoville WA, Bernard H: Cryoprecipitate reversal of opsonic α_2 surface binding glycoprotein deficiency in septic surgical and trauma patients. Science 201:622, 1978
14. Fuenfer MM, Scott K, Polk HC Jr: Evaluation of the phagocytic-bactericidal capacity of neutrophils: A current review. J Surg Res 21:207, 1976
15. Babior BM: Oxygen-dependent microbial killing by phagocytes. N Engl J Med 298:659, 1978
16. Heck E, Edgar MS, Masters BS, Baxter CR: The role of NADH-NADPH oxidase activity in leukocyte function of burned patients. J Trauma 19:49, 1979
17. Ninnemann JL, Fisher JC, Wachtel TL: Thermal injury associated immunosuppression: Occurrence and in vitro blocking effect of convalescent serum. J Immunol 122:1736, 1979
18. Constantian MD: Association of sepsis with an immunosuppressive polypeptide in the serum of burn patients. Ann Surg 188:209, 1978
19. Schoenenberger GA: Immunological evidences of the occurrence of a specific antitoxic IgG-fraction in serum of severely burned patients. In Koslowski L, Schmidt LK, Heitich R (eds): Burn Injuries: Local Treatment, Toxic Factors, and Infusion Therapy. Verlag, Stuttgart, F.K. Schattauer, 1979
20. Wilmore DW, Aulick LH: Metabolic changes in burned patients. Surg Clin North Am. 58:1173, 1978

21. Meakins JL, McLean AP, Kelly R, et al.: Delayed hypersensitivity and neutrophil chemotaxis: Effect of trauma. J Trauma 18:240, 1978
22. Munster AM: Immunologic manipulation of the injured patient: Looking into the future. In Ninnemann JL (ed): Traumatic Injury: Infection and Other Immunologic Sequelae. Baltimore, University Park Press, 1983
23. Warden GD: The use of plasma exchange in the management of thermally injured patients. In Ninnemann JL (ed): Traumatic Injury: Infection and Other Immunologic Sequelae. Baltimore, University Park Press, 1983

PART II
Initial Therapy

CHAPTER 4
Resuscitation

James W. Thornton

Fluid resuscitation for the patient with a burn greater than 20 percent total body surface area (TBSA) is a controversial issue. This chapter will cover (1) historical events associated with this area of burn care, (2) multiple burn fluid protocols currently advocated, and (3) a discussion of electrolyte changes associated with burn trauma.

HISTORY

Prior to 1940, burn shock was reviewed as purely a disturbance in the circulation. In 1863, Baraduc maintained that poor blood flow was the most probable cause of death with burns, secondary to increased viscosity of the blood. It had been observed for some time that following a major burn, fluid was lost from the circulation and plasma volume was reduced, leading to higher concentration of erythrocytes in the bloodstream and therefore increased viscosity. The early doctrine of fluid loss in burn patients was based on the incorrect notion that large amounts of fluids were lost through the surface of the burn and replacements were guided from this assumption.[1]

Not until the 1940s was the pathophysiology of burn fluid losses determined. In 1942, the Coconut Grove Fire in Boston turned the attention of Cope[2] and Moore[3] to look more closely at fluid losses through the burn surface. It was their observation that fluid loss was negligible through the burn surface of dry flame burns associated with a black leathery eschar, yet patients with this type of burn lost large quantities of intravascular fluid.

Using radioactive tracer techniques, Moore demonstrated that extracellular fluid volume increased massively during the first 48 to 72 hours postburn and then gradually decreased back to normal over the next 7 to 10 days. Furthermore, Moore showed that the extent of burn edema equalled approximately 10 percent of the patient's weight, the maximum extent to which the extracellular space can expand after a major burn, and that this fluid shift occurred most rapidly in the first 12 hours postburn. Analysis of this extracellular fluid demonstrated it to be essentially plasma.[2,3] This is the basis for the use of colloid in the resuscitation formulas proposed by Moore, Evans, and others.[2-6]

More recently, Monafo, Moylan, and Baxter have suggested that the total amount of sodium ion infused is the critical factor for successful resuscitation.[1,7-10] Others have presented evidence that colloid solution administered during the first 24 hours postburn is no more effective in maintaining plasma volume than hypertonic saline or lactated Ringer's solution, and therefore proposed the use of crystalloid solution until capillary integrity is restored.[7,8,11,12] This is the basis for the Parkland Formula, the current Brooke Formula, and the Hypertonic Formula.

BURN FORMULAS

At the outset of this discussion, it needs to be emphasized that formulas are merely guidelines for initiating resuscitation. Burn resuscitation formulas should not be viewed in a vacuum, and the need for consistent monitoring and examination of the patient cannot be neglected.[3,4,7,11,12]

Evans Formula

The Evans Formula as originally described in 1951[13] was designated to be a simple formula for estimating fluid requirements of the burn patient. Resuscitation is based on the surface area burned, times weight of the patient, plus insensible losses. The Evans Formula calls for (1) colloid—1 cc per percent burn per kg weight, (2) 0.9 percent saline—1 cc per percent burn per kg weight, and (3) 5 percent dextrose in water—2000 cc (for adults) for insensible loss per day. During the second 24 hours, one-half of the first 24 hours crystalloid and one-half of the colloid requirement of the first 24 hours are administered alone with replacement of insensible losses. Incorporated into this formula is the "Rule of 50." Patients over 50 years old or patients with burns more extensive than 50 percent TBSA should not receive more than 4000 ml of colloid or 4000 ml of saline solution in a 24-hour period. This formula functions well for burns up to 50 percent TBSA but complications of fluid overload with resultant postresuscitation pulmonary edema may occur, especially with pediatric burns or patients with cardiac or pulmonary complications (Table 4–1).[14]

TABLE 4–1. BURN RESUSCITATION FORMULAS

	First 24 hours	Second 24 hours
Evans Formula: "Rule of 50"	Colloid—1 cc/% burn/kg wt Saline—1 cc/% burn/kg wt D_5W for insensible losses (2000 cc)	½ of 1st 24 hr crystalloid ½ of 1st 24 hr colloid D_5W for insensible losses
Brooke Formula	2 cc/% burn/kg weight (adult)—lactated Ringer's 3 cc/% burn/kg weight (children)—lactated Ringer's ½ in the first 8 hr ½ each of next 8 hr	Colloid 0.3–0.5 cc/% burn/kg weight
Parkland Formula	4 cc/% burn/kg weight ½ first 8 hr ¼ each next 8 hr	Colloid 0.3–0.5 cc/% burn/kg weight
Hypertonic Formula	300 mEq Na, 200 mEq D, L lactate, 100 mEq Cl infused at a rate sufficient to maintain a urine output of 30 ml/hr	⅓–½ of first day requirements

HALFD Formula	1. 240 mOsm sodium, 120 mOsm of each chloride and lactate
	2. 1.5 g albumin/liter infused at a rate sufficient to maintain mean arterial pressure of 60 ton
	End point of resuscitation—urine output 40 ml/hr
	  pulse pressure ≥40 torr
	  declining serum lactate
	  abrupt rise in serum sodium
	  abrupt drop in serum potassium
	Postend point resuscitation
	  ¼ normal saline with 12.5 g albumin/liter	

Brigham Burn Budget	10% body weight with colloid
	  ½ first 12 hr
	  ¼ second 12 hr
	  ¼ second 24 hr
	Renal 1200 cc/day ½ nl saline)
	Pulmonary loss 1500–5000 cc/day (D_5W)
	Skin loss 1000–4000 cc/day (Ringer's lactate)	

Brooke Formula

The original Brooke Formula recommended the following fluids during the first 24 hours: (1) 0.5 ml of colloid, (2) 1.5 ml electrolyte solution (lactated Ringer's solution) per percent burn per kg body weight, and (3) 2000 ml of 5 percent dextrose in water per 24 hours to cover insensible losses. Half of this amount was to be administered during the first 8 hours. During the second 24 hours, half of the colloid and electrolyte requirements of the first 24 hours were recommended. With burns greater than 40 percent TBSA and burns to children, a larger amount of colloid and a decreased amount of electrolyte solution were recommended.

More recently a revision of the Brooke Formula has occurred (see Table 4-1). The new formula is based on the importance of sodium concentration and transcapillary fluid movements. A regression line generated from measurements of plasma volume lost rate on fluid infusion rate during the first 24 hours and second 24 hours postburn was calculated. From analysis of these data, the rate of fluid administration and the time of colloid infusion is expressed in the current Brooke Formula. This formula calls for: (1) 2 ml per percent burn per kg body weight (adult), or 3 ml per percent burn per kg body weight (child) of lactated Ringer's solution during the initial 24 hours postburn with administration of one-half in the first 8 hours and one-fourth of the estimated volume during each of the succeeding 8-hour periods; (2) *second 24 hours,* infusion of colloid (heat-treated plasma, fresh frozen plasma or albumin) at a rate between 0.3 to 0.5 ml per percent burn per kg body weight to correct plasma volume deficit; and (3) dextrose and water with electrolytes as needed to meet metabolic needs and replace evaporative water loss and sodium excretion.

Proponents of the Brooke Formula report excellent results with this form of resuscitation. Cardiac output has been reported to be depressed using this formula until the second postburn day when plasma volume is restored.[8,12]

Parkland Formula

Studies conducted by Baxter[7,8] led to the conclusion that successful resuscitation of patients with burns greater than 20 percent TBSA required 0.52 mEq of sodium per percent burn per kg body weight. Furthermore, colloid administration during the first 24 hours postburn was no more successful in restoring plasma volume than crystalloid, and fluid loss with major burns was underestimated by prior formulas. The Parkland Formula is derived from the above information and equals: (1) 4 cc per percent burn per kg body weight of lactated Ringer's solution with one-half given in the first 8 hours and an additional one-fourth in each of the next two 8-hour periods. During the second 24 hours postburn, resuscitation is completed by the infusion of plasma sufficient to restore the plasma volume. Colloid (heat-treated plasma, fresh frozen plasma, or albumin) is infused at a rate of 0.3 to 0.5 cc per percent burn per kg body weight. Insensible losses are replaced with 5 percent dextrose in water plus potassium as needed to meet physiologic needs. Baxter reports from over 10 years of experience using this formula that its predictive value is 70 percent accurate in providing fluid requirements for adults and 98 percent accurate in pediatric burns. Failures which he does observe occur in burns 80 percent or greater TBSA, especially in patients over 45 years old (see Table 4–1).[7,8]

Hypertonic Formula

Monafo introduced the use of hypertonic solution (300 mEq Na, 200 mEq racemic mixture of D, L lactate, and 100 mEq Cl) in the early 1970s for resuscitation of burn patients (see Table 4–1). The hypertonic solution is administered during the first 24 hours postburn at a rate sufficient to maintain urine output of 30 ml per hour and proportionately less in children. This solution can be administered intravenously or orally. During the second 24 hours postburn, one-third to one-half of the hypertonic solution is administered. Hypertonic Formula results in approximately one-half to two-thirds of the fluid volume necessary with standard formulas such as the Brooke Formula with similar or lower sodium loads.

The success of hypertonic solution in maintaining organ perfusion without leading to marked edematous states is based on intracellular dehydration as a result of the sodium ion concentration infused and the resultant osmotic gradient.

Clinical experience with the Hypertonic Formula indicates that a serum sodium concentration of 165 mEq or serum osmolity of 320 mOsm is associated with cerebral complications and decreased urinary output. Furthermore, intracellular function may be impaired with a 15 percent dehydration. Proponents, therefore, recommend careful monitoring of urine output, serum osmolity, and serum sodium concentration, and implementation of isotonic or hypotonic crystalloid solutions if the above parameters occur. The use of 0.5 percent silver nitrate topical treatment is often recommended to leach out sodium ion from the burn tissue to help prevent dangerous elevation of serum sodium concentration and serum osmolity.[11,12]

Advantages of hypertonic solution resuscitation include: (1) less edema, (2) increased urine output and natruresis (as long as serum sodium ion concentration remains less than 165 mEq), (3) similar or lower sodium loads as compared with other crystalloid resuscitation formulas, (4) decrease in the incidence of postburn ileus, and (5) earlier wound healing.[1,9,10,12,15,16]

HALFD Formula

The HALFD method of fluid resuscitation simply stated is the use of hypertonic sodium (240 mOsm of sodium, 120 mOsm each chloride and lactate) with 1.5 g of albumin per liter. HALFD: Hypertonic, Albuminated Fluid-Demand Resuscitation. This solution is given at a rate sufficient to maintain mean arterial pressure at 60 torr or better. The end point of resuscitation is a mean urine volume of approximately 40 ml per hour, a pulse pressure of greater than 40 torr, declining serum lactate, and an abrupt rise in serum sodium and an abrupt drop in serum potassium. The exact timing of such physiologic changes is dependent on the individual patient and extent of vasoconstriction. At the "end point," fluid resuscitation is switched to one-quarter normal saline in which 12.5 g of albumin is added and administered at a rate sufficient to maintain 30 to 50 ml per hour urine output and 70 to 110 mm Hg diastolic pressure (see Table 4–1).[8]

BRIGHAM BURN BUDGET

With the knowledge that a burned patient undergoes a sequestration of plasma-like fluid in the extracellular space, as well as external losses of fluid from the lungs, the burn surface, and the kidney, Moore designed a formula to restore the fluid losses, maintain blood volume and circulation, and maintain fluid and oncotic pressure so as to preserve intact brain, lung, and kidneys.[3]

In any full thickness burn over 20 to 25 percent of body surface, the size of the patient determines the size of the burn edema. This will require approximately 10 percent of the body weight in colloid solution during the first 48 hours, half of that during the first 8 to 12 hours with the rest administered over the next 36 to 40 hours. Colloid replacement may be accomplished with stored bank plasma, plasmanate, or reconstituted albumin at 5 percent concentration.

Daily urinary production is approximately 1200 ml per day (for a 70-kg adult) replaced with a half normal saline solution. Burn surface fluid losses range between 1000 and 400 ml per day (dependent on the wetness and size of the wound and surface treatment), and should be replaced with a balanced salt solution. The replacement of insensible losses from the lung (dependent on lung injury, tracheostomy, fever, dypsnea, or tachypnea) is accomplished with free water in an amount ranging between 1500 to 500 ml per 24 hours (see Table 4–1).

A modification of the Brigham Burn Budget employed at the University of California, Irvine, Burn Center designed to be utilized with an occlusive wound dressing (silver sulfadiazine, which minimizes fluid loss from the wound surface), has been successful in the resuscitation of burn patients for over 10 years. It calls for the infusion of colloid (5 percent albumin, 130 mEq/L Na, 100 mEq/L Cl). The colloid solution infusion is titrated to maintain normal perfusion (a mean arterial pressure of 80 mm Hg, pulse rate less than 120 per minute, urine output of greater than 20 cc per meter^2 per hour, Hct 45–55, and CVP of less than 5 cm H_2O with no metabolic acidosis). Daily water requirements are provided with a 5 percent dextrose solution, usually requiring approximately 2000 cc per day for an adult, or 1000 cc per meter^2 for pediatric patients (Fig. 4–1).

Mannitol is employed in those patients where hemoglobin or myoglobin

```
Continuous Infusion           to              Sustain
   of Plasma                              Adequate Perfusion
⎡ 5% Albumin    ⎤                       ⎡ BP 80 (120/70)         ⎤
│ 130 mEq/L Na  │        ⟶               │ Pulse < 120            │
⎣ 100 mEq/L Cl  ⎦                       │ Urine > 20 cc/m²/hr    │
                                        │ No metabolic acidosis  │
                                        │ Hct 45–55              │
                                        ⎣ CVP < 5 cm H₂O         ⎦

                              plus
                                  ⎧ 6% mannitol
        Daily water requirement as ⎨      or
                                  ⎩ 5% dextrose

        Usually requires  5% of initial weight in first 12 hours
                                       and
                          5% in next 36 hours
```

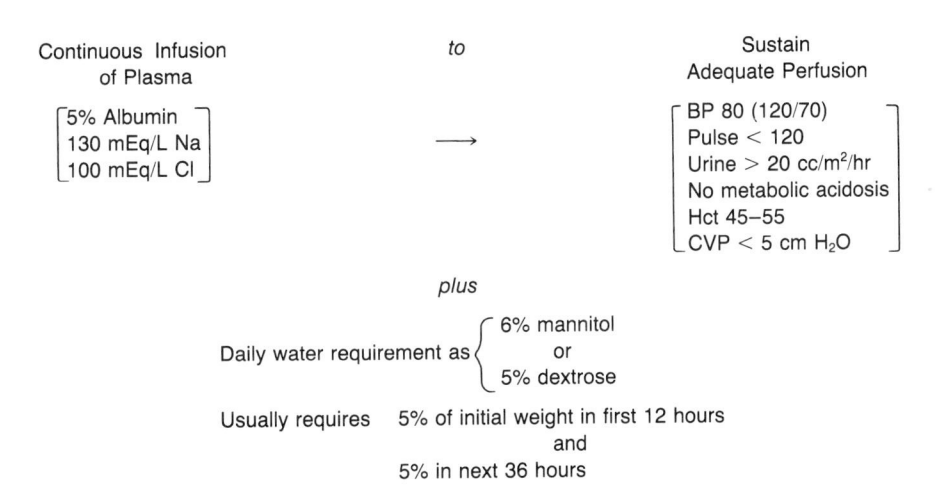

Figure 4–1. U.C.I. Burn Center fluid resuscitation formula. *(Based on Brigham Burn Budget.)*

is in the circulation as the result of the burn trauma. Osmotic diuresis (mannitol) is instituted to prevent acute renal failure secondary to pigmented casts.

The Brigham Burn Budget is designed to prevent pulmonary edema, cerebral edema, or renal failure. Fluids are administered at a rate based on the initial patient weight in an attempt to maintain plasma volume, oncotic pressure, cardiac output, and vital organ perfusion. Fluids utilized are those which are lost and a budget of fluid balance can be tabulated to guide further needs.[2-4]

MONITORING OF THE BURN PATIENT

The importance of careful monitoring of the burn patient cannot be overemphasized. For the patient with extensive burns who is under the age of 45 and has normal renal, pulmonary, and cardiac function, management should include hourly urine output measurements, daily electrolyte measurements, daily blood gas determination, continuous ECG monitoring, and central venous pressure (CVP) monitoring in addition to the standard intensive care units (ICU) care which includes hourly measurements of the vital signs, daily weight determination, and repeat physical examinations. Pulmonary artery and pulmonary capillary wedge pressure measurements should be instituted in patients with cardiac or pulmonary disease, and fluids should be titrated to a pulmonary artery diastolic pressure of 20 mm Hg or a wedge pressure of 15 mm H₂O (Fig. 4–2).[4]

The hematocrit is possibly the best guide to successful resuscitation of a burn patient. Titration of fluids to maintain a Hct of 45 to 50 will assure adequate volume replacement without fluid overload.[2-4,7,12]

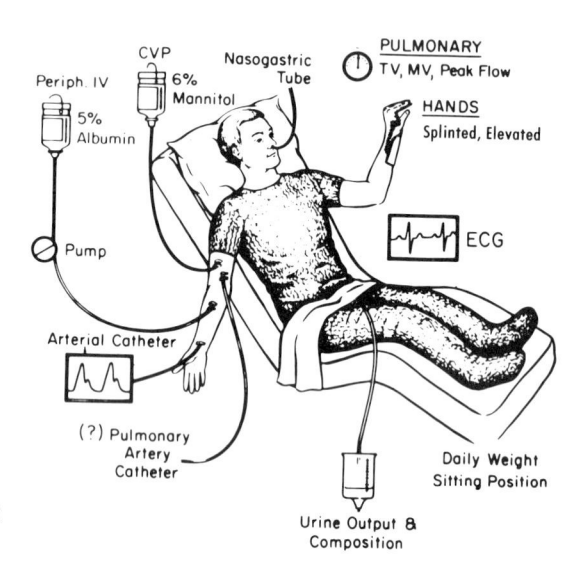

Figure 4-2. Initial management and monitors.

THE DIURETIC PHASE

The onset of the diuretic phase of burn resuscitation occurs at some point between 2 and 5 days after injury. The diuresis occurs as a result of the reabsorption of the edema fluid and its excretion by the kidneys. With the formulas discussed, fluid administration is tapering off during the second postburn day, and the onset of diuresis is not indicated so much by a massive sudden increase in urine output as it is by a maintained good urine flow in the face of drastically reduced fluid intake. Body weight decreases as the edema fluid is reabsorbed and excreted. The most dramatic effect of this diuresis, for example, is the loss of burn edema with the return of normal facial contour.

As with the initial fluid resuscitation, the diuretic phase deserves careful monitoring of the patient. Fluid overloading can occur with a sudden and marked elevation of CVP and congestive heart failure. This is especially true in the older patient with diminished cardiovascular reserve. Treatment requires drastic reduction or even termination of fluid therapy and the use of a diuretic such as furosemide to increase urinary excretion.

The diuretic phase presents no true therapeutic problems so long as it is recognized. The occurrence of the diuretic phase represents a recovery from the circulatory challenge produced by a severe burn injury.[3,4,12]

ELECTROLYTE DISTURBANCES

Hyper- and hyponatremia make up the most common electrolyte disturbance in burn patients. The most frequent cause of hypernatremia is inadequate replacement of insensible losses. Close monitoring of body weight, serum and urinary osmolality, and sodium concentration will help make the diagnosis and guide fluid replacement. Other causes of hypernatremia include salt loading especially with hypertonic resuscitation, sepsis (not usually a problem until later in the burn period), hyperglycemia, and glucosurea, and rarely secondary to a diabetes insipidus-like syndrome (Table 4–2).[3,4,7,12]

Hyponatremia is seen most commonly after the third day postburn. The use of hypotonic resuscitation formulas (lactated Ringer's), overestimation of free water requirements, and wound debridement with daily tubbing (loss of sodium through the wound surface into tubbing water) are the most common causes of this electrolyte disturbance. The former are treated by discontinuation of hypotonic fluids, the latter by sodium supplementation. Other causes of hyponatremia include: (1) use of silver nitrate wound dressing, (2) sepsis, (3) inappropriate antidiuretic hormone syndrome (low serum sodium concentration with less than maximally dilute urine), and (4) sick cell syndrome (inadequate energy supply impairing the ability of cells to exclude sodium) (see Table 4–2).[3,4,7,12]

Diagnosis and institution of appropriate therapy depends on measurement of serum and urinary electrolytes, serum and urinary osmolity, and examination of the patient.

Hyperkalemia of a moderate degree is not uncommon during the first day's postburn secondary to tissue destruction with release of intracellular potassium stores. Hyperkalemia in association with metabolic acidosis implies inadequate organ perfusion and reassessment of fluid needs as well as examination of the patient is needed (see Table 4–2).[3,4,7,11,12]

Hypokalemia is much more frequent in occurrence. With maximum aldosteronism, urinary loss of potassium can be impressive especially in association with respiratory alkalosis. Between 80 to 200 mEq of potassium may be required per day to maintain a normal serum potassium (see Table 4–2).[3,4,7,11,12]

Low serum calcium concentration often occurs with burn trauma; however, it is rarely necessary to institute calcium replacement.[4,7,11,12]

Hypomagnesium may insidiously occur postburn. Magnesium require-

TABLE 4–2. ELECTROLYTE DISTURBANCE

Hypernatremia	**Hyponatremia**
Inadequate insensible loss replacement	Hypotonic resuscitation
Salt loading	Wound treatment—tubbing
Sepsis	Silver nitrate wound dressings
Hyperglycemia and glucoseurea	Sepsis
Diabetes insepidas	Inappropriate ADH syndrome
	Sick cell syndrome
Hyperkalemia	**Hypokalemia**
Tissue destruction	Aldosterone
Metabolic acidosis	Respiratory Alkalosis

ments range between 16 to 30 mg per day. Prophylactic administration of magnesium sulfate has been proposed to avert hypomagnesium.[7,11,12]

SUMMARY

Any resuscitation method which supplies sufficient fluid to maintain normal hemodynamics will be successful. The Brigham Burn Budget is based on the administration of a colloid solution with the rate of administration determined by the initial weight of the patient, and the replacement of insensible fluid losses (kidney, lungs, burn surface) with crystalloid solutions. The Evans Formula also calls for the use of a colloid solution in combination with normal saline with the rate of administration determined by both the body weight and percent surface area burned. The current Brooke Formula recommends crystalloid (lactated Ringer's) for fluid resuscitation at a rate of 2 ml per percent burn per kg body weight during the first 24 hours postburn, and then the use of colloid during the second 24 hours postburn once the capillary integrity has been restored. The Parkland Formula is similar to the Brooke Formula in that it also recommends the use of crystalloid (lactated Ringer's), but at a rate of 4 ml per percent burn per kg body weight for the first day postburn and the use of colloid during the second day postburn. The Hypertonic Saline Protocols call for the infusion of a hypertonic sodium solution at a rate to maintain adequate urine output and blood pressure without causing dangerous hypernatremia or hyperosmotility.

Electrolyte fluctations need to be monitored routinely with the institution of the appropriate treatment as needed. Care should be directed especially toward potassium changes and the complications of hypernatremia or hyponatremia.

Monitoring of the burn patient with titration of fluid administration to CVP, pulmonary artery pressure or pulmonary capillary wedge pressure, blood pressure, urinary output, and, very importantly, hematocrit help to fine tune fluid and electrolyte therapy for the individual burn patient.

The acute care of the burn patient may last for weeks with the events, such as fluid administration that occurs during the first days of care, having a significant effect on the morbidity associated with the burn injury.

REFERENCES

1. Monafo WW: The treatment of burn shock by the intravenous and oral administration of hypertonic lactated saline solution. J Trauma 10:575, 1970
2. Cope O, Moore FD: The redistribution of body water and the fluid therapy of the burned patient. Ann Surg 126:1010, 1947
3. Moore FD: The body weight burn budget. Surg Clin North Am 509:1249, 1970
4. Bartlett RH, Tavis MJ: Burn Management Manual, 2nd ed. Orange, Calif., U.C.I. Burn Center, 1977

5. Carvajal HF: A physiologic approach to fluid therapy in severely burned children. Surg Gynec Obstet 150:379, 1980
6. Hilton JG: Effects of fluid resuscitation on total fluid loss following thermal injury. Surg. Gynec Obstet 152:441, 1981
7. Baxter CR: Problems and complications of burn shock resuscitation. Surg Clin North Am 58:1313, 1978
8. Baxter CR, Burke JF, Jelenko C, et al.: Supportive therapy in burn care. J Trauma 19:864, 1979
9. Moylan JA, Mason AD, Rogers PW, Walker HL.: Postburn shock: A critical evaluation of resuscitation. J Trauma 13:354, 1973
10. Moylan JA, Reckler JM, Mason AD: Resuscitation with hypertonic lactate saline in thermal injury. Am J Surg 125:580, 1973
11. Munster AM: The early management of thermal burns. Surgery 87:29, 1980
12. Pruitt BA: Fluid and electrolyte replacement in the burned patient. Surg Clin North Am 58:1291, 1978
13. Holleman JH, Gabel JC, Hardy JD: Pulmonary effects of intravenous fluid therapy in burn resuscitation. Surg Gynec Obstet 147:161, 1978
14. Evans EI, Purnell OJ, Robinett PW, et al.: Fluid and electrolyte requirements in severe burns. Am Surg 135:804, 1951
15. Shimazaki S, Yoshioka T, Tanaka N, et al.: Body fluid changes during hypertonic lactated saline solution therapy for burn shock. J Trauma 17:38, 1977
16. Yoshioka T, Maemura K, Ohhashi Y, et al.: Effect of intravenously administered fluid on hemodynamic changes and respiratory function in extensive thermal injury. Surg Gynec Obstet 151:503, 1980

CHAPTER 5
Monitoring

Kenneth Waxman

PRINCIPLES OF MONITORING

Tremendous progress has been made in critical care medicine over the past several decades. A large number of technical advances have allowed sophisticated bedside physiologic monitoring to be readily available. However, the large number of such monitoring devices available does not necessarily improve patient care. To have an impact on improving outcome for burn patients, physiologic monitoring must be selected that addresses those physiologic parameters that are relevant to burn patients' outcomes.

During the early phases of burn management, these parameters relate to optimal titration of fluid therapy for burn shock. Optimal therapy must address not only survival during this shock period, but must also address prevention of subsequent complications.

If monitoring is to improve the patient's outcome from burn shock, it must be directed toward those physiologic problems which are fundamental to the shock state. It must be clearly understood that shock may no longer be defined as low blood pressure; shock can be present with a low, normal, or high systemic arterial pressure. Shock cannot be defined in terms of low cardiac output; shock may be present with a normal or high cardiac output, as during sepsis. Rather than a pressure or flow phenomenon, shock is a consequence of inadequate oxygenation of the tissues. Only by addressing this cellular oxygenation deficit can we successfully monitor the basic physiologic deficits in shock states.

In burn shock, several factors contribute to inadequate tissue oxygenation. The most important of these factors, particularly in the early burn phase, is an inadequate circulating blood volume. This inadequate blood volume results in decreased preload, which causes low cardiac output relative to the tissues' circulatory needs. Further, during the early burn phase, there are a large number of circulating and local vasoactive substances. These include catecholamines, kinins, histamines, and prostaglandins. Each of these substances has local effects on the microcirculatory vessels which may directly interfere with microcirculatory blood flow and, thus, interfere with cellular oxygenation and nutrition. Another factor which may contribute to burn shock is tissue edema. Edema represents salt and water in the interstitial space, which will result in an increased perfusion distance between capillary and cell. This perfusion distance may contribute to the inadequate cellular oxygenation and nutrition of the shock state. Finally, sepsis may contribute to burn shock, especially during the postresuscitation period. Sepsis may exacerbate shock in several ways: First, sepsis causes an additional disturbance of the microcirculatory blood flow, perhaps by shunting blood past the capillary bed by precapillary arteriovenous shunts. Second, sepsis has been shown to directly affect mitochondrial function such that the cell does not utilize oxygen in its normal fashion. Additionally, sepsis interferes with biochemical pathways essential for adequate cellular nutrition and, thus, predisposes to malnutrition and thereby prevents recovery from the burn shock.

VITAL SIGNS

In every intensive care unit, the vital signs are closely and frequently monitored. Therefore, they represent familiar and accessible parameters to follow. The vital signs are only indirectly related to the pathophysiologic deficits in shock stages. Therefore, overreliance on vital signs leads to significant errors in patient management.

Systemic arterial blood pressure is dependent on cardiac output and on peripheral vascular resistance. Since increases in peripheral vascular resistance can maintain normal arterial pressure, even in the presence of very significant hypovolemia or cardiac dysfunction, the systemic arterial pressure loses value as a means to follow blood flow. In fact, a normal systemic arterial pressure should *not* be interpreted to mean that the patient is adequately perfusing his tissues. Blood volume deficits and decreases in cardiac output of up to 50 percent may be compensated, so that the systemic pressure remains unchanged.[1] On the other hand, decreased systemic arterial pressure does have significance. This implies a very significant blood volume deficit, cardiac dysfunction, or sepsis. Accordingly, monitoring of mean arterial pressure remains an important aspect of critical care. In general, however, physiologic deficits should be appreciated early, by other physiologic monitoring, before decreases in systemic pressure occur.

Similarly, the heart rate represents a complex physiologic response which may be difficult to interpret. While increases in heart rate usually occur under circumstances of hypovolemia and decreased cardiac output, increases in heart rate may also occur in the absence of these phenomena and may represent pain or stress. The absence of tachycardia does not insure that a low flow state is not present. Patients with pre-existing coronary artery disease, severe shock, and decreased coronary blood flow, anesthesia, and patients who are hypothermic may not respond with tachycardia, even under severe low flow states. Therefore, the heart rate, like the systemic arterial pressure, needs to be interpreted cautiously.

Continuous monitoring of systemic arterial pressure and of the heart rate can be achieved with an indwelling arterial catheter connected to a transducer and displayed on a bedside monitor. Catheters may be placed in the radial artery, the axillary artery, the femoral artery, the dorsalis pedis artery, or the superficial temporal artery.[2-4] Arterial catheters not only provide constant information on systemic pressure and heart rate, they also provide access for arterial blood sampling. Indwelling arterial catheters are particularly useful in patients with burns to the extremities, in whom cuff arterial pressure, venipuncture, and arterial puncture may be difficult to achieve.

Respiratory rate is another vital sign that is routinely monitored, although not always accurately. Accurate monitoring of the respiratory rate is a useful, though not specific, index of severe illness. An increase in the minute ventilation is a normal physiologic response to a major burn, since as the metabolic rate increases so, too, does carbon dioxide production. Burn patients normally have increased tidal volume and respiratory rates. Further increases in respiratory rates may be caused by hyperthermia, metabolic acidosis, respiratory burns, sepsis, or the onset of respiratory failure. Therefore, an additional increase in their respiratory rate may be a relatively early warning sign of complications.

Monitoring temperature is a very important aspect of burn care. A large amount of heat may be lost through burned surfaces and hypothermia may result. Enzyme systems do not work normally during hypothermia and compensatory physiologic responses will be markedly blunted. Hypothermia following burns needs to be prevented and treated aggressively. An elevated temperature following burns is a normal phenomenon in noninfected burn patients. However, a persistent fever may be an indicator of sepsis and this should be evaluated.

URINE OUTPUT

Since the vital signs are not particularly sensitive as early indicators of inadequate tissue perfusion, additional monitoring becomes quite important. Perhaps the most useful monitoring approach in the majority of patients is the measuring of hourly urine output. In patients with normal renal function, production of normal quantities of urine implies that renal perfusion is adequate. This further implies that cardiac output is relatively normal. Decrease in hourly urine output, below ½ to 1 cc/kg/hr, implies inadequate renal perfusion, implying inadequate cardiac output. Therefore, urine output monitoring is a very useful tool for following adequacy of fluid resuscitation following major burns. Hourly urine output should be monitored in every patient whose burns require admission and fluid resuscitation.

Several limitations do exist, however, on interpretation of urine output. All patients cannot be assumed to have pre-existing normal renal function. This is particularly true of patients with pre-existing atherosclerotic vascular disease, renal insufficiency, and diabetes. Further, patients with very extensive burns, or patients with blunt injury in addition to their burns, may have a significant amount of hemolysis, rhabdomyolysis, or both, which will alter renal function. Additionally, patients with very severe injuries and burns, whose resuscitation may have been delayed, may already be in a state where acute renal dysfunction has occurred and, under these circumstances, urine output will not adequately reflect renal perfusion. Finally, medications, such as hyperosmotic agents for intracranial pressure control, diuretics, or intravenous contrast agents, may cause a diuresis which will make hourly urine output an invalid indicator of cardiac output. In the most severely burned and injured patients, in whom accurate monitoring for severe shock and resuscitation is most urgent, hourly urine output is most likely to be a misleading indicator of cardiac output. More invasive monitoring becomes necessary.

CENTRAL VENOUS PRESSURE MONITORING

In major burns, particularly those with associated injuries and those in whom urine output may not be adequate, a more direct assessment of cardiac preload is very useful. Central venous pressure (CVP) catheters may be placed percutaneously through the jugular, subclavian, femoral, or upper extremity veins or may be placed by direct cutdown into the antecubital vein. Catheters are advanced into the superior vena cava, inferior vena cava, or right atrium and give an indication of right atrial pressure. Normal CVP in healthy individuals is between 0 and 5 cm of water. Therefore, a low CVP does not necessarily imply hypovolemia. Titrating fluid therapy to maintain CVPs in the range of 5 to 10 cm of water is helpful. A patient who is not responding as expected to fluid therapy should have a volume challenge performed (i.e., 1 unit of blood, 1000 cc crystalloid, or 500 cc colloid infused within 5 minutes). By monitoring CVP before and after such a volume challenge, it should become clear whether the problem is continuing fluid loss and hypovolemia or a problem with myocardial response despite increasing preload.

There are some pitfalls with CVP monitoring. Several conditions make filling pressures of the right heart different than the filling pressures of the left heart. Cardiac output may not be directly influenced by CVP in patients with left ventricular dysfunction due to either pre-existing organic heart disease, severe acute illness, anesthetic agents, or to myocardial contusion. Under these circumstances, left atrial pressure may exceed the CVP. Under other conditions, CVP may exceed left atrial pressure. These conditions are pulmonary embolism and acute respiratory failure, where the afterload against which the right ventricle must work is increased. Under any of these circumstances, all of which are common in severely burned patients, CVP will inadequately reflect preload of the left ventricle, which usually determines cardiac output.[5]

PULMONARY ARTERY MONITORING

Pulmonary artery catheterization is now an easily performed bedside procedure utilizing flow-directed balloon catheters (Swan–Ganz).[6] Placement of these catheters can be performed at the bedside utilizing either cutdown or percutaneous techniques. Pulmonary artery catheters allow continuous monitoring of pulmonary artery pressure, as well as intermittent determination of pulmonary artery occlusion pressure (wedge pressure). Furthermore, utilizing pulmonary artery catheters with thermistors, thermodilution measurement of cardiac output is possible. Although there are definite risks associated with the placement of pulmonary artery catheters, these risks are probably not significantly greater than those associated with placement of central venous catheters, especially if appropriate precautions are taken. Specific indications for placement of pulmonary artery catheters in burn patients are listed in Table 5–1.

Especially useful information is obtained by monitoring pulmonary wedge pressure.[7] This provides an estimate of left atrial pressure, which should reflect left ventricular end-diastolic pressure in most patients. This is especially important in those critically ill patients in whom left ventricular end-diastolic pressure may differ from CVP. Measurement of wedge pressures allows titration of fluids to provide optimal preload in order to achieve optimal cardiac output. Additionally, monitoring of the wedge pressure provides criteria for limiting intravenous fluids to prevent volume overload pulmonary edema. In general, wedge pressures of greater than 10 mm Hg are desirable to optimize cardiac performance, unless increased pulmonary capillary permeability pulmonary edema is present. Wedge pressures of greater than 18 mm Hg should be avoided in order to prevent volume overload pulmonary edema.

TABLE 5–1. INDICATIONS FOR PULMONARY ARTERY CATHETERIZATION IN BURN PATIENTS

1. Patients with pre-existing cardiac, respiratory, or hepatic disease
2. Patients with extensive burns in association with major blunt or penetrating trauma
3. Patients who develop complications, i.e., respiratory failure, renal failure, or systemic sepsis
4. Patients who are not responding to resuscitation as expected, utilizing less invasive monitoring

CARDIAC OUTPUT DETERMINATION

Monitoring of cardiac output can now be routinely performed utilizing a thermistor attached to a Swan–Ganz catheter. Injection of 10 cc of dextrose solution into the right atrium will change the temperature in the pulmonary artery depending on the magnitude of flow past the pulmonary artery catheter. Utilizing bedside computers, calibrated for this purpose, this information can be translated into cardiac output determination. This takes only seconds to perform and can be repeated as often as desired. Sequential bedside measurements of cardiac output can thus be easily obtained.[8,9]

It is particularly useful in the critically ill burned patient to measure cardiac output. The more extensive the burn and associated injuries, the greater the need for increased circulation if the patient is to recover. A normal cardiac output may not be sufficient in extensively burned patients who may require cardiac outputs of twice normal if they are to survive.[10,11] Therefore, measurement of low or even normal cardiac output, in this setting, is of great concern and therapeutic steps should be taken quickly to correct this. The most easily performed therapeutic step involves giving additional intravenous fluids, using wedge pressure determinations and cardiac output to determine at what wedge pressure cardiac output is optimized. Other therapeutic approaches can also be optimized by monitoring cardiac output, including afterload reduction, and the use of contractility and vasoconstrictor drugs. Cardiac output determinations are especially valuable when pressor drugs are being utilized, as inappropriate use of these agents might decrease, rather than increase, cardiac output. Cardiac output measurements become essential when respiratory failure complicates the burn, as ventilatory therapy, including positive end-expiratory pressure (PEEP) can impair cardiac output.

OXYGEN DELIVERY AND OXYGEN CONSUMPTION

Table 5–2 lists formulas of some derived variables that are quite useful in advanced cardiopulmonary monitoring of critically ill burned patients. Any of these derived variables are quite easily calculated, using a handheld programmable calculator, programs for which are now commercially available. Of the physiologic parameters that are useful to follow in critically ill burned patients, among the most useful are calculations of oxygen delivery and oxygen consumption.[10]

Oxygen delivery is the product of three variables. It is dependent upon cardiac output, hemoglobin concentration, and hemoglobin saturation. It is especially useful to monitor oxygen delivery when therapeutic maneuvers are performed which may alter one or more of these variables. For example, when PEEP is being increased, there may be an increase in hemoglobin saturation, but, at the same time, there may be a decrease in cardiac output. The net effect on the patients is best determined by calculating oxygen delivery.[12]

TABLE 5–2. PHYSIOLOGIC VARIABLES USEFUL IN MONITORING BURN PATIENTS

Variable	Formula	Normal Value	Units
Mean arterial pressure (MAP)	Measured	82–102	mm Hg
Urine output	Measured	½–1	cc/kg/hr
Pulmonary artery pressure (PAP)	Measured	25/10	mm Hg
Mean PAP (MAAP)	Measured	12–15	mm Hg
Pulmonary artery wedge pressure (WP)	Measured	0–5	mm Hg
Central venous pressure (CVP)	Measured	0–4	mm Hg
Cardiac index (CI)	Cardiac output / body surface area	2.8–3.6	L/min · M²
Systemic vascular resistance (SVR)	79.92 (MAP − CVP)/CI	1760–2600	Dyne · sec / cm⁵ · M²
Arterial O₂ content (Cao₂)	Measured or hemoglobin concentration × arterial hemoglobin saturation × 1.39	18–20	ml/dl
Mixed venous O₂ content (Cvo₂)	Measured or hemoglobin concentration × venous hemoglobin saturation × 1.39	13–16	ml/dl
Oxygen delivery (O₂del)	Cao₂ × 10 × CI	520–720	ml/min · M²
Oxygen consumption (VO₂)	CI × (Cao₂ − Cvo₂) × 10	100–180	ml/min · M²

Oxygen consumption is calculated using the Fick equation. Oxygen consumption may also be directly measured using a Douglas bag technique; however, these techniques are more cumbersome than using the Fick equation by measuring cardiac output, arterial and mixed venous oxygen contents. Determination of oxygen consumption allows titration of therapy to that level which the patient physiologically needs.[10] Normal cardiac output and normal oxygen deliveries may be inadequate for a severely burned patient. To what extent these parameters must be increased can only be assessed by measuring oxygen consumption. As oxygen is not stored in the body, any oxygen that is consumed may be assumed to be necessary for metabolism. Therefore, increases in cardiac output and oxygen delivery that result in increased oxygen consumption can be said to be necessary for that patient's metabolic state. Therapy can then be titrated to increase oxygen delivery to that point when oxygen consumption no longer increases. Again, normal levels of oxygen consumption may be inadequate for a severely ill burn patient. During the first several days following severe burns, oxygen consumption of 1½ to 2 times normal is frequently required.

COMPLICATIONS OF INVASIVE MONITORING

Sepsis is a very serious complication of invasive monitoring of burn patients.[13-16] Indwelling venous and arterial catheters have an increased risk of causing sepsis in burn patients for several reasons. First, burn patients have decreased immunologic defenses. Second, the increased concentrations of bacterial flora on the burn wound make catheter sepsis more likely. For these important reasons, indwelling catheters should only be utilized when the physiologic monitoring information obtained will be important to patient care and when it is felt that the potential benefit of these catheters outweighs the risk of sepsis.

Several principles should be followed in catheter placement. First, catheters should be placed through unburned areas, if at all possible. Although it is possible to successfully place a catheter through burned tissue, host defenses are markedly reduced with loss of epithelial barrier and catheter infections become much more likely. Second, percutaneous techniques are less likely to be associated with infections than are cutdown techniques. Arterial catheters and central venous catheters can be safely placed utilizing established percutaneous techniques; a variety of kits with guide wires are currently available to facilitate this. Third, very strict aseptic techniques must be used when inserting indwelling arterial or venous catheters and sterile techniques must be maintained during catheter care. Intravenous connecting tubing should be changed on a daily basis to prevent bacterial colonization. Lines should be disconnected as seldom as possible and, again, sterile technique should be emphasized when this is necessary. By utilization of these precautions, sepsis caused by intravenous lines can be minimized. However, intravascular catheters should be removed as soon as the information they provide is no longer essential to patient care.

Other complications are also associated with placement of central venous catheters. Minor arrhythmias, as well as pneumothorax and hemothorax, frequently occur, and life-threatening arrhythmias are reported.[17] These complications should be largely preventable when experienced personnel place the catheters and when patients are positioned correctly. Another complication that is specifically reported with the use of pulmonary artery catheter is pulmonary infarction caused by allowing the balloon to remain inflated for long periods of time; this is a preventable complication. Other complications associated with the Swan–Ganz catheter include knotting of the catheter, pulmonary embolism, and cardiac arrhythmias. These are recognized risks of the procedure that must be considered when assessing the risk and benefit ratios for a particular patient.

TRANSCUTANEOUS OXYGEN MONITORING

One alternative to invasive cardiorespiratory monitoring, with its attendant risks, are noninvasive techniques. Of a variety of noninvasive monitoring techniques currently available, one that has shown promise in monitoring critically ill burn patients is the transcutaneous oxygen monitor. Transcutaneous oxygen is monitored with a heated oxygen electrode placed over an unburned portion of the patient's skin. Heating the skin makes the stratum corneum permeable to oxygen and, thereby, a continuous monitoring of tissue oxygenation becomes possible. Transcutaneous oxygen values are dependent on both adequate arterial oxygen content and also cardiac output. Therefore, a decrease in transcutaneous oxygen implies that either the patient is hypoxic or that cardiac output has decreased. These two possibilities can be quickly distinguished by drawing an arterial blood gas. Therefore, transcutaneous oxygen is a continuous monitor of tissue blood flow, which is sensitive to both arterial oxygen and cardiac output. As such, it represents a useful, noninvasive monitor of patients' cardiorespiratory status.[18]

OTHER DIRECT AND INDIRECT ASSESSMENTS OF BLOOD VOLUME

In addition to cardiorespiratory monitoring, there are other techniques that are commonly utilized to assess blood volume. Perhaps the most frequently used, and also the most inaccurate, is assessment of the intake and output. It is frequently assumed that because the intake far exceeds the output the patient must have adequate or supernormal circulating blood volume. This is, of course, not the case as a huge amount of fluid in the burn patient is lost through the burned surface area. Further, that fluid which is retained within the body is, to a large extent, not within the vascular space but is distributed through the interstitial and intracellular spaces. Therefore, intake and output records give very little clue as to the status of the blood volume. This is true during the acute resuscitation phase, during which time a great deal of fluids in excess of output must be given to maintain a reasonable blood volume, and also during the recovery phase, in which time a great deal of fluid is mobilized in comparison to the amount of fluids administered to the patient. As a corollary to this, daily weights are also not helpful in assessing the adequacy of the circulating blood volume, for the same reasons.

Therefore, other indirect hemodynamic measurements must be utilized to assess the blood volume, unless a direct measurement of blood volume is made. This is quite possible, utilizing either chromium-labeled red cell techniques or radioiodine-labeled albumin techniques. Although these direct measurements of blood volume are seldom used in clinical practice, they do represent a reproducible and accurate assessment of the blood volume and, perhaps, deserve wider clinical application.[19]

MONITORING RESPIRATORY FUNCTION

The arterial blood gases are basic to adequate monitoring of the respiratory status of seriously burned patients. Probably, every patient with burns serious enough for admission should have a baseline arterial blood gas measurement both to determine the possibility of respiratory burns and also to establish a baseline against which subsequent blood gases might be compared. An indwelling arterial line has the advantage of facilitating sequential blood gas sampling.

The recent introduction of pulse oximetry has added greatly to our ability to monitor pulmonary status. These continuous and noninvasive monitors, placed on an unburned digit, reliably indicate whether adequate arterial oxygen saturation is maintained, and quickly indicate changes in arterial oxygenation.

Arterial $Paco_2$ values provide an excellent indication of the adequacy of ventilation. Perhaps the only shortcoming of a $Paco_2$ monitoring is that it must be done intermittently. A continuous method of analyzing the adequacy of ventilation is available with the infrared monitoring of end-tidal CO_2, which normally is nearly equivalent to a $Paco_2$. These monitoring devices, though somewhat expensive, are quite useful for monitoring patients with borderline ventilatory function.

The oxygenating capacity of the lungs is indicated by a Pao_2 measurement. However, interpretation of an isolated Pao_2 value may be somewhat difficult, particularly if the patient is receiving supplemental oxygen. A more reliable indicator of oxygenating status is the alveolar–arterial difference in oxygen gradient (A–aDo_2 gradient). Even the A–aDo_2 gradient, however, has shortcomings in that it too will vary when the inspired oxygen concentration is varied and, in addition, it may depend on cardiac output. An even better estimation of pulmonary oxygenation is the venous admixture or shunt determination. Calculation of venous admixture allows a determination of the status of the patient's oxygenation that can be following through different ventilatory adjustments, different inspired oxygen concentrations, and changing cardiac output (Table 5–3).

The patient's acid-base status is also assessed, utilizing arterial blood gas

TABLE 5–3. PHYSIOLOGIC VARIABLES USEFUL FOR MONITORING RESPIRATORY FUNCTION

Variable	Formula	Normal Value	Units
Arterial O_2 tension (Pao_2)	Measured	80–100	Torr (mm Hg)
Arterial O_2 saturation (Sao_2)	Measured	95–99	%
Arterial CO_2 Tension ($Paco_2$)	Measured	36–44	Torr
Alveolar–arterial difference in O_2 gradient (A–aDo_2)	$PAo_2 - Pao_2$	0–100 (Fio_2 1.0) 0–20 (Fio_2 0.2)	Torr
Pulmonary venous admixture or shunt (O_s/O_t)	C capillary O_2 – Cao_2 / C capillary O_2 – Cvo_2	0–8	%

sampling. It is essential in critically ill patients to correct both respiratory and metabolic acidosis and alkalosis. In particular, metabolic acidosis may be an excellent indicator of inadequate tissue oxygenation. Correction of this acidosis should not usually require bicarbonate administration, but should be accomplished by improving the patient's hemodynamic status. Alkalosis is important to recognize and treat, not only because of the underlying disorders that may be responsible, but also because an alkalosis causes a shift of the oxyhemoglobin dissociation curve such that the tissues may be inadequately oxygenated.

The chest x-ray is often relied upon to indicate the status of the lungs. This is often misleading, as chest x-ray changes may occur many hours following the occurrence of significant pulmonary pathology, including respiratory burns, aspiration pneumonia, pulmonary contusion, and even pulmonary edema. Therefore, overreliance on chest x-rays is an error and more faith should be placed upon physiologic measurements of pulmonary function. A more accurate method of determining the degree of pulmonary edema has recently been developed. This is the lung water measurement, utilizing a double indicator technique. A catheter is placed into the aorta, with sensors for thermodilution and for green dye determination. An injection of cold green dye is made into the pulmonary artery and, by comparison of the thermodilution and green dye curve, a quantitative estimation of the amount of lung water can be made. This measurement has been made in several studies in critically ill patients, including burn patients, and, in general, has indicated an increase in lung water in these ill patients. However, there has not been good correlation between the amount of lung water, as indicated by this test, and any physiologic assessment of pulmonary function, such as venous admixture.[20] Further, lung water determination requires the placement of a large bore arterial catheter as well as pulmonary artery catheter and is, perhaps, too invasive for routine clinical utilization.

SUMMARY OF MONITORING APPROACHES

Monitoring of physiologic parameters in burn patients is extremely important. These patients can be critically ill and optimal titration of therapy and early recognition of complications is essential. Several principles should be kept in mind when choosing appropriate monitoring for a burn patient. First, monitoring devices that provide relevant information upon which therapeutic decisions can be made should be selected. Second, when alternative, noninvasive monitoring devices are available, these should be utilized. Third, information that is obtained from monitoring should be frequently recorded, and therapy should be continuously titrated based upon information generated. Finally, invasive monitoring devices should be removed as soon as they are no longer necessary.

REFERENCES

1. Asch MJ, Feldman RM, Waller HL, et al.: Systemic and pulmonary hemodynamic changes accompanying thermal injury. Am J Surg 178:218, 1973
2. Downs JS, Rackstein AD, Klein EF Jr, et al.: Hazards of radial artery catheterization. Anesthesiology 38:283, 1973
3. De Angelis J: Axillary arterial monitoring. Crit Care Med 4:205, 1976
4. Williams CD, Cunningham JN: Percutaneous cannulation of the femoral artery for monitoring. Surg Gynec Obstet 141:773, 1975
5. Wilson JN, Owens J: Pitfalls in monitoring central venous pressure. Hosp Med 6:86, 1978
6. Swan HJ, Ganz W, Forrester J, et al.: Catheterization of the heart in man with use of flow-directed balloon-tipped catheter. N Engl J Med 283:447, 1970
7. Lappas D, Lell WA, Gabel JC, et al.: Indirect measurement of left atrial pressure in surgical patients—pulmonary capillary wedge and pulmonary artery diastolic pressures compared with left atrial pressure. Anesthesiology 38:394, 1973
8. Ganz W, Swan HJ: Measurement of blood flow by thermodilution. Am J Cardiol 29:241, 1972
9. Sorenson MB, Bille-Brahe NE, Engell HC: Cardiac output measurement by thermodilution. Reproducibility and comparison with dye dilution technique. Ann Surg 183:67, 1976
10. Shoemaker WC: Pathophysiologic basis of therapy for shock and trauma syndromes. Semin Drug Treat 3:211, 1973
11. Shoemaker WC, Matsuda T, State D: Relative hemodynamic effectiveness of whole blood and plasma expanders in burned patients. Surg Gynec Obstet 144:909, 1977
12. Walkinshaw M, Shoemaker WC: Use of volume loading to obtain preferred levels of PEEP. Crit Care Med 8:81, 1980
13. Nichols WW, Nichols MA, Barbour H: Complications associated with balloon tipped slow-directed catheters. Heart Lung 8:503, 1979
14. Elling T, Reno D: Septicemia rates using Swan–Ganz catheters: Influence of duration of catheterization. Crit Care Med 6:129, 1978
15. Ehrie M, Morgan AP, Moore FD: Endocarditis with the indwelling balloon-tipped pulmonary artery catheter in burn patients. J Trauma 18:664, 1978
16. Wilson JA: Infection control in intravenous therapy. Heart Lung 5:430, 1976
17. Cairns JA, Halder D: Ventricular fibrillation due to passage of a Swan–Ganz catheter. Am J Cardiol 35:1589, 1975
18. Tremper K, et al.: Continuous transcutaneous oxygen monitoring during respiratory failure, cardiac decompensation, cardiac arrest, and CPR. Crit Care Med 8:377 1980
19. Shippy CR, Appel PL, Shoemaker WC: Reliability of clinical measurements to assess blood volume in critically ill patients. Crit Care Med 10:219, 1982
20. Tranbaugh RF, Elings VB, Christensen J, et al.: Determinants of pulmonary interstitial fluid accumulation after trauma. J Trauma 22:820, 1982

PART III
Care of the Burn Wound

CHAPTER 6
Treating the Burn Wound

Bruce M. Achauer

Since ancient times care of a burned patient focused on what was put on the burn. Tannic acid was one of the oldest[1] burn dressings and was reintroduced in the early 20th century. The systemic dangers of tannic acid and of the burn injury itself were not pointed out until the Second World War. Turpentine and liquor of pickled cabbage were mentioned as efficacious by Kentish in 1817.[2] A warmed, oiled frog was the prescription given in the Papyrus Ebers in 1500 BC.[3] The first effective topical antibiotics were 0.5 percent silver nitrate soaks[4] and 10 percent mafenide, both introduced in the mid-1960s.[5] Both are still used but less frequently than silver sulfadiazine which was introduced a few years later.[6] Silver sulfadiazine has two major advantages over mafenide: it is not painful nor does it produce metabolic acidosis (mafenide inhibits carbonic anhydrase). However, mafenide penetrates the eschar more effectively than silver sulfadiazine. Leukopenia has been observed secondary to silver sulfadiazine. The leukopenia has not been associated with increased infection rates. Silver nitrate solution can produce electrolyte disturbances. Silver nitrate also requires bulky dressings and stains the surroundings black. The major characteristics of the three most commonly used topical antimicrobials are listed in Table 6–1.[7]

The antibiotic creams can be "buttered" onto the patient or placed on the patient via gauze strips coated with the medication. In either case, an evening reapplication is usually indicated. With the latter technique, an elastic "suit" can be tailored for the patient with various sizes of elastic tubular dressing. The patient can then be active and comfortable. This technique is also well suited for outpatients.

TABLE 6-1. COMMONLY USED TOPICAL ANTIMICROBIAL BURN WOUND AGENTS

	Mafenide Acetate Cream (Sulfamylon Burn Cream)	Silver Nitrate Soaks	Silver Sulfadiazine Cream (Silvadene)
Form of treatment	Exposure	Occlusive dressings	Exposure or single layer dressing
Concentration of active agent (%)	11.1	0.5	1.0
Advantages	Penetrates eschar; wound readily visible; compatible with treatment of associated injuries; no gram-negative resistance identified; motion of involved joints is maintained.	No hypersensitivity; painless except at time of dressing change; no gram-negative resistance; reduces heat loss from wound; most compatible with hypertonic resuscitation regimen	Painless on application; wound readily visible when cream is applied without dressings; compatible with treatment of associated injuries; motion of involved joints is maintained
Limitations	Painful for 20–30 minutes after application to second degree burns; accentuates postburn hyperventilation; hypersensitivity noted in 7% of patients; delays spontaneous eschar separation	No penetration of eschar; marked transeschar loss of Na^+, K^+, Ca^{++}, and Cl^-; methemoglobinemia (rare); dressings limit motion of involved joints; discolors unburned skin of patient, skin of attending personnel and any environmental objects in contact	Poor penetration of eschar; bone marrow suppression with neutropenia; hypersensitivity (infrequent); resistance of many *Enterobacter cloacae* and of some *Pseudomonas* sp.; delayed eschar separation

(From Pruitt BA, 1979, reproduced with permission.[7])

SURGICAL MANAGEMENT OF THE BURN WOUND

A number of excellent options are now available to the burn surgeon as far as time and method of eschar excision and skin grafting. There has been a dramatic increase in the application of early excision. These techniques are now a standard part of the burn surgeon's armamentarium. Some of the more common approaches are outlined.

Sequential Excision

The most frequently used method of surgical management of the burn wound involves daily removal of loose debris during hydrotherapy coupled with repeated sharp excisions of eschar with guarded skin graft knives once or twice weekly. Ketamine anesthesia is ideal for the major sessions. Delayed, spontaneous separation of eschar is a natural consequence of improved bacterial control. Therefore, aggressiveness is required to make this technique successful. No more than 3 weeks should pass before an acceptable surface for grafting is obtained. When burn depth is in question and less than 40 percent of the body is burned, this conservative method is most appropriate. Burns of the face, palms, soles, and perineum are particularly suited for this technique. However, wound care must be vigilant. If the debridements are not adequate, more than 3 weeks will pass before the wound is ready for grafting and morbidity and mortality will become excessive. The main advantages of this method are that no decision is required as to burn depth, no viable tissue is excised, and no surgery is required during the unstable early period of resuscitation. Disadvantages include a longer period of time before skin grafting and, therefore, an increased risk of sepsis. Also, granulation tissue is scar tissue and, therefore, the possibility of subsequent hypertrophic scarring and contractures may be increased.

Escharectomy

Some burn surgeons excise the obvious full thickness burn about 10 days postburn followed by immediate application of autografts. Relatively moderate bleeding is encountered and the separation between viable and nonviable tissue is apparent. A disadvantage associated with this schedule is greater bacterial concentrations found beneath the eschar. Advantages are that the burn wound is well demarcated and fluid resuscitation problems are stabilized.

Tangential Excision

This method involves shaving the eschar with guarded skin graft knives to bleeding tissue followed by immediate application of autografts or allografts. It is usually done 48 to 72 hours postburn.[8] Advantages include intervention before wound sepsis and coagulation problems develop. The patient may not be ideally stabilized at this stage. However, proponents feel that tissue in the zone of stasis can be salvaged at this stage when covered by viable skin grafts. A great deal of surgical judgment and technical expertise is essential to make this method routinely successful. If the excision is not deep enough, precious autografts will be lost. Clinical judgment is required to assess burn depth. Intravenous fluorescein will stain viable tissue and has been used as an adjunct. It is also possible to measure the amount of fluorescein by fluorometry.[9] Blood loss can be prodigious, a total body exchange transfusion may be necessary for a 20 percent body surface area (BSA) excision. An experienced team of nurses, surgeons, and anesthesiologists is necessary. Burns of the dorsum of the hand are well suited to this technique. The heated Shaw scalpel fitted with a Goulian blade may also help to reduce blood loss.[10] Topical agents such as thrombin or epinephrine are applied to the bleeding surface. Intravenous vasopressin is an intriguing possibility.[11] Subcutaneous injections of Neo-

Synephrine or epinephrine are also used. Great care must be taken to maintain body temperature.

Beneficial effects of early tangential excision include reduced mortality,[12,13] shorter hospital stays, less sepsis, fewer surgeries, and better wound healing.[14] Burns greater than 40 percent BSA are a high priority for initial excision because they cannot be entirely covered in one skin grafting procedure. High risk individuals (concomitant medical conditions, advanced age) should be treated in this fashion if at all practical.[15] This procedure is covered in detail by Heimbach and Engrav.[16]

Primary Excision

Excision to the fascial level is done acutely (48 to 72 hours). This is an old technique recently experiencing a successful revival due to improved techniques.[17] An electrocautery, heated scalpel, or carbon dioxide laser is used to excise burned skin and subcutaneous tissue to the level of the superficial fascia. There is less blood loss than with tangential excision and no question about grafting onto viable tissue. Judgment about depth of injury is less critical. An excellent bed for grafts is produced with good graft take expected. A greater deformity is produced and, therefore, this technique is not used for the face, hands, or feet. It is relatively contraindicated for the female breast (complicated reconstruction would be required) and lower leg (hyperkeratosis of skin grafts may occur years later). This method will be most frequently used for trunk, arm, and thigh burns in an attempt to salvage a patient with a high expected mortality. Any type of excision may have to be done in several stages. Usually about 20 percent of the body surface will be excised in one

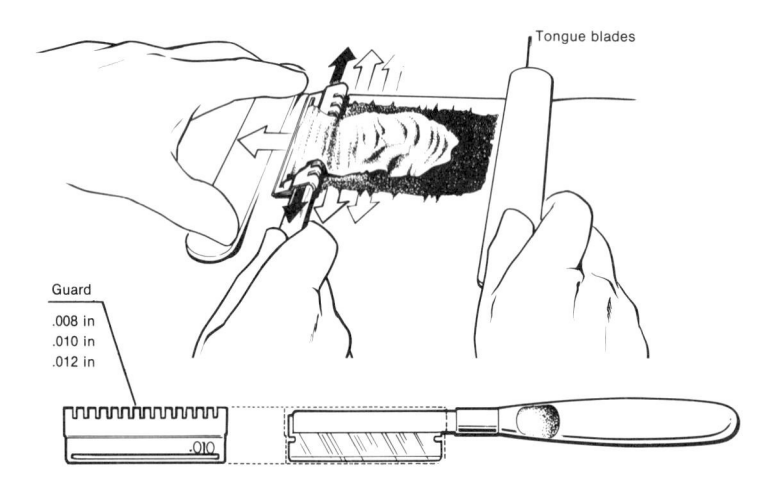

Figure 6–1. These razor blade dermatomes are very useful for small grafts and for tangential excision of burn wounds.

procedure. Excised areas as much as 40 percent can be done if felt to be essential by an experienced excision team. Excised areas should be covered with autograft (allograft or synthetic skin if autograft is unavailable). The procedure can be repeated in a few days during which donor sites may have healed providing more autographs.

Autografting

Dermatomes are either of the hand, drum, or power variety. An example of each is demonstrated in Figures 6–1 through 6–3. Hand skin graft knives require the most skill to use. They are essential for tangential excisions. They are also very useful for rapid skin graft harvesting and for obtaining grafts from small or irregular areas.

The small instrument (see Fig. 6–1) has guards of three different thicknesses and uses commonly available razor blades. Larger knives are of many designs (Watson, Cobbett), are either right- or left-handed, and require special blades.

There are two popular types of drum dermatomes—the Padgett and the Reese. The Reese is diagrammed. The Padgett is similar; however, it does allow changing the graft thickness while harvesting skin (much more difficult to do with the Reese). A rubber backing is available for the Padgett, although not part of the original design. In some techniques (postage stamp grafts), the rubber backing is quite useful.

Drum dermatomes usually yield a wider graft which have a more uniform thickness than power dermatomes. Drum dermatomes are also very useful over convex surfaces since the basic technique involves pulling the skin up from the underlying tissue (the opposite is the case with hand and power dermatomes). Injections of saline over bony prominences are also helpful in obtaining skin grafts in these situations (see Fig. 6–2).

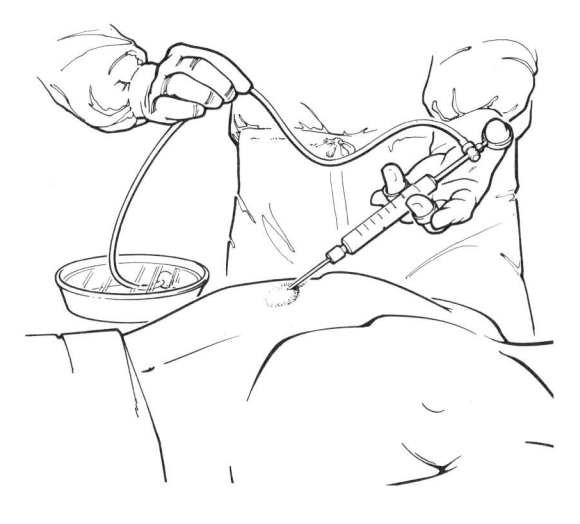

Figure 6–2. Injectable saline infiltrated over bony prominences with the Pitkin syringe makes harvesting skin grafts from the scalp, chest, and iliac crests technically easier.

98

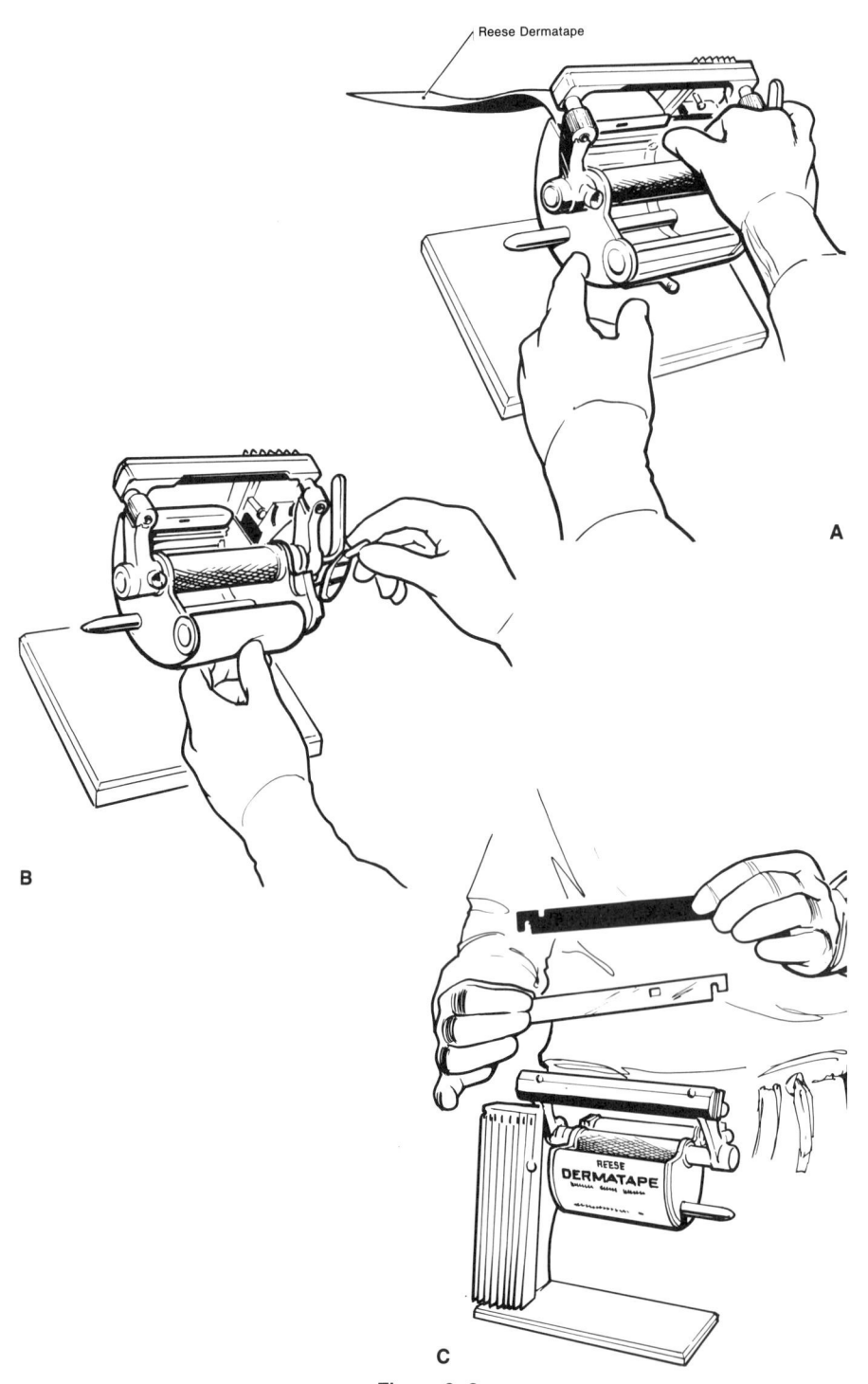

Figure 6-3

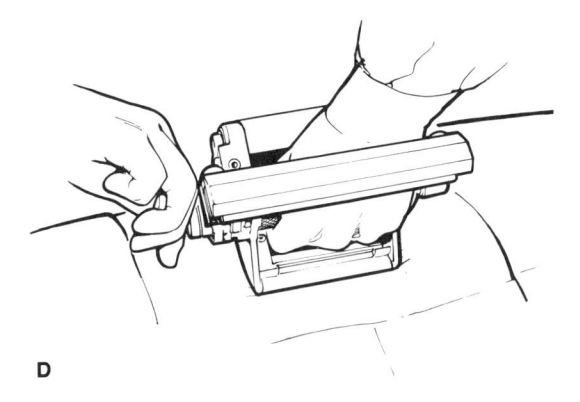

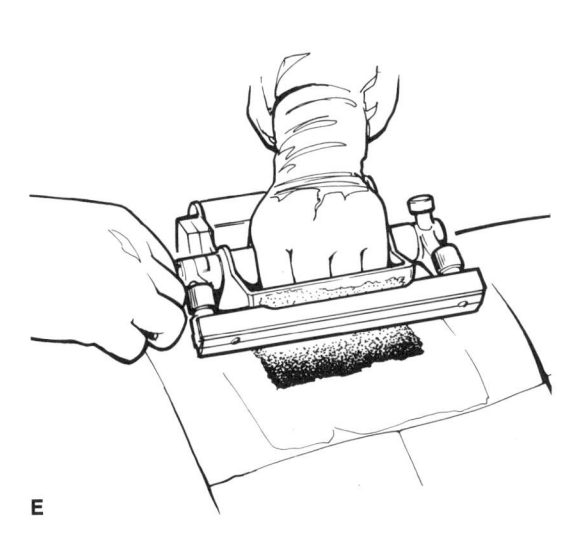

Figure 6-3. Use of the Reese dermatome. **A.** The dermatape is first placed on the drum. **B.** The tape is tightened as much as possible with the key. **C.** The appropriate spacer is chosen. Thinner grafts (8 to 14 ten thousandths of an inch) are used for covering burn wounds. Thicker grafts (16 to 20) are used for reconstructive procedures to minimize contracture. A uniform thickness is possible with the drum-type dermatome. **D.** After the protective covering has been moved from the adhesive part of the tape, it is applied to the glue which has been painted on the skin. **E.** The leading edge of the drum is then elevated. The bar of the dermatome is moved back and forth to slice the skin graft.

Drum dermatomes (see Fig. 6-3) are tedious to use for harvesting large areas of grafts since the skin must first be thoroughly cleaned of surface oils, glue must then be applied, and the drum prepared (either glue for the Padgett or tape for the Reese).

The Brown dermatome (either electric or gas driven) is the most popular type of dermatome in use in the United States. It can be used successfully by relatively inexperienced surgeons and permits rapid harvesting of large areas of skin. Irregular grafts are the most frequent complications.[18] The Padgett electric dermatome is the most effective dermatome for burn surgery (see Fig. 6-4). With little preparation, large areas of uniform thickness graft can be obtained by the most junior member of the burn team.

Skin grafts to the face and usually to the hands are applied as sheets. Most other areas are grafted with an expanded graft. This is done for two reasons: drainage is allowed around or through the graft, and a graft can be

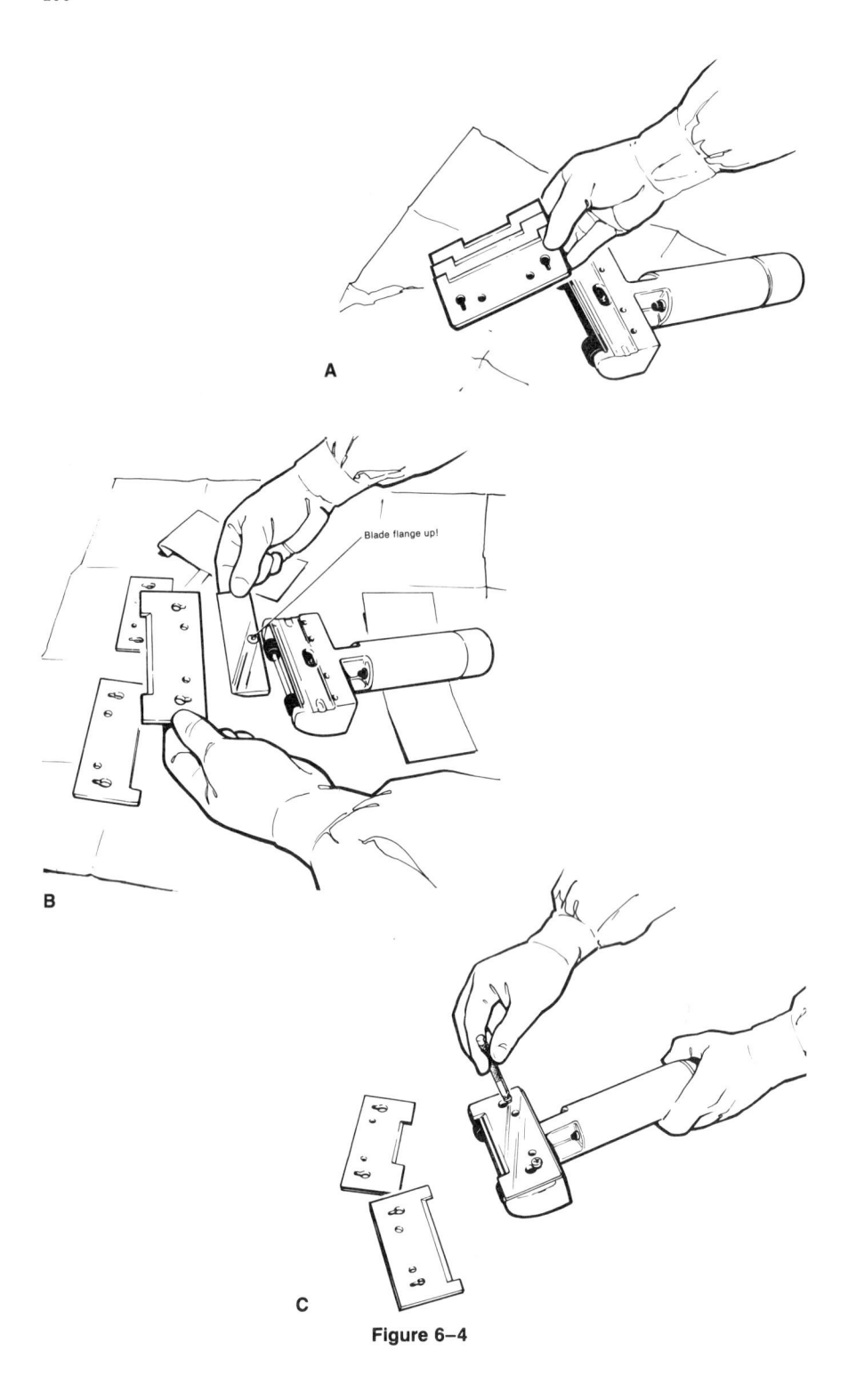

Blade flange up!

Figure 6-4

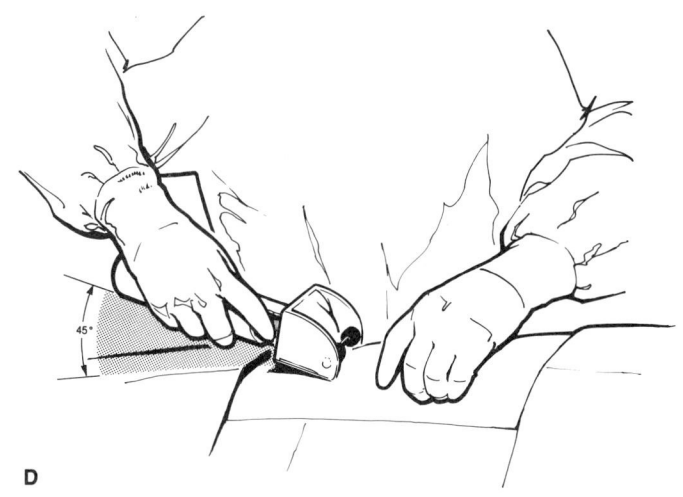

Figure 6-4. Use of the Padgett dermatome. **A.** The Padgett electric dermatome has a choice of three widths. **B.** The blade is first inserted with the blade flange up. The proper width is then selected. The medium width is most suitable for the Tanner mesher and will be the most commonly used size. **C.** The metal plates are secured with a screwdriver. **D.** The dermatome is held at a 45-degree angle from the patient. The skin is lubricated with mineral oil. Constant pressure is applied. It is not necessary to retrieve the skin from the head of the dermatome while the skin graft is being taken.

used for a larger area (1½ to 9 times the size of the donor area). Expanding the graft is essential for coverage of large burns where donor sites are limited and desirable in smaller burns to minimize donor site morbidity. Expansion can be done by meshing (Fig. 6-5) or postage stamp technique. Three types of meshers are currently available; the most common is illustrated. An inexpensive model using a handheld roller is acceptable for occasional use (Padgett). A French model (Genetic Laboratories, Inc.) does not require skin graft carriers; however, only one ratio of graft is possible with each instrument. Postage stamps are secured with nylon netting which is secured by staples. Mesh grafts are stapled and then covered with nylon netting, antibiotic dressing, synthetic skin, xenograft, or allograft.[19]

Skin expansion techniques have been used extensively in China.[20] Large sheets of full thickness allograft are secured to a freshly excised wound. Holes are then cut and small (1 to 2 cm^2) pieces of autograft are intermingled with the allograft. As the allograft progresses to rejection, the autographs epithelialize and eventually join each other. This method has been used to salvage extensively burned patients. Alexander et al. have proposed a similar technique[21] using widely meshed autograft which is then covered with allograft. Yet another technique involves the application of strips of autograft (3 to

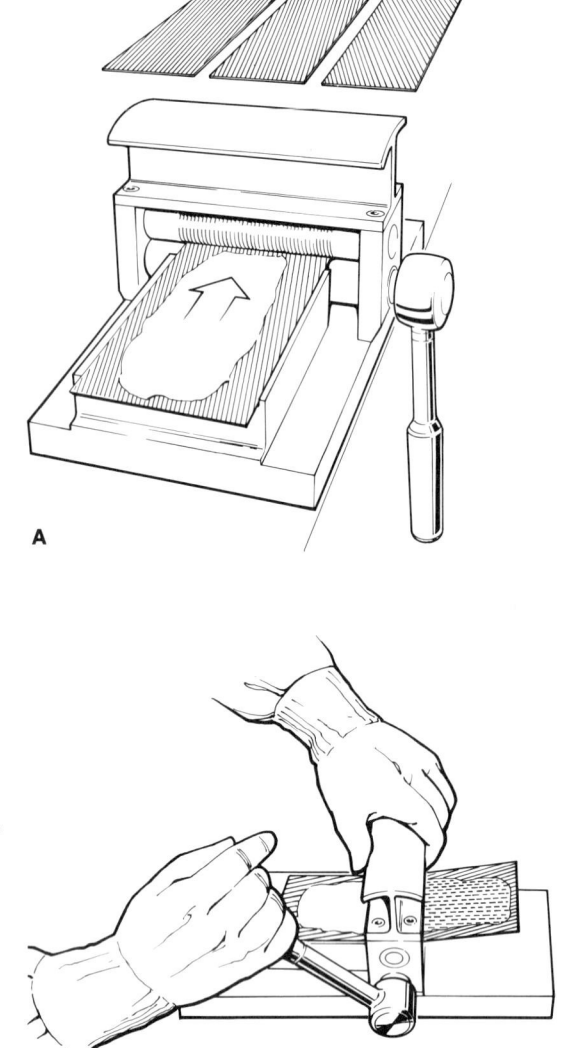

Figure 6–5. Use of the Tanner mesher. **A.** Tanner mesher carriers have a predetermined ratio of 1½:1, 3:1, 6:1, and 9:1 selection. It is crucial that the skin be placed on the grooved side. The skin can be placed either epidermal side or dermis side up depending on the operator's preference. **B.** The skin graft and carrier are then passed through the blades of the mesher.

4 mm wide) alternating with strips of allograft (15 to 22 mm wide). The allograft is gradually replaced by adjacent autografts which spread out by epithelialization.[22] Attempts have been made to grow a patient's own skin in tissue culture thereby greatly expanding the surface area of harvested skin. These have been successfully applied to burn patients, but thus far have had limited clinical application.[23]

Areas that cannot be covered by autograft and that do not require further debridement should be covered with a temporary covering. The best of these materials is allograft. This is not widely available and is expensive. Skin banks have been established in various locations throughout the country. Harvested skin is stored in liquid nitrogen and can be maintained for several months. Donor programs need to be greatly expanded to ensure a more reliable supply of this useful material. Burke et al. have reported combining allografts and immunosuppression.[24] Salvage of extensively burned children was possible. This technique required strict isolation because of the increased risk of sepsis and is no longer used. A new immunosuppressive drug, cyclosporine, primarily affects T cells, therefore allowing the organism to resist bacterial invasion. This drug shows great promise in the experimental stage for burn patients. It may soon be possible to use allografts for extended periods of time, replacing them with autografts weeks or months after the burn.[25] The first successful clinical case has been reported.[26]

Researchers have devoted a great deal of effort to develop acceptable substitutes for skin. Ideal properties are listed in Table 6–2. Alternatives now available include xenograft (porcine skin), amnion, and synthetic materials. Physiologic dressings are used (1) to cover partial thickness burns, (2) to test for autograft take, (3) as a temporary cover following debridement or excision, (4) to cover granulation tissue between crops of autograft in massive burns, and (5) to cover donor sites (which represent a large wound for the burn patient and require greater consideration). Beneficial effects include a decrease in evaporative water loss and protein loss. They should serve as a bacterial barrier and reduce pain. Xenografts differ from allografts in that they are not vascularized.[27] Viability does not appear to be a key element in a physiologic dressing.[28] Porcine xenografts have been reported to have properties very similar to allografts as far as preventing water–vapor loss, promoting epithelialization, and adherence to granulating wounds. Pigskin is available in several forms. Lyophilized pig skin graft is not recommended. Newer preparations are available meshed and with silver sulfadiazine. Amniotic membranes are readily available and inexpensive. Technical problems include dessication (requiring occlusive dressings) and less secure bed adherence.[29] Biobrane is a trilaminate of thin silicone, nylon fabric, and collagen peptides.

TABLE 6–2. IDEAL PROPERTIES OF A SKIN SUBSTITUTE

Adherence
Safety (sterile, hypoallergenic, nontoxic, nonpyrogenic)
Controls evaporative water loss
Flexible
Durable—stable on various wound surfaces
Bacterial barrier
Ease of application and removal
Availability—easy to store
Cost effective
Hemostatic

(From Woodroof EA; Biobrane: A biosynthetic skin prosthesis. In Wise DL (ed): Burn Wound Coverings. New York, CRC Press, 1984, reproduced with permission.)

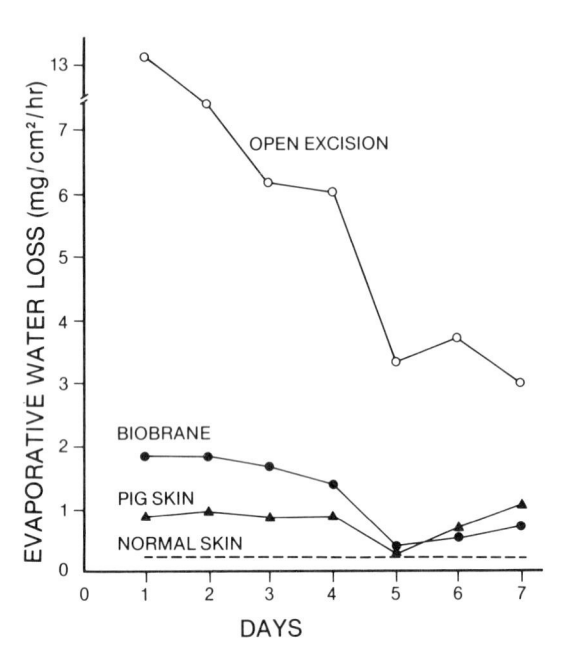

Figure 6-6. Evaluation of evaporative water loss. Coverage of 20 percent full thickness wounds with Biobrane or pigskin reduced evaporative water loss compared to the open wound. *(From Woodroof EA: Biobrane: A biosynthetic skin prosthesis. In Wise DL (ed): Burn Wound Coverings. New York, CRC Press, 1984, reproduced with permission.)*

It has excellent adherence, water–vapor control (Fig. 6–6), and is commercially available and practical to use. Frank et al. have reported excellent control of bacterial proliferation as well (Fig. 6–7).[30]

A collagen–chondroitin sulfate–silicone skin substitute has been described. This material is resorbed and a thin skin graft applied to the wound.[31] This product has been used on a number of extensively burned patients. Further refinements are underway and commercial production contemplated. This may be a great help to burn surgeons in the future. Tissue culture of autogenous epithelium has also been making great progress. This technique will also become much more widely available.[32]

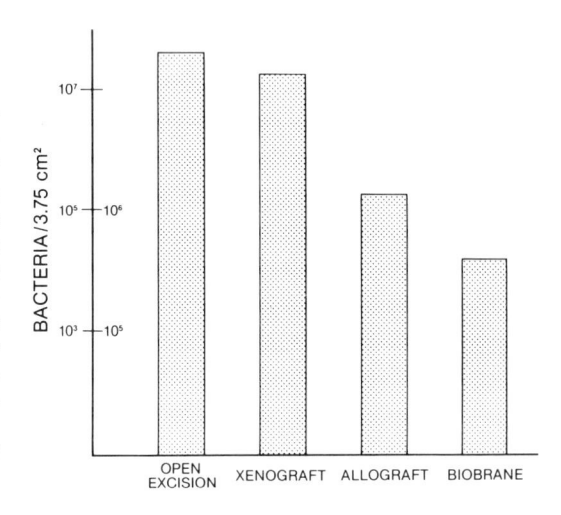

Figure 6-7. Evaluation of bacterial presence subadjacent to Biobrane, xenograft, or allograft, or from open wound surface, 7 days postexcision. Sample area was 3.75 cm. The bars represent the mean value of bacteria per swab area. Biobrane controlled bacterial proliferation better than the other dressings. *(From Woodroof EA: Biobrane: A biosynthetic skin prosthesis. In Wise DL (ed): Burn Wound Coverings. New York, CRC Press, 1984, reproduced with permission.)*

Donor Sites

In burn patients, donor sites become quite important because of the magnitude of surface area involved. It is highly desirable to minimize evaporative water and protein loss. Pain control is also important. Biologic materials (allograft, xenograft, and amnion) are not useful for donor sites. There has been tissue ingrowth of the dressing into the donor site causing chronic inflammatory reactions. Synthetic materials (Biobrane, Tegaderm, and OpSite) seem best suited to the burn patient.

Unusual donor sites may be necessary for severely burned patients. Typically, the scalp and plantar surfaces of the feet are not burned. These make excellent donor sites and can be reharvested in a few days.

Burn Wound Sepsis

Burn patients are at risk for burn wound sepsis until skin grafting is complete. Daily vigilance is required. Signs of wound infection include: conversion of partial to full thickness injury, focal black, dark brown, or violaceous areas, hemorrhagic discoloration or superficial ulceration of unburned skin at wound margins, erythematous nodular lesions in unburned skin, and vesicular lesions in healed burns.[7] Any of these changes should prompt a wound biopsy. Part of the biopsy is sent for culture and part for histology. The presence of a bacterial invasion into unburned areas is diagnostic of burn wound sepsis. Greater than (1×10^5 power) of organisms per gram of tissue is also felt to be indicative of wound sepsis. Even though less diagnostic, surface cultures give qualitative information and are useful for surveillance and epidemiologic control. Aggressive action is required once burn wound sepsis has been diagnosed. Extensive debridement, systemic antibiotics, and a change in topical antibiotics are indicated. Blood cultures must be monitored and intravascular lines changed. Other foci must also be excluded. Examples include suppurative thrombophlebitis and pneumonia. *Pseudomonas* species, resistant Staphylococcus organisms, and fungi are common predators of the burn victim. In addition to practical advances in wound care, immunologic evaluation and manipulation are becoming possible. These efforts may be very helpful to burn patients (see Chap. 3). Subeschar injections of antibiotics has been proposed,[33] but should not be considered a substitute for definitive surgical management.

REFERENCES

1. Meeuws WA: The Progress of Plastic Surgery. New York, Oxford Press, 1982
2. Kentish E: Essay on Burns. London, Longman, Hurst, Rees, Orme and Brown, 1817
3. Jackson DM: A historical review of the use of local physical signs in burns. Br J Plast Surg 23:21, 1970
4. Moyer CA, Brentano L, Gravens DL, et al.: Treatment of large human burns with 0.5% silver nitrate solution. Arch Surg 90:812, 1965

5. Moncrief JA, Lindberg RB, Switzer WE, et al.: The use of a topical sulfonamide in the control of burn wound sepsis. J Trauma 6:407, 1966
6. Fox CL, Roppole BW, Stanford W: Control of Pseudomonas infection in burns by silver sulfadiazine. Surg Gynec Obstet 128:1021, 1969
7. Pruitt BA: The burn patient. II. Later care and complications of thermal injury. Curr Prob Surg, 16:5, 1979
8. Janzekovic Z: A new concept in the early excision and immediate grafting of burns. J Trauma 10:1103, 1970
9. Gatti J, LaRossa D, Silverman G, Hartford C: Evaluation of the burn wound with perfusion fluorometry. J Trauma 23:202, 1983
10. Levenson SM, Gruber PK, Gruber C, et al.: A hemostatic scalpel for burn debridement. Arch Surg 117:213, 1982
11. Keogh EJ: The use of ornithine-8-vasopressin in the management of burn eschar in children. Burns 1:314, 1975
12. Moberg AW, Maldonado A, Tobin G, Weiner L: The comparative advantages of early tangential excision and grafting (TEG) in burn wound management. Abstract 109:197 Plast Surg Forum 1982
13. Wolfe RW, Roi LD, Flores JD, et al.: Mortality differences and speed of wound closure among specialized burn care facilities. JAMA 250:763, 1983
14. Heimbach DM, Engrav LH: Burn wound excision. Curr Conc Trauma Care, 4:14, 1981
15. Deitch E, Clothier J: Prospective study of early surgery in the elderly. Abstract 74, p. 76, Ann Meet Am Burn Assoc, 1983
16. Heimbach DM, Engrav LH: Surgical Management of the Burn Wound. New York, Raven Press, 1985
17. Burke J, Quinby W, Bondoc CC: Primary excision and prompt grafting as routine therapy for the treatment of thermal burns in children. Surg Clin North Am 56:477, 1976
18. Rudolph R, Fisher J, Ninnemann J: Skin Grafting. Boston, Little Brown, 1979
19. Edlich RF, Rodeheaver G, Carucci D, et al.: Technical considerations in mesh grafting. J Burn Care Rehab 3:6, 1982
20. Yang CC, Shih TS, Chu TA, et al.: The intermingled transplantation of auto- and homografts in severe burns. Burns 6:141, 1980.
21. Alexander JW, MacMillan BG, Law E, et al.: Treatment of severe burns with widely meshed skin autograft and meshed skin allograft overlay. J Trauma 21:433, 1981
22. Zawacki BE, Asch MJ: A technique for autografting very large burns from very limited donor sites. Surgery 74:774, 1973
23. Nicholas E, O'Connor JB, Mulliken B, et al.: Grafting of burns with cultured epithelium prepared from autologous epidermal cells. Lancet 1:75, 1981
24. Burke JF, Quinby WC, Bondoc CC, et al.: Immunosuppression and temporary skin transplantation in the treatment of massive third-degree burns. Ann Surg 182:183, 1975
25. Achauer BM, Hewitt CW, Black KS, et al.: Cyclosporine prolongs skin allografts in a rat burn model. Transplant Proc 15:3073, 1983
26. Achauer BM, Hewitt CW, Bloch KS: Long term skin allograft survival after short-term cyclosporin treatment in a patient with massive burns. Lancet 1:14, 1986
27. Silverstein P, Currerri PW, Munster AM: Evaluation of fresh viable porcine

cutaneous xenograft as a temporary burn wound cover. U.S. Army Inst Surg Res Anl Res Prog Rep, Sec. 51, B.A.M.C., Ft. Sam, Houston, Texas, 30 June 1971

28. Luterman A, Kraft E, Bookless S: Biologic dressings: An appraisal of current practices. J Burn Care Rehab 1:18, 1980
29. Robson MC, Krizek TJ, Koss N, et al.: Amniotic membranes as a temporary wound dressing. Surg Gynec Obstet 136:904, 1973
30. Frank DH, Wachtel TL, Frank HA: Comparison of biobrane, porcine, and human allograft as biological dressings for burn wounds. Surg Forum 31:552, 1980
31. Burke J, Yannas I, Quinby W, et al.: Successful use of physiologically acceptable artificial skin in the treatment of extensive burn injury. Ann Surg 194:413, 1981
32. Gallico GG, O'Connor NE, Compton CC, et al.: Permanent coverage of large burn wounds with autologous cultured human epithelium. New Eng J Med 311:448, 1984
33. Baxter CR, Curreri PW, Marvin JA: The control of burn wound sepsis by the use of quantitative bacteriologic studies and subeschar cylsis with antibiotics. Surg Clin North Am 53:1509, 1973

CHAPTER 7
Outpatient Burns

Suzanne E. Martinez

OUTPATIENT MANAGEMENT

As a rule, patients with burn injuries less than 20 percent of total body surface area (TBSA) can be treated on an outpatient basis. Shuck[1] notes that in specialized burn centers, the team approach can be utilized for minor burns being treated totally in the outpatient department or for follow-up of patients who have been discharged from a burn center. The burn center team includes physicians and nurses as well as physical and occupational therapists, a dietitian, social worker, psychologist, and recreational therapist. The physician members of the team include representatives from general surgery, plastic surgery, and pediatrics when indicated.

The American Burn Association has established criteria for classification of burn injuries (see Table 1-2). Patients with minor and moderate burns are usually candidates for outpatient care. Major burns require admission to a burn unit.

Poor risk patients are those with pre-existing or concurrent medical disease such as diabetes, seizure disorders, musculoskeletal, cardiac or pulmonary disease, or psychiatric disturbances. Patients are at risk if the burn accident has resulted in an unexpected and irreversible change in social or economic status. Most common examples of these situations are loss of one's home to fire, loss or incapacitation of one's method of transportation, death or injury to another—family member or loved one.

Burns to the face require admission to a burn unit because of possible damage to the eyes or inhalation injuries. The resultant periorbital edema from facial burns may, of itself, be adequate cause for admission until the edema subsides and vision is clear. Burns to the hands or feet, regardless of extent of damage, may pose functional problems in activities of daily living and ambulation and necessitate a brief hospital stay.

WOUND CARE

Treatment of the burn wound is best done in an aggressive and meticulous manner. Patients who meet the criteria for outpatient care return to the burn unit daily for hydrotherapy, debridement, and dressing changes. In our unit, the hydrotherapy area is staffed with registered nurses, vocational nurses, and physical therapists with expertise in burn care. They follow the patient's progress and wound healing and refer to the physician only when problems arise.

Burn wounds are immersed in a dilute Clorox–Betadine solution with whirlpool agitation (Clorox 1:240, Betadine 1:1000) for 15 to 20 minutes, followed by gentle washing to remove any residue of Silver Sulfadiazene cream and loosened eschar or proteinaceous material which has collected and coagulated on the burn surface. Washing is done with cotton pads (the type used in the operating room work well). These have been found to be the softest and most effective tool for efficient cleaning of the burn surface (Fig. 7–1).

Following whirlpool, burn wounds are dressed in a semi-closed manner.

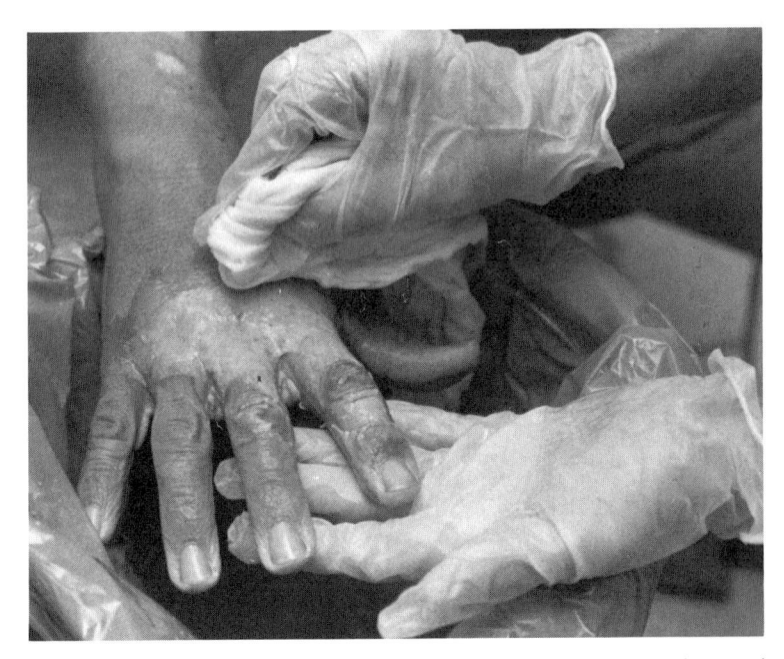

Figure 7–1. Burn wounds are cleansed following whirlpool to remove loosened eschar or exudate. Cotton pads are effective because of their soft texture.

Silver Sulfadiazene (SSD) is the surface agent most widely used. SSD may be impregnated on fine mesh gauze and applied to the burn wound (Fig. 7–2). To prevent a constricting effect on a fresh burn with edema, the gauze is not wrapped but cut in strips and placed in succession on the affected part. Additional SSD cream is applied to the impregnated gauze after it is placed on the wound (Fig. 7–3). Tubular net bandage is then applied to help hold the gauze in place (Fig. 7–4). Tubular net comes in a variety of sizes to fit all body parts from fingers to the trunk. Experienced burn nurses become increasingly adept and creative in the use of tubular net. Turtle neck shirts, bolero jackets, and panty hose can be fashioned to accommodate burn dressings on any body part.

All burn wounds are cultured on a weekly basis and systemic antibiotics are prescribed based on these reports. Wound cultures may be done more frequently if the appearance of the burn surface suggests bacterial contamination.

MEDICATIONS

A vital part of successful outpatient case is adequate pain control. Patients in their own environment will eat better, sleep more soundly, and develop a more positive attitude toward total recovery, but not if their pain is out of control.

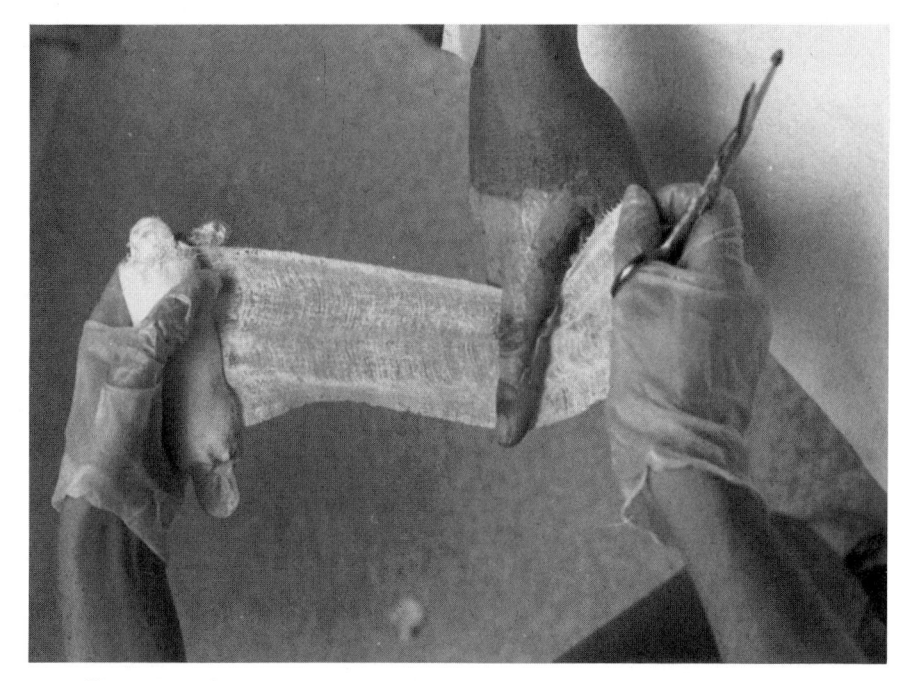

Figure 7–2. Silvadene cream impregnated on fine mesh gauze is applied to the burn surface.

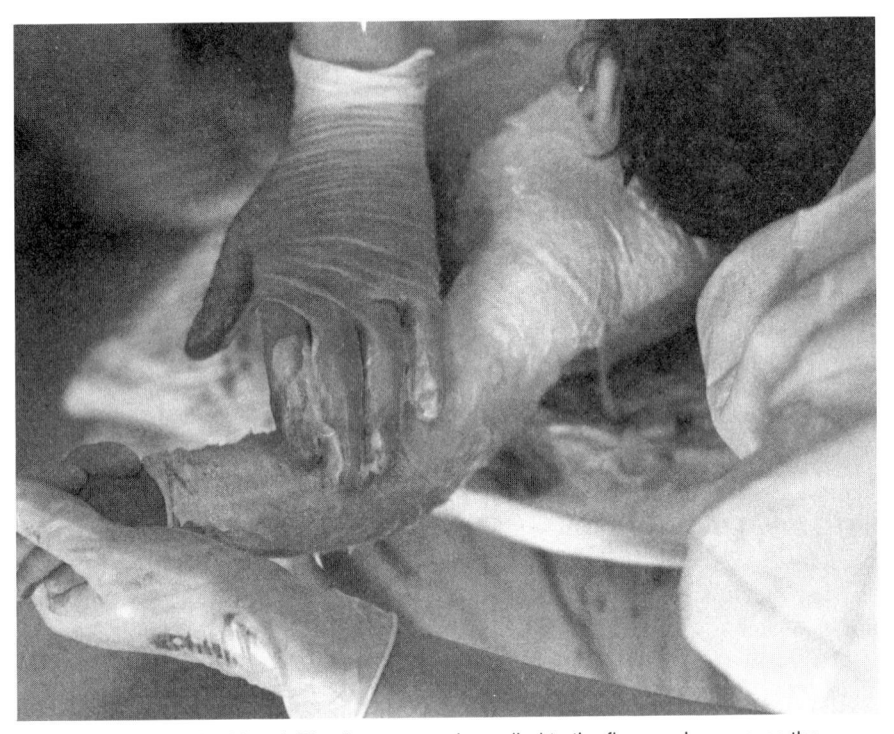

Figure 7-3. Additional Silvadene cream is applied to the fine mesh gauze on the burn wound.

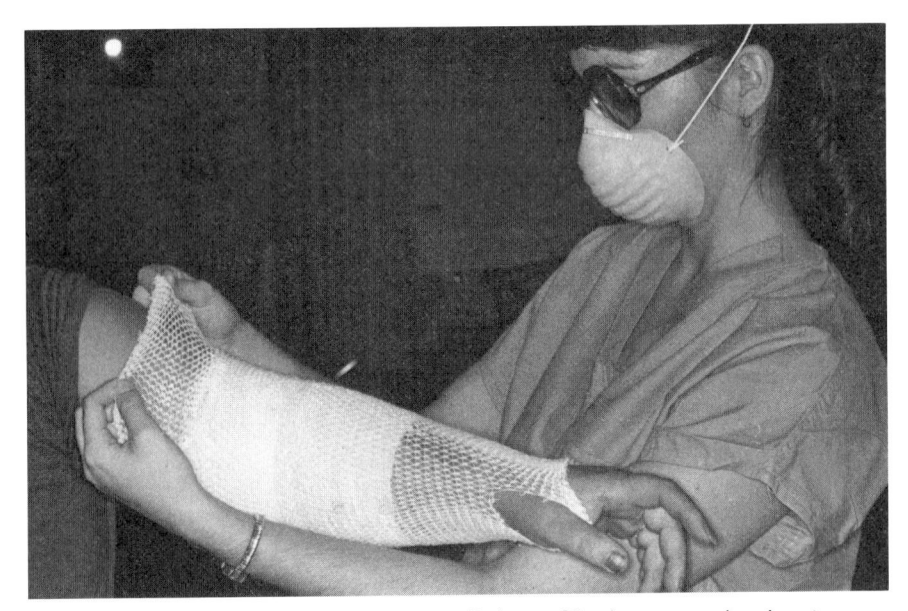

Figure 7-4. Tubular net bandage is applied over Silvadene gauze dressings to hold them in place.

Oral analgesics are prescribed for all patients and they are instructed to take one dose prior to arrival at the hospital. Vicodin (hydrocodone bitartrate and acetaminophen) or acetaminophen with codeine are commonly used. As healing progresses, patients also receive oral antihistamines (diphenhydramine hydrochloride, hydroxyzine) for pruritus. The patients and their families need to be aware of all medications that are prescribed as well as the amount to be taken and the frequency. Patients are taught the names of their medications and the reasons for taking them. Specific side effects and precautions are also explained to the patients and their families. Outpatients are instructed to take pain pills before coming to the hospital for dressing changes and therapy. Patients are also advised to notify the staff when they are left with a 1-day supply of pills. Since a physician may not be available at the time of their appointments, this will allow time for new prescriptions to be written and filled without causing undue suffering from delays in processing.

THE TEAM CONCEPT

Patients with burns to the lower extremities wear elastic bandages for support and to prevent venous stasis. Gauze wraps may be used over the tubular bandage prior to wrapping the elastic bandage to prevent soaking it with SSD. Patients with minor or moderate burns of the lower extremities can usually tolerate ambulation if begun in minimal amounts, such as to the bathroom and to the car. Gradual increases in activity, coordinated with healing, promote rapid return to the preburn level. When indicated, physical therapists work with the patient to increase muscle strength and endurance. Most patients who qualify for outpatient care can maintain mobility at an optimal level.

Patients with hand burns are seen by the burn unit occupational therapist prior to or following whirlpool. These patients are evaluated for splinting and exercise throughout the course of wound healing. The occupational therapist is also available for exercise and splinting in other areas as needed, such as axilla, elbow, or neck.

When possible, coordination of other hospital appointments is accomplished so that the patient can take care of all business during one trip to the hospital. Other appointments may include visits with the burn unit social worker or psychologist, occupational therapist, or with other medical specialists.

The physician–nurse relationship is strong in all aspects of burn care, but especially so in outpatient management. Patients are seen on a daily basis by the nursing staff. The physician sees the patient for medications (analgesics, antibiotics, or antihistamines), for specific adjustment problems affecting physical well-being (dehydration, nausea, or insomnia), or delayed healing. Those patients with unhealed burns after 2 weeks are seen by the physician to establish the need for surgery and to coordinate the time when grafting will take place. It is the nurse whose daily assessment of the patient and his or her burn who keeps the physician informed of the patient's progress and problems. The nurse's observations and recommendations based on first-line patient contact provide valuable input in planning the course of treatment.

DEBRIDEMENT

Patients with small full thickness injuries (less than 15 percent TBSA) may require debridement. This can be done on an outpatient basis. Ketamine (ketalar) anesthesia is used. Its popularity is due to its short action and the fact that intubation is not necessary as with other anesthetic agents.

Ketamine is a nonbarbiturate anesthetic agent. It is rapid acting and produces an anesthetic state characterized by deep analgesia, normal pharyngeal–laryngeal reflexes, normal or slightly enhanced skeletal muscle tone, cardiovascular and respiratory stimulation. Bosomworth[2] describes this as dissociative anesthesia which appears to selectively disrupt association pathways of the brain before producing somesthetic sensory blockade. Drain and Shapely[3] explain this phenomenon as selectively blocking pain conduction and perception, leaving those parts of the central nervous system that do not participate in pain transmission free from the depressant effects of the drug.

Sage and Laird[4] advocate the use of Ketamine for burn surgery and cite advantages for its use which include: (1) unimpaired pharyngeal–laryngeal reflexes which preclude the necessity of intubation and allow access to the head and neck when necessary, (2) protection against hypotension due to cardiovascular stimulation, and (3) the absence of postoperative anorexia.

Bosomworth[2] adds to the list of advantages by including ease of administration, rapid onset, brevity of action, modest and usually no adverse respiratory and circulatory side effects, compatibility with other agents when used concurrently, wide safety margin, no apparent hepatic or renal damage, no immunosuppressive effects, and minimal gastrointestinal effects.

The main side effect of Ketamine anesthesia is hallucinations. These can be minimized by supplemental administration of diazepam or other antianxiety medication. Careful predebridement preparation and explanation to the patient are also helpful in decreasing these adverse reactions.

Patients who will be debrided are instructed to take nothing by mouth after midnight on the day of debridement and to plan on staying in the burn unit longer than usual. The drug is given intramuscularly (4 mg/kg). This dose can be repeated after 20 minutes, but for minor debridements it is usually not necessary. Tangential excision of burn eschar with the Goulian knife accelerates the healing process and hastens the time of grafting for minor or moderate deep partial thickness or full thickness burns. An electrocautery unit is available as needed.

Following debridement and redressing in hydrotherapy, the patient is taken to the subacute area of the burn unit for recovery. Vital signs are monitored and the burn dressings are observed for bleeding. The patient usually sleeps for 2 to 3 hours postdebridement and awakens without difficulty. After the patient is completely awake, is taking fluids without difficulty, and is able to void, he or she is released to go home with instructions to return the following day for further hydrotherapy.

It is often necessary to increase the type and dosage of pain medication following debridement since the vigorous cleansing of the wound may result in hypersensitivity of exposed nerve endings. It may be necessary to administer an intramuscular injection prior to the next hydrotherapy treatment. This can be planned and available as needed.

The debridement procedure has proved to be an extremely useful adjunct to outpatient burn care.

EDUCATION

Patient and family teaching continues on a daily basis throughout the course of wound healing. Reinforcement and encouragement are essential. Family members are instructed to reapply a thin layer of SSD cream to the gauze and under the tubular net. This should be done in the evening prior to retiring to be sure that the dressings stay moist.

Family members must also be taught the proper application of elastic wraps and splints and the routine care and cleaning of these.

Both patient and family are informed of the importance of nutrition to wound healing. The patient is encouraged to eat a high protein, high carbohydrate diet. The patient's weight should be monitored during daily visits. Most patients with burns that can be treated outside the hospital can usually consume enough food to maintain adequate nutrition.

INPATIENT TO OUTPATIENT CARE

In many instances patients who require admission to a burn unit may still be considered for outpatient management. Following fluid resuscitation, hemodynamic stabilization and resolution of edema, patients with uncomplicated burns up to 35 percent TBSA may be treated on an outpatient basis. Warden et al.[5] point out that the hospital setting does not provide a normal environment for burn patients. Irregular sleeping hours, constant unit activity, noise level, foreign diet, and limited contact with family members place the patient in an even more stressful situation.

It is commonly agreed that patients' progress will be more rapid at home. Their nutritional status will be enhanced by home cooked food, and they will be more relaxed and less anxious in familiar surroundings. The need for pain medication may be decreased if the patients are returned to the comfort of their homes and loved ones. Unfortunately, there is seldom an ideal situation or a smooth transition from inpatient care to outpatient management in the early postburn period. Thus, patient teaching and continuous reinforcement of positive events are of extreme importance.

Social factors must be re-evaluated in depth at this time. If the patient's house has burned, he or she may not have a place to live. If the car has been damaged, transportation to and from the hospital for outpatient care may not be possible. The burn unit social worker can be helpful in locating temporary housing or alternative modes of transportation.

Frequently, family members are less willing than the patient to begin home care. Thorough patient and family education, tempered with understanding and concern for all the anxiety providing incidents which can and will occur during the first few days following discharge, are of utmost importance.

Reinforcement of positive behavior and any or all successes must continue through the entire course of outpatient care. Any of the changes that occur must be dealt with as another first and nurtured to success or mastery by the patient and family. The change may be as small as scheduling the outpatient appointment at a different time to accommodate an additional appointment with the social worker. That seemingly small change may raise enormous problems for the patient involving transportation, meals, or child care.

After the initial anxiety has been overcome, patients are followed in the outpatient department in a routine manner. Readmission for skin grafting, if necessary, is coordinated as with other outpatients.

Family members of patients who are being treated on an outpatient basis sometimes need a healthy measure of support for themselves. In spite of extensive teaching and planning, the first night is usually sleepless or, at least, sleep is interrupted many times. Concerns over eating, sleeping, medications, or ambulation must be repeatedly addressed.

As the patient and family become more comfortable with their situation and uncomplicated healing is assured, treatment may be extended to every other day with the patient or family assuming responsibility for bathing and dressing changes on alternate days. This routine may continue until the patient will return to the hospital only once or twice a week during the last stages of healing.

OTHER TECHNIQUES

Another dressing technique for use in outpatient burn wound management is biosynthetic dressing (Biobrane). The advantages of this type of dressing are that the wound is clearly visible. Exudate can escape through the barrier and bacterial growth is inhibited. Since these dressings can remain in place for extended periods, the inconvenience of daily hospital visits is eliminated. These dressings allow mobility and increased patient comfort due to less frequent dressing changes. Since they contain no antimicrobial agent, this type of dressing is limited to use on clean, light partial thickness wounds. Topical antimicrobial agents such as SSD can be used with these barrier dressings, but in these instances there is no advantage over aggressive cleaning and daily dressing changes.

7. OUTPATIENT BURNS 117

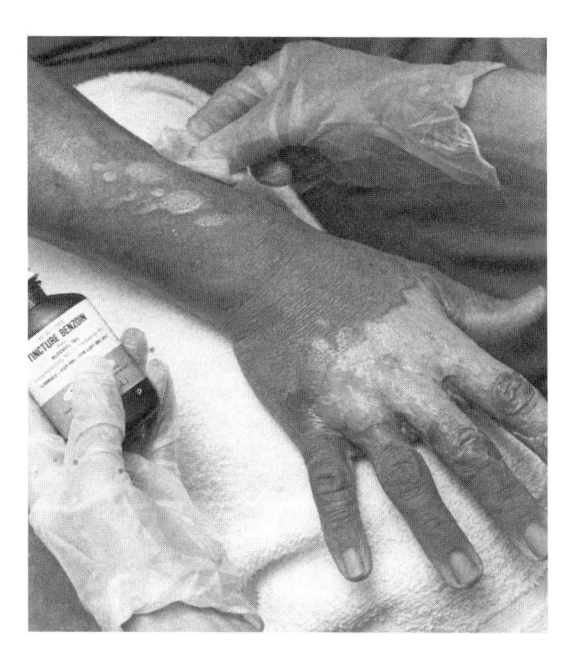

Figure 7-5. Tincture of benzoin can be used on undamaged skin to facilitate application of Biobrane.

Biobrane is applied to the superficial burn wound after cleaning and removal of loose tissue. Tincture of benzoin may be applied to undamaged skin to enhance adhesion (Fig. 7-5). The Biobrane is placed shiny side up and wrinkle free over the burn surface (Fig. 7-6). Steri-Strips may be used to hold the Biobrane in place. A gauze wrap may be used in the first 24 hours to

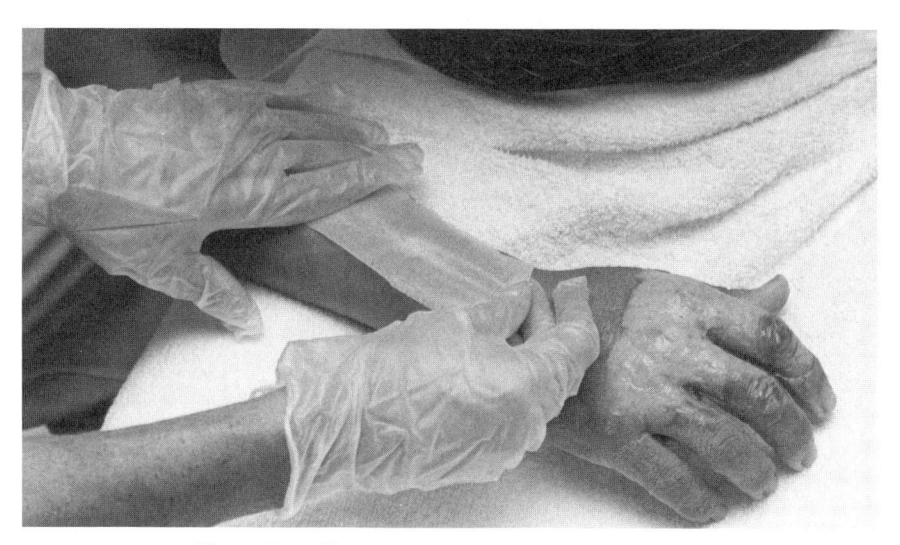

Figure 7-6. Biobrane is applied to the wound surface.

provide added pressure until adherence to the burn wound is achieved. Once adherence is complete and there is no sign of infection, the dressing may remain in place until healing has occurred.

Biobrane may also be used for patients following skin grafting as a dressing for small open areas (Fig. 7–7). The use of Biobrane in these situations is advantageous since continued use of other topical agents may cause breakdown of newly healed skin.

HEALING AND BEYOND

As healing progresses, different approaches become appropriate. Healed areas need lubrication with a moisturizing or lanolin-based lotion. This will prevent drying and cracking of newly healed skin and facilitate movement of the affected part.

Newly healed skin must be protected from direct exposure to sunlight. Caps or hats to protect faces and long sleeves and pants are recommended to minimize the danger from exposure of burned areas to sun and heat.

Long-term outpatient management for all burn victims may continue in a weekly clinic setting where all disciplines can see the patient together. The

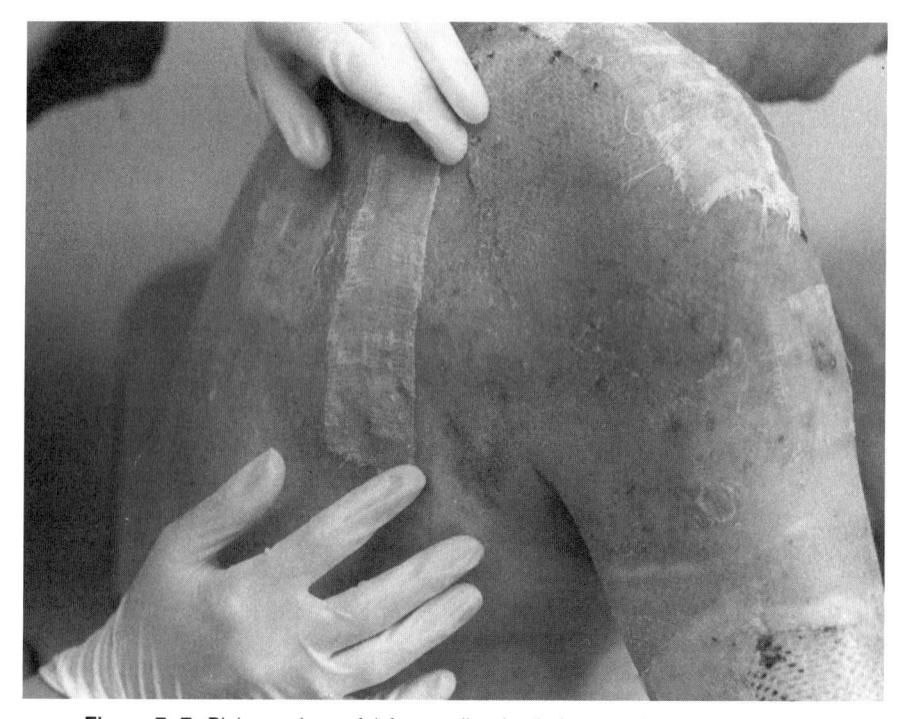

Figure 7–7. Biobrane is useful for small unhealed areas that remain following skin grafts.

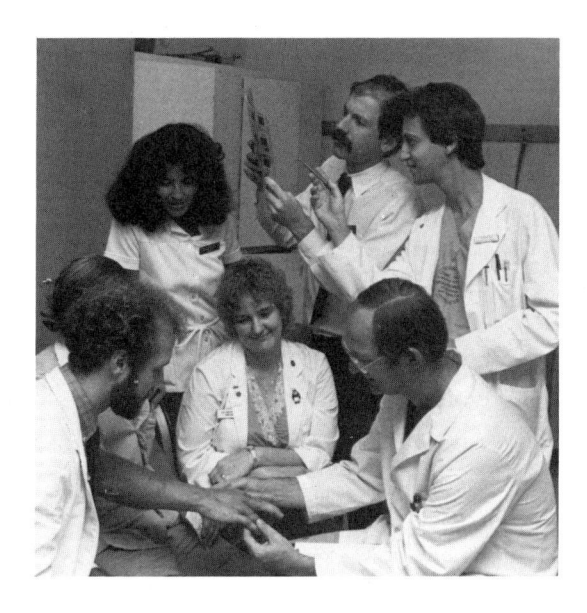

Figure 7-8. Follow-up appointments for long-term outpatient management are conducted in a clinic setting where all members of the burn care team can discuss and coordinate further intervention with the patient.

patients meet with the physician, nurse, occupational therapist, social worker, and psychologist to discuss their progress, adjustment, and plans for the future. Thus, the team approach to burn care continues throughout the entire rehabilitation phase. These visits then occur monthly and advance to semi-annually, then annually as the patient returns to work or school at an optimal functional level (Fig. 7-8).

APPLICATIONS FOR THE NONBURN CENTER FACILITY

The techniques of burn care described are those that have evolved over the years in our burn center. Each emergency department, doctor's office, or community hospital will want to modify burn care to suit their situation. For example, the doctor would want to inspect the wound more frequently in the absence of experienced burn nurses. It should be emphasized that if there is deterioration in healing, some change should be made (e.g., antibiotics started, the patient hospitalized, or extensive debridement performed). If a wound is not healed in 3 weeks, generally grafting is recommended. Wounds taking longer than this will often produce hypertrophic or unstable scars and certainly an undesirable end result.

REFERENCES

1. Shuck JM: Outpatient management of the burned patient. Surg Clin North Am 58:1107, 1978

2. Bosomworth PP: Ketamine symposium—Comments by moderator. Anesth Anal Curr Res 50:471, 1971
3. Drain CB, Shapely SC: The Recovery Room. Philadelphia, Saunders, 1979, pp. 160–163
4. Sage M, Laird SM: Ketamine anesthesia for burn surgery. Postgrad Med J 48:156, 1972
5. Warden GD, Kravitz M, Schnebly A: The outpatient management of moderate and major thermal injuries. J Burn Care Reconstr 2:159, 1981

CHAPTER 8
Extremities
Bruce M. Achauer

Three important decisions must be made about the burned hand in the first 24 hours. Splints need to be fitted, a decision reached about immediate surgical intervention and, in circumferential burns, escharotomies must be considered.

ESCHAROTOMY

Burned tissue is unyielding and can become a tourniquet if the deep tissues are expanding secondary to fluid accumulation. Vascular compromise may be severe resulting in arterial compression and loss of palpable or Doppler pulses. Clinical signs associated with this problem include cyanosis, decreased capillary filling, and neurologic changes. The Doppler has been noted to be more sensitive to early compression than clinical judgment.[1] Changes in photoplethymographic tracings have also been useful.[2] Since edema is maximal 36 hours postinjury, any evaluation of an extremity must be repeated until a decision about escharotomy is reached. Concern about vascular compromise has centered around limb survival. Recently, more objective studies have emphasized the importance of lymphatic, venous, and capillary flow. It is possible to have intact pulses (arterial pressures are over 100 mm Hg) and severe muscle ischemia (capillary perfusion pressure is on the order of 30 mm Hg). Therefore, the most sensitive and objective method of assessing the burned limb is tissue pressure measurements. These are not difficult to do (Fig. 8–1). A wick catheter is inserted into a muscular compartment (or be-

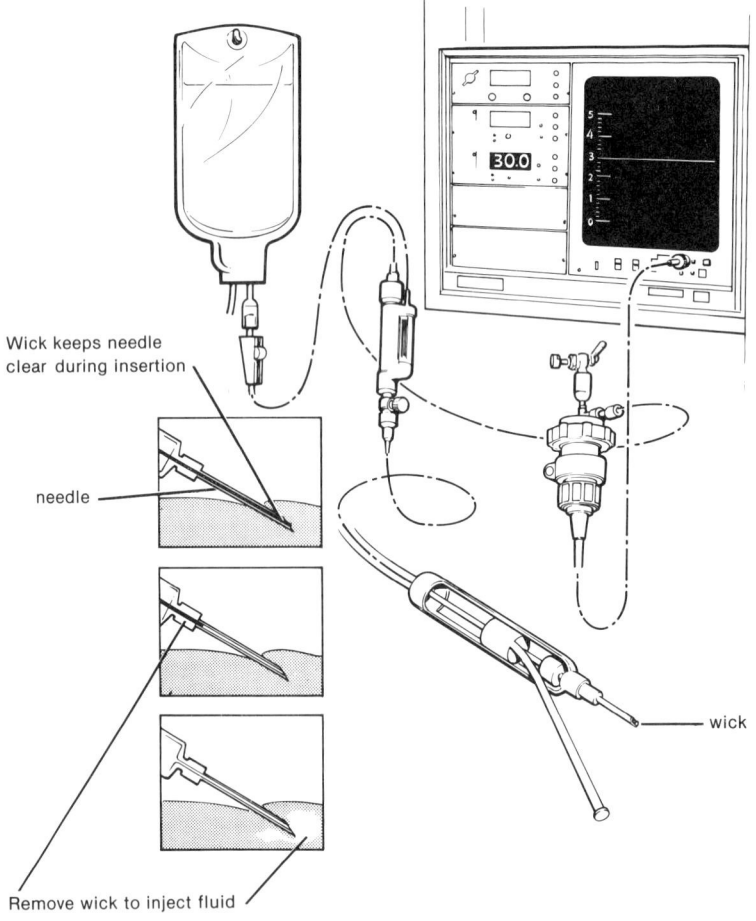

Figure 8–1. Wick catheters. A catheter is inserted into the subcutaneous tissue, either subeschar or subfascial. The wick in the system prevents tissue from plugging the needle. The wick is withdrawn and the system filled with fluid. The system is then connected to a transducer or a manometer. Readings are taken at regular intervals, usually each hour for the first 36 hours. If two readings are above 30 mm Hg, an escharotomy is indicated.

neath the eschar), the line filled with fluid and connected to a pressure transducer. Readings are taken every 1 to 2 hours during the first 36 hours. If there are two readings above 30 mm Hg, escharotomies are done.[3] An additional advantage of tissue measurements is that the effectiveness of the escharotomy can also be documented. If a medial incision does not lower the pressures, lateral ones or deeper incisions or fasciotomies are made. The preferred sites for escharotomies are shown in Figure 8–2. Escharotomies can often be done without anesthesia. Sedation with morphine, some local anesthetic, or a single intramuscular (IM) injection of ketamine may sometimes be

HAND — On one side of each digit

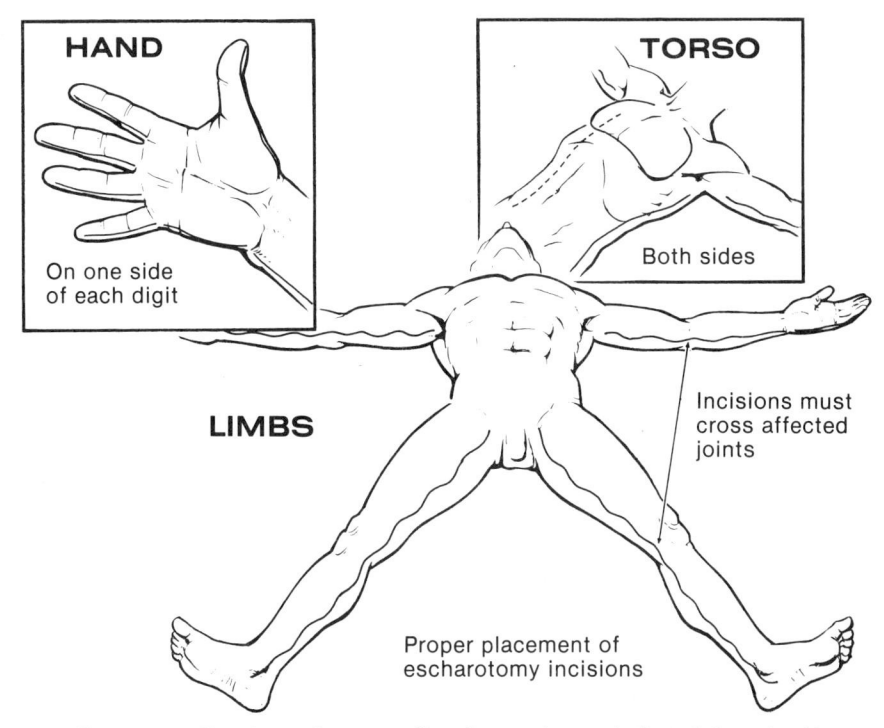

TORSO — Both sides

LIMBS — Incisions must cross affected joints

Proper placement of escharotomy incisions

Figure 8–2. Sites for escharotomy. If escharotomies are indicated, they should be placed so that scar contracture bands are not produced. In the hand this is the midaxial part of the fingers and the ulnar, or radial border of the hand and the radial, or ulnar border of the forearm and arm. Usually escharotomy of one side of a digit or extremity is sufficient to relieve pressure. The catheter measurements should be continued during their release to judge its effectiveness. Burn escharotomy may well be required for the chest to permit adequate ventilation.

required. The electrocautery unit or heated scalpel are preferred for the incision. Interestingly, the frequency of escharotomies has decreased since the introduction of tissue pressure measurements. In severe hand burns, the incision should be extended onto the fingers to relieve intrinsic muscle pressure.[4]

HAND POSITION

Proper position of the hand is crucial to any method of burn care. The position of comfort for the common dorsal hand burn is metacarpophalangeal extension, proximal interphalangeal (PIP) joint flexion, wrist flexion, and thumb adduction. These are also the positions of deformity and will lead to a claw hand. The claw hand deformity is preventable with proper positioning and therapy. Most hand burns involve the dorsum of the hand and therefore the thin skin overlying the extensor mechanism, particularly over the PIP joints. This factor, coupled with the greater strength of the flexor tendons, may lead to rupture of the extensor tendon and exposure of the joint. The metacarpophalangeal joints are eccentric in their axis of rotation, hence the collateral ligaments are relaxed in extension and stretched in flexion. If the joints are not flexed, these ligaments permanently contract producing an extension deformity. The thenar muscles also tend to contract and fibrose, resulting in an adduction deformity. The strong wrist flexors tend to produce wrist flexion deformities. All of these forces must be overcome. The hand must be positioned in the antideformity (anticlaw) position (see Chap. 15). In severe burns, it may not be possible to maintain the hand in the antideformity position with splints. Small Kirschner wires can be placed across the PIP joint to gain control of the hand (Fig. 8–3). With these joints immobilized, M-P flexion is easy to obtain and the risk of extensor tendon rupture from repeated flexion is minimized. There is a risk of joint sepsis and joint stiffness. How-

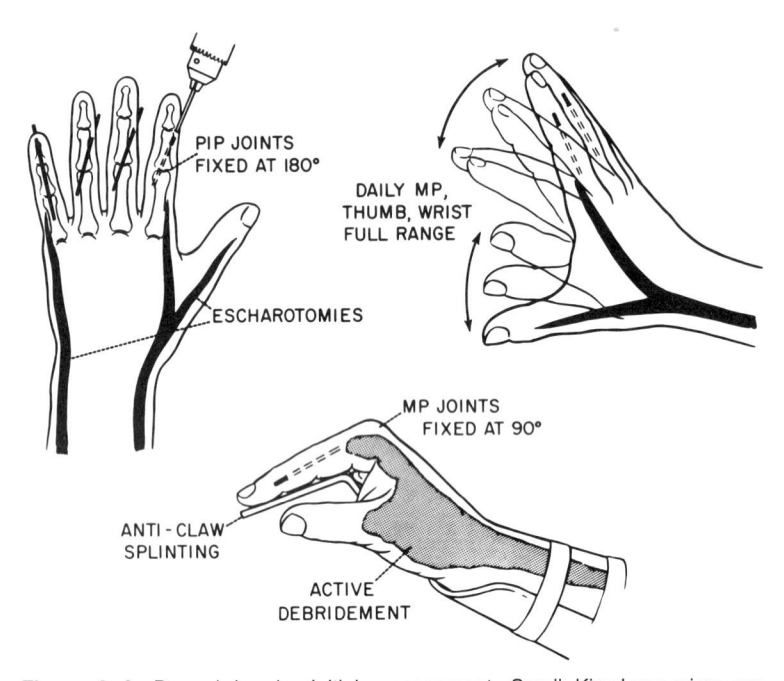

Figure 8–3. Burned hands: Initial management. Small Kirschner wires are placed across the PIP joints to control the position in severe hand burns. This maneuver allows the wrist and M-P joints to be properly positioned. The M-P joints may be moved as much as desired. This method prevents early rupture of the extensor tendons, thus protecting the PIP joint. Complications of this technique are directly proportioned to the length of time the wires are in place. (Three weeks should be absolute maximum.) *(From Achauer BM, et al., Internal fixation in the management of the burned hand. Arch Surg 108:815, 1974, reproduced with permission.)*

ever, these can be avoided with careful wound care and prompt removal of the pins after grafting. This technique is usually reserved for joints that are likely to progress to exposure and eventual fusion. Splinting techniques are discussed in Chapter 15.

PRIMARY EXCISION

There are reports demonstrating excellent results with early tangential excision of hand burns.[5-8] Earlier techniques involved a meticulous dissection. Later, the techniques of Janzekovic[9] were adapted to hand excision. Guarded skin graft knives are used to remove the burn eschar. Devitalized skin is removed in layers until viable tissue is reached (Fig. 8–4). The best quality graft available, usually sheets, is carefully applied and secured. The hand must be immobilized to ensure graft take. Internal fixation (Fig. 8–5) allows open graft treatment. Splints and fingernail hooks are widely used as are bulky compression dressings. Intravenous fluorescein has been recommended as an aid in assessing depth.[10] Enzymatic debridement with sutilains enzyme has been combined with early excision.[11]

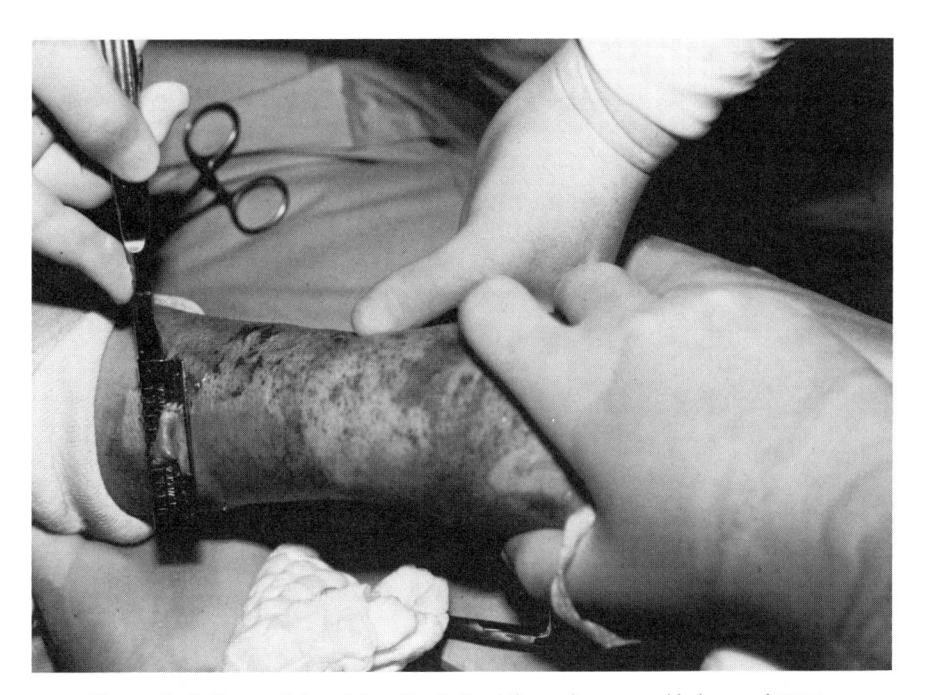

Figure 8–4. Tangential excision. Devitalized tissue is removed in layers. Intravenous fluorescein, appearance of bleeding, and gross appearance of the tissue are used to judge the depth of excision. See Chapter 7 for further details on use of Goulian knife.

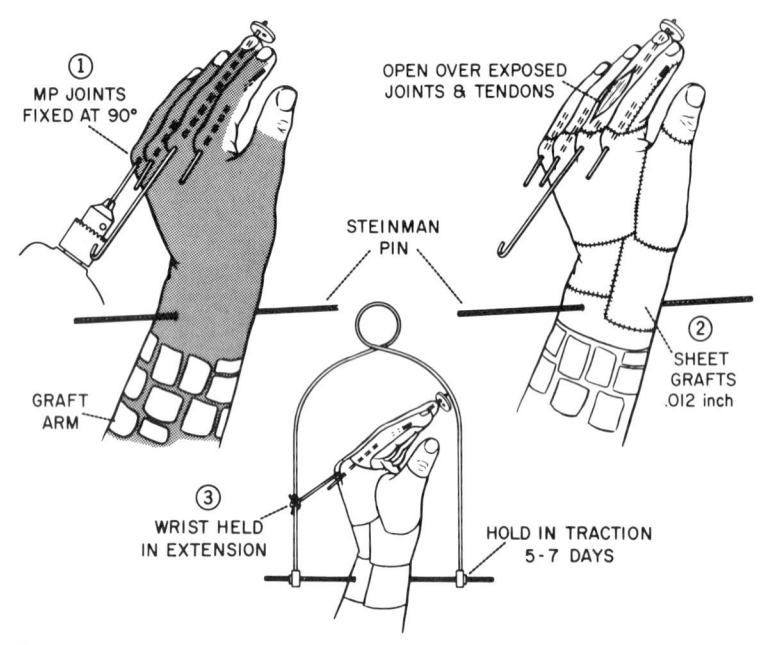

Figure 8–5. Burned hands: Grafting. Internal fixation may be used to immobilize the hands for a 5-day period following grafting. Long pins can be passed through the M-P joints into the PIP and distal interphalangeal (DIP) joints. A larger pin is placed through the distal radius. The hand is suspended from this pin. Wires are placed through the finger and attached to the suspension bow to further position the hand. Grafts can be treated by the open method, thus maximizing graft take. *(From Achauer BM, et al., Internal fixation in the management of the burned hand. Arch Surg 108:815, 1974, reproduced with permission.)*

Although it has been demonstrated that early excision (first 72 hours) can produce excellent results when employed by experienced surgeons, no one has demonstrated the superiority of primary excision over good burn care and grafting 2 to 3 weeks after injury. Salisbury and Wright[12] found no difference in randomized groups treated with early excision, routine grafting, or spontaneous healing.

INTERMEDIATE CARE

A very important phase of burned hand care begins after the wound has healed. A therapist experienced in burn care is crucial. Motion should be begun as soon as practical and pursued vigorously. Incipient contractures must be fought with appropriate splints and hypertrophic scars combated with pressure garments. Details of these treatments are outlined in Chapter 15. The number of late reconstructive procedures required is inversely propor-

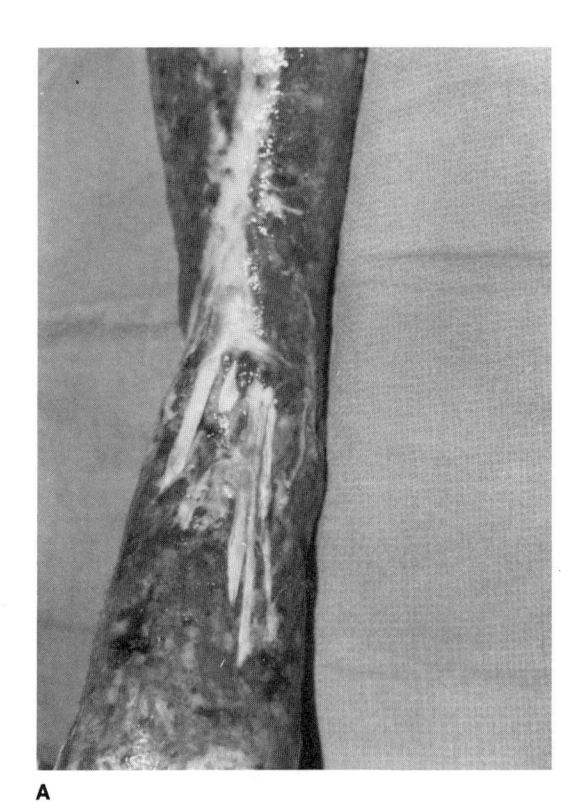

Figure 8–6. Cross-leg myocutaneous gastrocnemius flap. **A.** Exposed tendon and ankle joint. Flap coverage required. **B.** Cross-leg gastrocnemius myocutaneous flap with external fixater.

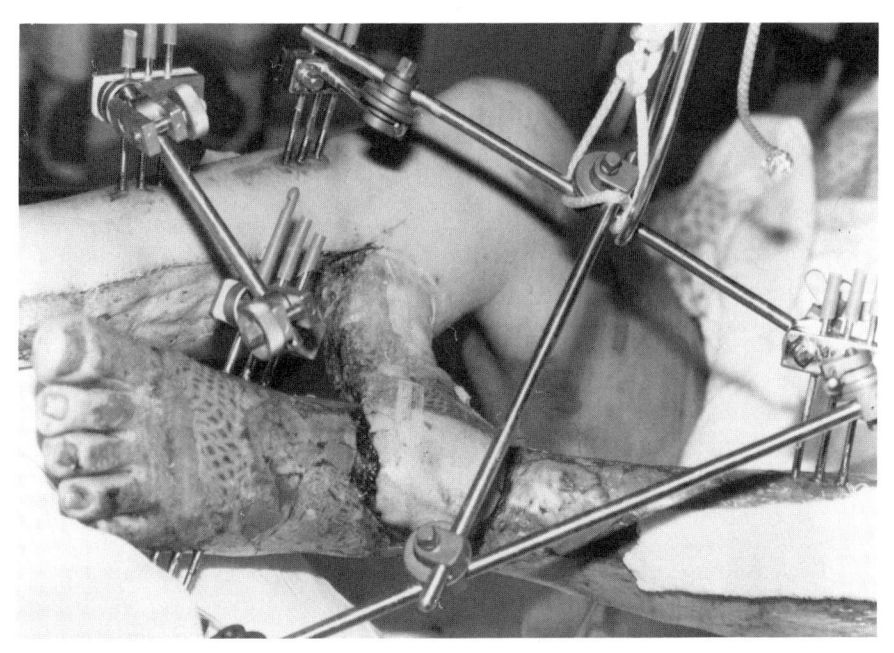

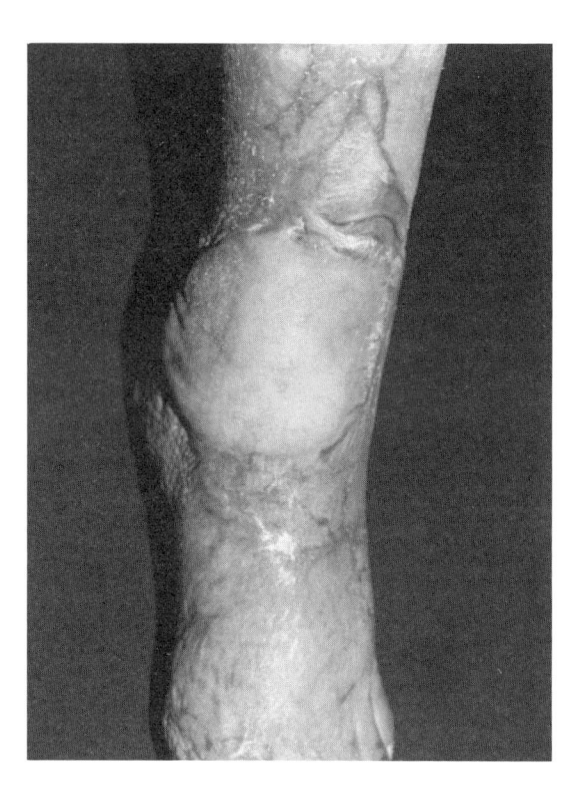

Figure 8-6. C. Final result after flap division.

tional to the quality of care and patient compliance during the period of scar maturation (6 to 12 months postburn).

LOWER EXTREMITY BURNS

Although little has been written about lower extremity burns, they do deserve special attention.[13] Morbidity can often be excessive.[14] Wounds of the legs and feet do not do well if the patient is ambulatory. This is especially true of skin grafts. Patients with leg burns will have greater pain and pruritis and typically are slower to return to work. They should not be labeled as malingerers. The increased tissue pressure seems to result in greater discomfort as well as delayed healing.

Molten metal burns are a common form of foot thermal injury. They are almost always full thickness. Immediate tangential excision is usually indicated to reduce morbidity. Early physical therapy is required for rapid rehabilitation. Pressure garments will certainly be required.

Escharotomies are often indicated and tissue pressure monitoring is recommended for circumferential burns. In seriously ill patients, particularly elderly patients and patients with electrical injuries, urgent amputation may

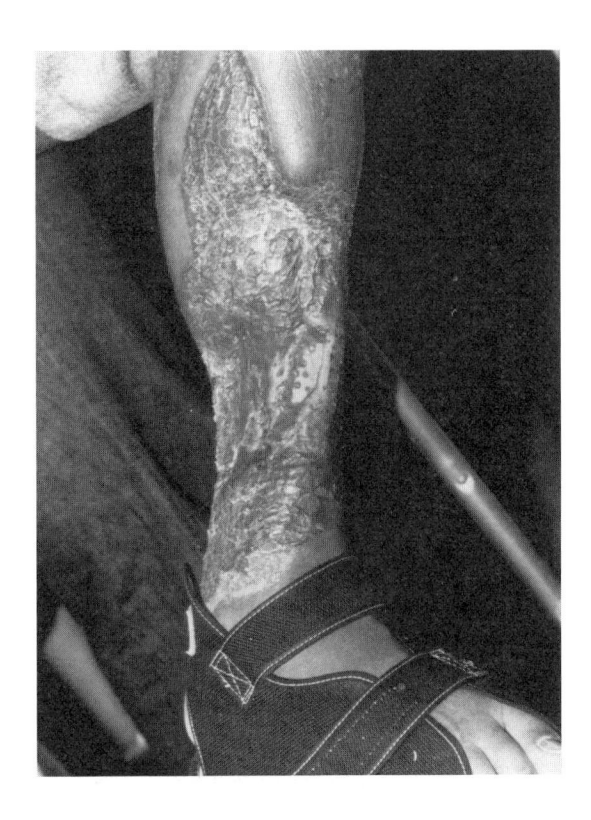

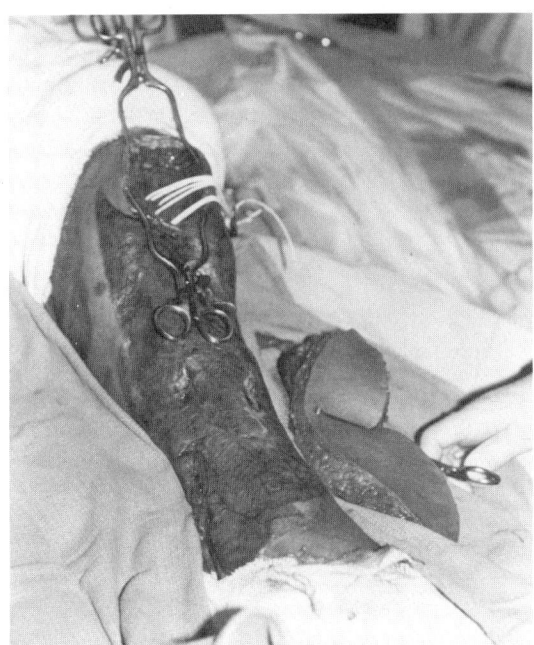

Figure 8-7. Innervated free latissimus dorsi flap. **A.** Exposed tibia following electrical burn. No active dorsiflexion of foot. **B.** Latissimus dorsi myocutaneous flap. Vessels will be anastomosed and the thoracodorsal nerve joined to the peroneal.

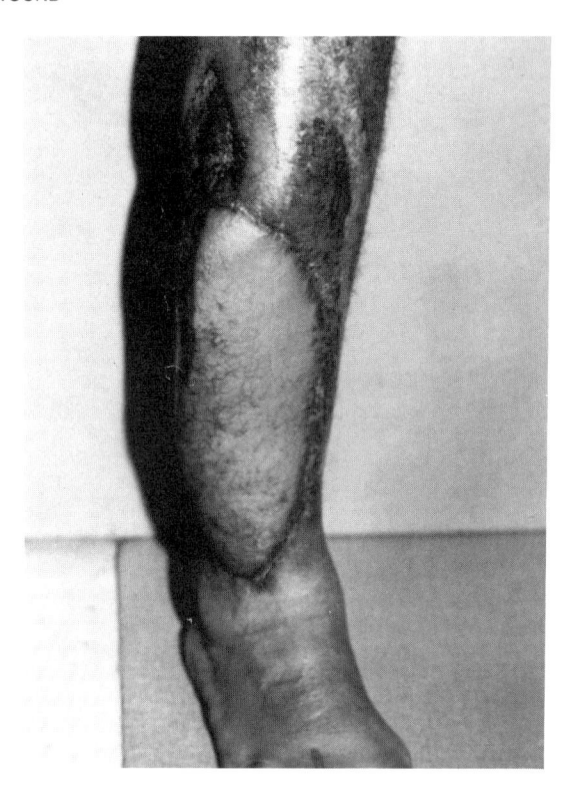

Figure 8–7. C. Final result. Active contracture of latissimus muscle prevents foot drop. Orthosis no longer needed.

be lifesaving. Flaps are required for salvage of deeper burns involving tendons or bone (Fig. 8–6). As much surface as possible should be covered with skin grafts. Local muscle or fasciocutaneous flaps are the next order of priority. If local tissue is not available, a cross-leg fasciocutaneous or myocutaneous flap or a free flap is required (Fig. 8–7).

REFERENCES

1. Moylan JA, Inge WW, Pruitt BA: Circulatory changes following circumferential extremity burns evaluated by the ultrasonic flowmeter: An analysis of 60 thermally injured limbs. J Trauma 11:763, 1971
2. Bendick PJ, Mayer JR, Glover JL, Park HM: A photoplethysmographic technique for detecting vascular compromise: A preliminary report. J Trauma 19:398, 1979
3. Saffle JR, Zeluff GR, Warden GR: Intramuscular pressure in the burned arm: Measurement and response to escharotomy. Am J Surg 140:825, 1980
4. Salisbury RE, McKeel D, Mason A: Ischemic necrosis of the intrinsic muscles of the hand after thermal injuries. J Bone Joint Surg 56-A:1701, 1974
5. Moncrief J, Switzer W, Rose L: Primary excision and grafting in the treatment of third-degree burns of the dorsum of the hand. Plast Reconst Surg 33:305, 1964

6. Burke J, Bondon C, Quinby W, Remensynder J: Primary surgical management of the deeply burned hand. J Trauma 16:591, 1976
7. McDowell F: Accelerated excision and grafting of small deep burns. Am J Surg 85:407, 1953
8. Hunt JL, Sato R, Baxter CR: Early tangential excision and immediate mesh autografting of deep dermal hand burns. Ann Surg 189:147, 1979
9. Janzekovic A: A new concept in the early excision and immediate grafting of burns. J Trauma 10:1103, 1970
10. Leonard L, Munster A, Su CT: Adjunctive use of intravenous fluorescein in the tangential excision of burns of the hands. Plast Reconstr Surg 66:30, 1980
11. Gant TD: The early enzymatic debridement and grafting of deep dermal burns to the hand. Plast Reconstr Surg 66:185, 1980
12. Salisbury RE, Wright P: Evaluation of early excision of dorsal burns of the hand. Plast Reconstr Surg 69:670, 1982
13. Achauer BM, Bartlett RH, Wilson LF: Burns of the foot. J Foot Surg 15:43, 1976
14. Kahn AM, McCrady-Kahn V: Molten metal burns. West J Med 135:78, 1981

PART IV
Systemic Effects

CHAPTER 9
Nutrition

Linda Chilstrom Giel

Major thermal injury results in a hypermetabolic response which is proportional to the severity of the burn. Basal metabolism expenditure may be increased 40 to 100 percent above normal in patients with burns exceeding 30 percent of the total body surface area. This accelerated rate begins after fluid resuscitation is accomplished, reaches peak levels between the fifth and twelfth postburn day, then tapers but remains elevated until the burn is healed or covered by grafting.[1]

The increased energy expenditure is mediated by the neurohormonal response to stress. Following burn shock, the sympathetic nervous system triggers an increased plasma level of catecholamines that stimulate heat production and substrate mobilization. Severe catabolism occurs during the immediate postburn period which is characterized by protein mobilization, increased rates of gluconeogenesis, decreased levels of insulin, and increased plasma concentration of glucagon, reflecting an increased flow of glucose to the wound.[2] This increase of glucose production is reflected by increased urea production, therefore urinary urea nitrogen can serve as a basis for estimating nitrogen requirements. Failure to provide an exogenous source of energy to burned patients can result in a rapid depletion of endogenous fuel reserves with resultant weight loss and eventual morbid consequences associated with starvation such as muscle weakness, respiratory failure, sepsis, delayed wound healing, and even death.

Nutritional support for the burned patient should begin as soon as shock resuscitation is accomplished, usually within 24 to 48 hours postinjury. In order to maintain body cell mass and prevent excessive weight loss, careful attention to the nutritional requirements of the burned patient as well as to the appropriate methods of feeding and continual monitoring of his or her response to nutritional therapy is imperative. Optimal nutritional support requires the coordinated efforts of the patient, dietitian, nurse, and physician.

ASSESSING NUTRITIONAL STATUS

In determining the nutrient needs of the burned patient, consideration must be given to his or her existing nutritional status. Any patient with an extensive burn who has an already depressed nutritional status, as determined by anthropometric measurements and laboratory testing, is at a greater risk of having a complicated hospital course.[3]

Anthropometric measurements include the weight–height index, triceps skinfold (TSF) thickness, and midupper arm circumference (AC). The weight–height index can be determined by comparing the actual weight of the patient with the ideal value for a patient of the same height and gender using standard tables. It is important that the patient's preburn or usual weight be used as a baseline, as a burned patient's early postadmission weight may be elevated 12 to 15 percent as a result of edema associated with massive fluid administration. An index less than 80 percent of standard indicates moderate depletion, and below 60 percent, severe depletion.[4] Attempts should be made to correct any deficits.

As the accuracy of body weight in assessing nutritional status is limited in the obese or edematous patient, additional measurements are needed. TCF can be measured using large calipers and is useful in estimating body fat stores. Values below 60 percent of standard represent a significant nutritional problem, as depressed fat stores interfere with the body's ability to use endogenous fat for fuel in the starved or semistarved patient; body protein reserves must be used in the absence of appropriate nutritional therapy. A depletion in lean body mass (skeletal muscle protein) can be determined from TSF and AC to give an arm muscle circumference (AMC): AMC = AC − (π × TSF).[4] This measurement is particularly useful in burned patients with fluid retention, in whom the weight–height index underestimates protein–calorie malnutrition.

Visceral proteins are essential for wound healing, host defense, oncotic pressure, and many enzyme functions of the body. Deficiencies in visceral protein cannot be determined by visual inspection. These patients may appear well nourished or even obese despite severe malnutrition because of the edema which accompanies hypoalbuminemia. It is important to realize the rapidity with which visceral protein concentrations fall in the presence of thermal injury or any trauma when skeletal muscle protein and body fat reserves are depleted.[3] Visceral protein function can be assessed by determination of serum protein levels and immune response. Serum albumin is the most commonly measured serum protein, and values less than 3 g/dl suggest significant depletion. Serum transferrin levels are more sensitive indicators of visceral protein status because they have a shorter half-life than albumin. These tests are usually more expensive, however, and not available in all laboratory facilities. It should be noted that depressed serum proteins can occur in the presence of protein–calorie malnutrition. In response to injury or surgery, albumin increases in the estravascular spaces secondary to

TABLE 9-1. NUTRITIONAL ASSESSMENT GUIDE

Weight–Height Index

% Standard	Nutritional Status
> 90	Not depleted
80–90	Mildly depleted
60–80	Moderately depleted
< 60	Severely depleted

Triceps Skinfold Thickness (mm)

% Standard	Male	Female	
100	12.5	16.5	
90	11.3	14.9	Not depleted
80	10.0	13.2	Mildly depleted
70	8.8	11.6	Moderately depleted
60	7.5	9.9	↓ Severely depleted

Muscle Arm Circumference (cm)

% Standard	Male	Female	
100	25.3	23.2	
90	22.8	20.8	Not depleted
80	20.2	18.6	Mildly depleted
70	17.7	16.2	Moderately depleted
60	15.2	13.9	↓ Severely depleted

Visceral Protein Status

	Deficit		
	Severe	Moderate	Mild
Serum albumin (g%)	< 2.5	< 3–2.5	> 3.5–3
Transferrin (mg%)	< 160	< 180–160	> 200–180
Total lymphocyte count	< 900	< 1500–900	> 1800–1500

Skin Test Antigens

Deficit[a]		
Severe	Moderate	Mild
< 5–0 mm	< 10–5 mm	< 15–10 mm

[a] A patient with 15-mm response on any one test is considered immune competent.

wound edema or sodium retention resulting in depressed serum albumin independent of nutritional status. Serum albumin levels should, therefore, be drawn near to the time of trauma and again 10 days later to diagnose malnutrition.[3]

Hypoproteinemia is common during the early postburn course with as much as 50 percent of the circulating protein being lost within the first few hours. This trend generally reverses itself later as capillary permeability returns to normal, provided there is an adequate intake of protein and calories. Serum albumin levels consistently below 2.5 g/dl may cause decreased absorptive power of the intestinal villi and create a malabsorption state. Long-term parenteral administration of albumin may be beneficial in this case provided that adequate nutrient intake is given concurrently so that albumin is not needlessly converted to glucose for energy.[5]

Significantly higher rates of sepsis and mortality occur among patients with impaired cellular immune response.[1] This can be estimated from recall skin antigen tests and the total lymphocyte count (TLC). The recall antigens most commonly used for delayed hypersensitivity skin testing are *Candida albicans*, mumps, streptokinase–streptodornase (SK–SD), and tuberculin purified protein derivative (PPD). Induration of 5 mm or more 24 to 48 hours after intradermal injection is considered a positive response and reflects immune competence. A total lymphocyte count less than 800 cells/cc is considered indicative of severe malnutrition; 800 to 1500 cells/cc, moderate malnutrition. There appears to be a correlation between depressed TLCs and cell-mediated immunity, and the preoperative TLC has been shown to be a reliable and simple predictor of postoperative sepsis.[6] Immune functions of lymphocytes may be the first metabolic system to respond to nutritional support because of their high metabolic priority. Thus, periodic measurements of delayed hypersensitivity response may be of use in determining the effectiveness of nutritional therapy.

In summary, assessment of a burn patient's nutritional status can be determined by anthropometric measurements, plasma protein levels (albumin), and delayed hypersensitivity response. While each measurement has its own particular drawbacks and it is often not practical to perform all these tests in the extensively burned patient, their importance in assessing a patient's nutrient needs and response to therapy should be recognized. If deficiencies are realized, they can be corrected before they become manifest as delayed wound healing or decreased resistance to infection. Values for assessing nutritional status of patients are shown in Table 9–1.

SPECIFIC NUTRIENT REQUIREMENTS

To meet the increased metabolic demands caused by burn injury, intakes of two to three times the normal energy requirements are often necessary. Direct or indirect calorimetry is the ideal method of estimating individual caloric expenditure, but is expensive and usually not available to clinicians in burn centers. Curreri and his coworkers have developed the following formula for estimating daily caloric requirements for adult patients based on body size (preburn weight) and magnitude of burn up to 50 percent of total body surface area[7]:

$$25 \text{ kcal} \times \text{weight (kg)} + 40 \times \text{percent TBS burn}$$

A similar formula for estimating caloric needs of the burned child up to 12 years of age was developed by Sutherland[8]:

$$60 \text{ kcal} \times \text{kg} + 35 \times \text{percent TBS burn}$$

Additional calories should be added to the estimated level of caloric intake to allow for losses incurred during the initial resuscitation periods and before and after surgical procedures. Similarly, patients with a weight–height index significantly below standard may require calories above those estimated in attempts to improve the patient's overall nutritional status (Table 9–2). Patients who have a greater than ideal weight should not be placed on a reduced caloric intake at this time, as it may severely compromise their rate of recovery. In these cases, the goal of therapy should be to maintain the patient's preburn weight as well as a positive nitrogen balance to promote proper wound healing. Attempts toward weight reduction can begin once the patient has completely recovered from the burn injury.

Whatever method of determining energy needs is used, one must not lose sight of the fact that these are merely estimations. Variations in caloric requirements will occur from patient to patient depending on physical activ-

TABLE 9–2. ESTIMATING NUTRIENT NEEDS

Example 1: Adult	kcals = 25 × kg + 40 × TBSA		
Preburn weight		60 kg	
Percent burn		50%	
25 kcal × 60 =		1500 kcal	Estimate of preburn needs
40 kcal × 50 =		+ 2000 kcal	Increment for burn
		3500 kcal	Minimum calorie goal
Increment for		+ 1000 kcal	
energy losses		4500 kcal	Estimate of total energy needs to prevent weight loss
	(1 g × 60 kg) + (3 g × 50) = 210 grams Estimated protein needs		
Example 2: Child	kcals = 60 × kg + 35 × TBSA		
Preburn weight		10 kg	
Percent burn		30 %	
60 kcal × 10 =		600 kcal	
35 kcal × 30 =		+ 1050 kcal	
		1650 kcal	Minimum calorie goal
	(3 g × 10 kg) + 1 g × 30) = 60 grams Estimated protein needs		

ity, body tissue composition, and environmental temperature and humidity. These formulas do, however, provide the health care team with a baseline for developing a nutritional program designed to minimize weight loss.

Increased nitrogen losses in the burned patient, like energy expenditure, are due to the increased metabolic rate and are related to the size of the burn. Other factors involved in nitrogen catabolism include: loss of protein and water through the burn wound, extensive tissue breakdown, infection, and decreased anabolism because of impaired liver and pancreatic function.[9] Nitrogen excretion provides a reliable estimate of the actual protein losses: 1 g of urinary nitrogen reflects the loss of 30 g of lean body tissue, which is equivalent to 6.25 g of protein. In the severely burned patient, nitrogen losses may increase to 30 to 40 g per day, representing 190 to 250 g of metabolized protein.

Early correction of this protein deficiency is necessary in order to prevent deficiencies in the synthesis of tissue and blood proteins, lymphocytes, hormones, antibodies, and enzymes. Protein intake should comprise 20 percent or more of total calories. Protein requirements can be estimated from the following formulas:

1 g protein/kg body weight + 3 g/1 percent TBS for adults

3 g protein/kg body weight + 1 g/1 percent TBS for children[10]

Since energy as well as amino acids are necessary for achieving a positive nitrogen balance, it is imperative that a proper ratio of dietary protein and nonprotein calorie sources be achieved so that dietary proteins will not be used for energy rather than tissue building. Approximately 100 to 200 nonprotein calories per gram of dietary nitrogen are desired for proper metabolism in contrast to 350:1 ratio seen in normal subjects.[1,11] For a patient with renal failure associated with his or her injury, giving protein without adequate calories may be expected to cause a breakdown of endogenous protein stores and consequent rise in the blood urea nitrogen. In these cases, higher calorie to nitrogen ratios may be desired.

Once protein requirements have been determined, the remaining energy needs can be divided among carbohydrate and fat sources. Carbohydrates are the main source of energy for the body yielding 4 kcal/g. Body stores of carbohydrate, mainly glycogen, are small and are rapidly catabolized following burn injury. Carbohydrates prevent oxidation of body tissue because their reserves are drawn on first, sparing fat and protein stores. During the first few days after injury, carbohydrate may be the sole source of calories in the form of intravenous glucose solutions. Two to 3 liters of 5 percent glucose and water contain approximately 400 to 600 kilocalories. This may provide a mild protein-sparing effect initially, but falls extremely short of the energy needs of the burned patient and should not be continued for extended periods without further nutritional support. Approximately 50 to 60 percent of the total energy intake should be derived from carbohydrate. Intakes in excess of these amounts do not offer significant advantages and may even increase the risk of hyperglycemic complications such as fatty liver and a hyperosmolar state.[1]

Because of their high caloric density (9 kcal/g), fats have been incorporated into a number of oral and intravenous solutions. Recommended intakes are approximately 20 to 30 percent of total calories, however, only 1 to 3 percent is actually needed to prevent essential fatty acid deficiency. The rate of catabolism of fat increases in proportion to the severity of the burns to as much as 600 grams per day, thereby liberating more than 5000 kilocalories of energy.

VITAMIN-MINERAL REQUIREMENTS

It is generally agreed that supplemental vitamin therapy is indicated in the treatment of burns although exact requirements are not known. A number of enzyme systems are interfered with during the hypermetabolic state following burns, mainly because of increased protein catabolism. These enzymes depend on certain vitamins for their integrity, particularly vitamins A, C, and B complex. The B complex vitamins (thiamine, niacin, and riboflavin) are involved in many metabolic pathways.

Usual supplements recommended include ascorbic acid (2 g), riboflavin (50 mg), thiamine (50 mg), nicotinamide (500 mg), folic acid (1.5 mg), and vitamin B_{12} (4 mg). To meet these requirements, either two multivitamin capsules or two ampules of parenterally administered vitamin additive plus 2 g of ascorbic acid per day are needed.[9] In addition, vitamins A and D are essential for children and probably important for optimum healing in adults. Vitamin K is important in blood clotting and may be needed in certain situations.

Maintenance of a daily supply of minerals which will meet the recommended daily allowances (RDA) is important for many physiologic processes. Intake exceeding the RDA for zinc (i.e., 2 mg/liter parenterally, 440 mg zinc sulfate enterally) is recommended because of its importance in wound healing. Deficiency states of calcium, magnesium, phosphorus, and zinc can result in patients on total parenteral hyperalimentation for extended periods of time.

DELIVERY OF NUTRIENTS

Once the nutritional requirements of the burned patient have been established, the method of delivery of nutrients must be determined. A variety of feeding techniques may be incorporated into the nutritional care plan depending on the patient's initial and subsequent condition.

Within 48 to 72 hours postburn, most patients have recovered from postinjury paralytic ileus and should be able to take oral alimentation. The

TABLE 9-3. COMMERCIAL ENTERAL FEEDINGS[a]

Product Composition	Ensure (Ross)	Ensure Plus (Ross)	Isocal (Mead Johnson)	Travasorb MCT (Travenol)	Meritene Powder + Milk (Doyle)
Protein (g)	3.7	5.5	3.4	4.92	6.9
Protein source	Na[a] and Ca[b] caseinates, soy isolate	Na[a] and Ca[b] caseinates, soy isolate	Na[a] and Ca[b] caseinates, soy isolates	K$^+$ caseinate, lactalbumin	Cow's milk, nonfat dry milk
Fat (g)	3.7	5.3	4.4	3.3	3.5
Fat source	Corn oil	Corn oil	Soy oil MCT oil	MCT, sunflower oil	Cow milk fat
CHO (g)	14.5	19.7	13.0	12.3	11.9
CHO source	Corn syrup solids Sucrose	Corn syrup solids Sucrose	Corn syrup solids	Corn syrup solids	Lactose Corn syrup solids
kcal/100 cc	106	150	106	100[b]	107
Lactose (g)	0	0	0	0	5.6
mOsm/kg H$_2$O	450	600	300	314	690
Na$^+$ mEq/mg	3.2/74	4.6/106	2.3/52.1	1.52/34.96	4.1/96
K$^+$ mEq/mg	3.3/126.8	4.9/190	3.3/130	4.45/173.55	7.6/296
Nonprotein cal:N	153	146	167	102	71
Volume needed to meet 100% RDA for protein, vitamins and minerals	2000 cc	2000 cc	2000 cc	2000 cc	1200 cc
Comments	Flavored Tube or oral feeding	Flavored Tube or oral feeding	Unflavored Tube feeding, generally not accepted as oral feeding	Can be reconstituted to provide 1-2 cal/cc; unflavored tube feeding[b]	Oral protein-calorie supplement

[a]Composition data calculated from manufacturers' product information.
[b]Branched chain amino acids (valine, leucine, isoleucine).

dietitian and nursing staff play an important role in helping the patient to achieve an adequate oral intake. Efforts should be made to provide foods the patient is accustomed to eating. Whenever possible, treatments and tests should be scheduled so that they do not interfere with meal time. Equipment should be available in the burn unit, such as a refrigerator, microwave oven, and blender, for providing supplementary food stuffs to the patient whenever he or she wants them throughout the day. Fluids offered to the patient should all include calories, such as fruit juices, carbonated beverages, fortified milk drinks, and commercially prepared oral feedings. Beer and wine, when not contraindicated, are also used in some burn units to stimulate appetite and increase calories. The hospital diet may provide adequate calories, but often does not contain sufficient nitrogen. Various commercial protein supplements can be added to foods and beverages to increase nitrogen intake. There are

Vivonex HN (Eaton)	Amin Aid (McGaw)	Hepatic Aid (McGaw)	Polycose Liquid (Ross)	MCT Oil (Mead Johnson)	Casec (Mead Johnson)
4.2 Pure crystalline amino acids	1.9 Essential AA + histidine	4.3 Amino acids (high BCAA[b] low aromatic AA)	0 —	0 —	88 Ca[b] caseinate from skim milk curd
0.1 Safflower oil	4.7 Soy oil lecithin mono- and diglyceride	3.6 Soy oil, lecithin lecithin, mono- and diglyceride	0 —	93.3 MCT oil	2
21.0 Glucose Oligosaccharides	37.2 Maltodextrins Sucrose	28.7 Maltodextrins Sucrose	50 Modified cornstarch	0 —	0 —
100	198	164.5	200	775	370
0	0	0	0	0	0
810	850	900	850	NA	NA
3.4/77	Negligible	Negligible	2.7/62	0	6.5/150
1.8/70	Negligible	Negligible	< 1 mEq	0	0
124	830	225	NA	NA	NA
3000	Contains no vitamins or minerals	Contains no vitamins or minerals	NA	NA	NA
Elemental diet requires minimal digestion and absorption (unpalatable)	For chronic renal disease (unpalatable; recommended for tube feeding)	For hepatic failure (unpalatable)	Concentrated CHO source; mix with food or beverage	Modular fat calorie source	Concentrated protein calorie source; add to food or liquid

also many nutritionally complete oral supplements which can be planned into the patient's diet when protein and calorie intake is low. Table 9–3 is a partial listing of some of the commercially available formulas that are available for oral supplementation.

Patients with burns covering over 40 percent of the body surface area are seldom able to ingest enough voluntarily. Anorexia often accompanies burn injury thus making oral alimentation difficult. In such cases, nasogastric or nasoduodenal tube feedings are required to provide or augment caloric intake during periods of highest energy expenditure (Fig. 9–1). Tube feedings are particularly useful in patients who have burns of the face and mouth which prevent adequate oral intake. Since the advent of small bore, soft Silastic feeding tubes (i.e., Keofeed, Dobhoff) (Fig. 9–2), mechanical infusion pumps, and a variety of commercial formulas, tube feedings are a safe and effective

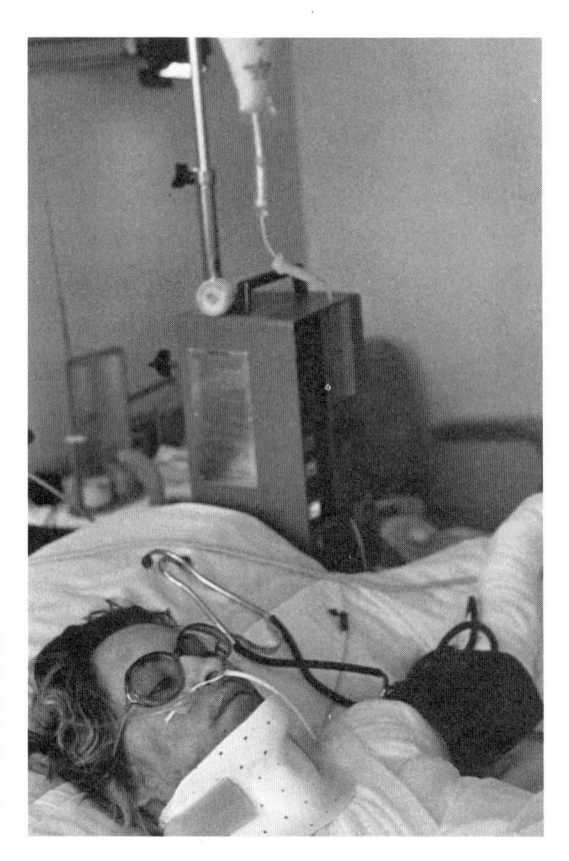

Figure 9-1. Patient with second and third degree burns over 40 percent of her body, requiring nasogastric enteral feedings. Patient is shown here receiving nasogastric feedings administered continuously via infusion pump.

means of hyperalimenting the burn patient. Tube feedings should always be viewed as a medical approach rather than a threat or punishment because the patient has not eaten enough. The patient should be allowed to continue oral intake as well.

A number of proprietary formulas are available for use as tube feedings (see Table 9-3). Nutritionally complete formulas with intact nutrients and without lactose are generally well tolerated by tube-fed patients. Caloric concentrations of 1 to 2 kcal/ml can be achieved in order to meet the nutritional needs of the patient. Modular systems using a variety of different ingredients are becoming popular as they allow greater flexibility in providing specific nutrients for each patient. Elemental formulas should be used in patients with gastrointestinal dysfunction, or in patients who have burns on the buttocks and thighs, to reduce contamination from fecal soilage. Disease-specific formulas for metabolic conditions such as renal or hepatic failure may also be useful. Adequate vitamins are provided in almost all commercial formulas, but many are deficient in sodium which must be supplemented. Commercial tube feeding preparations are not recommended for children under 1 year of age. Instead, infant formulas should be used and modified

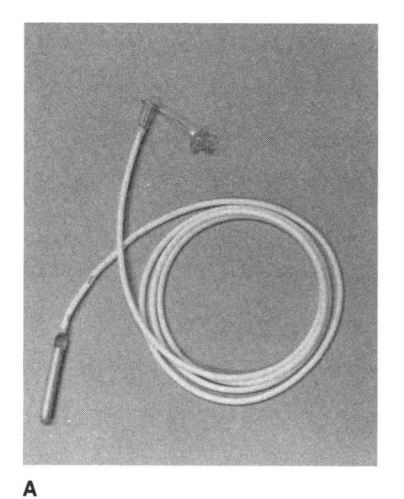

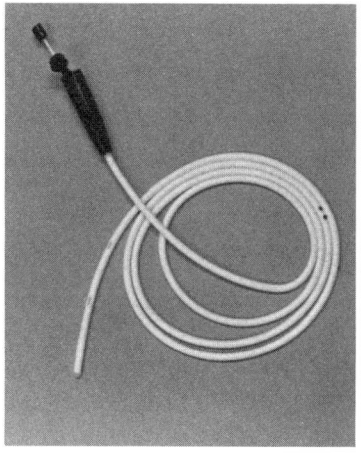

Figure 9-2. Sample enteral feeding tubes. **A.** Dobhoff tube manufactured by Biosearch Medical Products is made of polyurethane, comes in sizes 8 French, 43 inches long, has 7 g mercury-weighted bolus to assist in transpyloric passage of tube, and is radiopaque. **B.** Keofeed tube manufactured by IVAC Corporation is made of silicone, comes in sizes 7.3 to 18 French, 43 inches, has 1 to 5 g mercury-weighted bolus, and is radiopaque.

through the use of modular formulas to meet the specific nutrient needs of the burned infant.

Tube feedings are best tolerated if initiated via an infusion pump over a 24-hour period beginning at a slow rate of 25 to 50 ml per hour with increments of 25 ml per hour added every 8 hours as tolerance is established, until the desired flow rate is achieved. Volumes will be proportionately less in infants. (Formulas with an osmolality of 400 mOsm/kg water are often started at concentrations of 1 kcal/ml (half strength) and increased to full strength after volume increments have been achieved.) When using infant formulas, begin with 10 to 12 calories per ounce of feeding. Once half the desired total volume is achieved, increase to the desired concentration (20 to 24 kcal/ounce or more). Later, gradually work up to full volume.[12] It is important that concentration and rate increases are not made at the same time, as the cause of any complications will be unclear if both are advanced simultaneously.

To avoid vomiting and the danger of aspiration, residual gastric volume should be checked by the nursing staff every 4 hours. Tube feeding should be discontinued for a few hours if gastric residual volumes are greater than one and one-half times the hourly rate. If intermittent gravity feedings are given rather than continuous feedings, gastric residuals should be checked before each feeding and feedings held if residual is greater than 150 ml. Persistently high gastric residuals probably indicate delayed gastric emptying. This can occur for a variety of reasons, including prepyloric ulcers, bowel ileus, or gastric atony secondary to hyperglycemia. If feedings are continued into a closed system, a potentially dangerous complication of aspiration or even gastric rupture can occur.[12] To further reduce the risk of aspiration, frequent check of the tube's position and maintaining the patient's head of bed at least 30 degrees at all times is advised. Placement of tubes in the duodenum or jejunum may also be advantageous as both the gastroesophageal and pyloric sphincters are operating to prevent gastric regurgitation.

Common complications of tube feeding include diarrhea and hyperosmolar hyperglycemic nonketotic dehydration. Diarrhea can usually be treated by a temporary reduction in the concentration or volume of formula, although use of antidiarrheal agents may be necessary. Hyperosmolar syndromes caused by glucosuria can be treated by administration of exogenous insulin. Dehydration caused when excessive amounts of protein and electrolytes are given with inadequate fluids can best be treated by increasing free water intake.[5] Monitoring of intake and output, body weight, urinary sugar and acetone, stool volume and consistency, serum electrolytes, and sugar level is necessary while the patient is being tube fed to ensure optimal recovery.

Once the burns have been grafted, metabolic needs are generally decreased, and patients should be weaned off tube feedings. To accomplish this, feeding rates can be gradually decreased over a 24-hour period as oral intake increases. It is often helpful to shut continuous feedings off for a few hours before meals to encourage increased oral intake. In some cases, feedings can be given only at night. Whatever method is used, it is important to ensure adequate oral intake before tube feedings are discontinued altogether.

Whenever enteral feedings are inadequate, impossible or contraindicated, then intravenous feedings should be initiated, particularly in patients who had limited body fuel stores at the time of injury and for patients who experience persistent or recurrent paralytic ileus or intractable diarrhea. A combination of enteral and parenteral nutrition may be necessary to provide sufficient energy and nitrogen to patients with extensive burns. Whenever it is determined that the patient will be unable to receive enteral nutrition for greater than 2 to 3 days, central venous hyperalimentation is necessary.[13]

If parenteral alimentation is to be the sole source of nutrition, then it must be given via central vein. Adequate nutritional intake is difficult to achieve via peripheral vein. Solutions used for central hyperalimentation consist of 20 to 25 percent dextrose and 25 percent crystalline amino acids, providing approximately 7 g of nitrogen and 800 to 1000 kcal per liter. Water- and fat-soluble vitamins as well as trace elements and electrolytes must be added to parenteral feedings to prevent nutritional deficiencies. Up to 40 to 60 percent of the energy requirement can be achieved by intravenous fat emulsion. By using fat as the major calorie source in parenteral regimens, the dextrose and amino acids can be kept near isotonicity. Dextrose–amino acids–vitamin–mineral–electrolyte solutions must be delivered separately from the fat emulsion. This can be accomplished by infusing the two solutions into the same vein via a Y-connector located near the infusion site.

Anorexia often develops after a patient has been on prolonged central hyperalimentation. As soon as bowel function returns, enteral nutrition should be resumed. Oral feedings should be encouraged but tube feedings may be necessary initially if oral intake is not adequate to meet energy needs. Parenteral feedings should be decreased gradually during this time to prevent the complications of hypoglycemia which can occur with sudden cessation of hypertonic solutions.

Central venous hyperalimentation has considerable risk which is even greater in the burned patient, therefore, special precautions must be taken. Entrance sites of all intravenous catheters must be resterilized and redressed daily, and the catheters themselves should be changed at least once or twice a week to prevent sepsis and thrombosis. It should be realized, however, that for the patient who cannot eat, total parenteral nutrition can be lifesaving.

MONITORING NUTRITIONAL STATUS

To ensure optimal recovery following burn injury, nutritional monitoring is an important aspect of the patient's care. A number of clinical factors must be monitored closely wherever any supranormal dietary program is used. As already mentioned, serum electrolyte and glucose determinations must be obtained daily during the initial phase to guard against hyperglycemia, hypernatremic dehydration, and hypokalemia. Frequent checks for urine glucose is essential in protecting against the serious complications associated with glucosuria.[14]

In the absence of major fluid shifts, body weight is perhaps the best indicator of the effectiveness of the nutritional therapy. Weight loss is a common outcome of major thermal injury, however, attempts should be made to prevent weight loss of greater than 10 percent of a patient's preburn weight. Weight loss greater than 10 percent is associated with increased morbidity and mortality.[1, 14] Body weight should be recorded daily at the same time each day and without dressings. In conjunction with daily weights, an accurate record of the patient's food intake should be kept by the nursing staff and calculated by the dietitian. Whenever caloric intake is not sufficient to maintain body weight, the health care team must revise the nutritional care plan. On the other hand, an increase in body weight with a concomitant decrease in caloric intake may be an indication of other metabolic complications such as sepsis, heart failure, or renal failure. Again, re-evaluation of the feeding program is necessary.

Further evaluation of a patient's response to nutritional therapy can be accomplished by obtaining repeat anthropometric measurements, serum protein determinations, and skin testing with recall antigens, and nitrogen balance studies. Although somewhat difficult to obtain in burned patients because of the unmeasured amount of nitrogen lost through wound exudate, nitrogen balance studies are useful in assessing the adequacy of nitrogen and calorie intake. Urea excretion accounts for 90 percent of total urinary nitrogen loss, and most of daily nitrogen loss is excreted in the urine. Therefore, nitrogen balance can be computed as: nitrogen intake (from enteral and parenteral sources—24-hour urine urea nitrogen + 4). This 4 g factor accounts for stool and skin losses as well as nonurea urinary nitrogen losses. Losses from burn wound exudate may add an additional 2 to 5 g to the nitrogen deficit.[14] The therapeutic goal for patients with severe protein deficits is a +4 to +6 nitrogen balance (nitrogen intake exceeds nitrogen loss by 4 to 6 g per day).

Daily communication between the dietitian, nurse, and physician as to the nutritional status of each patient is essential. Nutritional care record sheets can be developed as a useful tool in accomplishing this goal.[11,15] Such records should be kept at the patient's bedside or in his medical record for the entire team to utilize. With the combined efforts of the entire burn team, a successful nutritional regimen should be able to be formulated that will result in maintenance of body weight, improved wound healing, and reduced morbidity and mortality among burned patients.

REFERENCES

1. Metabolic and nutrition support for trauma and burn patients. Abstracts from Nutrition Symposium sponsored by Mead Johnson Nutritional Division, 1982
2. Curreri PW, Luterman A: Nutritional support of the burned patient. Surg Clin North Am 58:1151, 1978
3. Blackburn GL, Harvey KB: Nutritional assessment as a routine in clinical medicine. Postgrad Med 71:47, 1982
4. Blackburn GL, et al.: Nutritional and metabolic assessment of the hospitalized patient. J Parent Ent Nutr 1:11, 1977
5. Kaminsky MV: Enteral hyperalimentation. Surg Gynec Obstet 143:12, 1976
6. Lewis RT, Klein H: Risk factors in postoperative sepsis: Significance of preoperative lymphocytopenia. J Surg Res 26:365, 1975
7. Curreri WP, Richmond D, Marvin J, et al.: Dietary requirements of patients with major burns. J Am Diet Assoc 65:415, 1974
8. Sutherland AB: The nutritional care of the burned patient. Br J Plast Surg 8:68, 1955
9. Crenshaw C: Nutritional Support for Burn Patients in Intake: Perspectives in Clinical Nutrition. Norwich, N.Y., Eaton Laboratories, 1973
10. Polk HC, Stone HH: Contemporary Burn Management. Boston, Little, Brown, 1971, p 151–167
11. McLaurin NK, Goodwin CW Jr, Zitzka CA, et al.: Computer-generated graphic evaluation of nutritional status in critically injured patients. J Am Diet Assoc 82:49, 1983
12. Cataldo CB, Smith L: Tube Feedings: Clinical Application. Columbus, Ohio, Ross Laboratories, 1980
13. Kaufman CS: Nutritional support of the trauma patient. Nutr Supp Serv 1:11, 1981
14. Schenk W, Moylan J: Nutritional aspects of burn care. In Practical Approaches to Burn Management. Deerfield, Ill., Flint Laboratories, 1973
15. Pennisi VM: Monitoring the nutritional care of burned patients. J Am Diet Assoc 69:531, 1976

CHAPTER 10
Pulmonary Management

Kenneth Waxman

With improved early care, burn shock is now routinely treated successfully and renal failure is uncommon. Respiratory failure has now emerged as the most common cause of early mortality in the hours and days following major burns. Further, respiratory failure frequently complicates sepsis in burned patients, and this combination is the most common cause of death in those patients who die in the subsequent weeks. If burn mortality is to be further reduced, it has become essential to focus on the effective diagnosis and therapy of respiratory complications.

Widespread interest in respiratory complications of burns came in the 1940s following the Coconut Grove night club fire in Boston. There were 114 casualties from this fire taken to Massachusetts General Hospital, and 75 of these were either dead on arrival or died within minutes. This group was felt to have died from carbon monoxide poisoning, inhalation of toxic vapors, or from airway obstruction due to upper respiratory tract damage. A second group of patients developed respiratory failure within a few hours, associated with pulmonary edema. A third group developed difficulty only after 24 hours; these patients had laryngeal edema. A final group of patients developed symptoms of late respiratory failure several days following burn. As a result of these respiratory complications, 36 of the 39 patients who survived initial therapy subsequently died.[1]

While modern respiratory therapy has made major progress, respiratory failure complicating burns remains a major problem. Pulmonary complications occur in 15 to 18 percent of patients admitted to burn centers.[2,3] When respiratory failure does occur, the mortality remains extremely high, i.e., 70 to 90 percent.[4-6]

PATHOPHYSIOLOGY

A number of quite different pathologic processes can cause respiratory failure following burn injury. This is often confusing, both conceptually and clinically, so it is best to separate these. Figure 10–1 schematically represents the various etiologies of respiratory failure following burns.

Carbon Monoxide Poisoning

Carbon monoxide is a gaseous component of smoke, yet, unlike other gaseous causes of smoke poisoning, does no physical damage to the lung. Carbon monoxide is toxic due to its high affinity for the oxygen-binding site of hemoglobin, forming carboxyhemoglobin. The affinity of carbon monoxide is 257 times that of oxygen for the hemoglobin-binding site; thus, when carboxyhemoglobin is formed, oxygen is displaced. The result is low circulating volumes of oxygen, despite normal partial pressures. This results in tissue hypoxia, inadequate cellular oxygenation, inadequate cellular and organ function, and eventually death. Because of the extremely high affinity of hemoglobin, small concentrations of carbon monoxide in inspired air result in severe physiologic impairments. Carbon monoxide levels of 0.1 percent in inspired air result in binding of over 60 percent of hemoglobin molecules and may be fatal.

Patients inhaling carbon monoxide develop symptoms depending on the amount of carboxyhemoglobin formed, thus leaving hemoglobin unavailable for oxygenation. In general, central nervous system and cardiovascular symptoms appear first, since brain and heart dysfunction are most apparent after

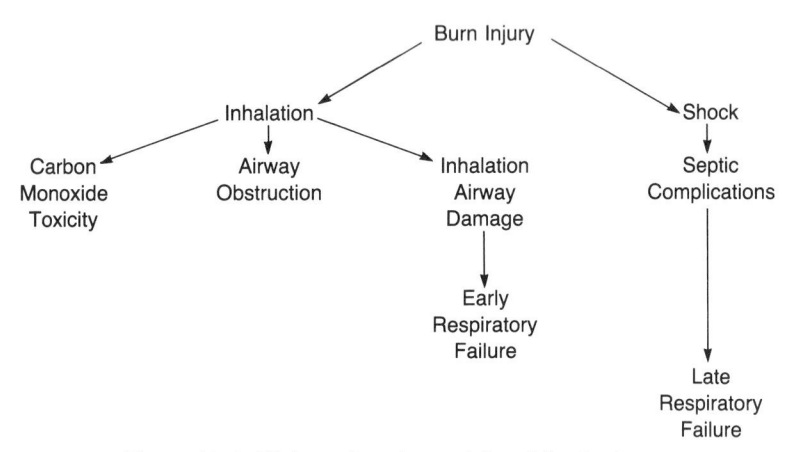

Figure 10–1. Etiology of respiratory failure following burns.

inadequate tissue oxygenation. The diagnosis can only be made by measuring carboxyhemoglobin concentrations in a blood sample (carboxyhemoglobin levels of 20 percent usually cause mild symptoms such as headache and irritability, levels of 50 percent are associated with marked confusion, shortness of breath, and cardiovascular collapse, and levels of 80 percent are usually rapidly fatal).

Circumferential Chest Wall Burns

Burns which encompass all or most of the circumference of the thorax may lead to ventilation difficulty due to restriction of chest wall expansion. Respiratory distress is often progressive over the first 24 to 48 hours in this circumstance as burn edema accumulates. This problem of circumferential thoracic burn causing ventilatory difficulty might be overlooked in the severely burned patient with other causes of pulmonary distress unless carefully considered. The significance of the chest wall restriction can be best quantitated and followed by measuring ventilatory compliance. If circumferential burns are present, and especially if decreased chest wall motion and respiratory difficulty is evident, early escharotomy needs to be performed (Figure 10-2).

Inhalation Injury

Inhalation injuries are caused both by the heat of inhaled smoke and by toxic chemicals inhaled into the respiratory tract. Heat and inhaled chemicals cause injury in different fashions.

Heat causes direct damage to the respiratory epithelium, resulting in

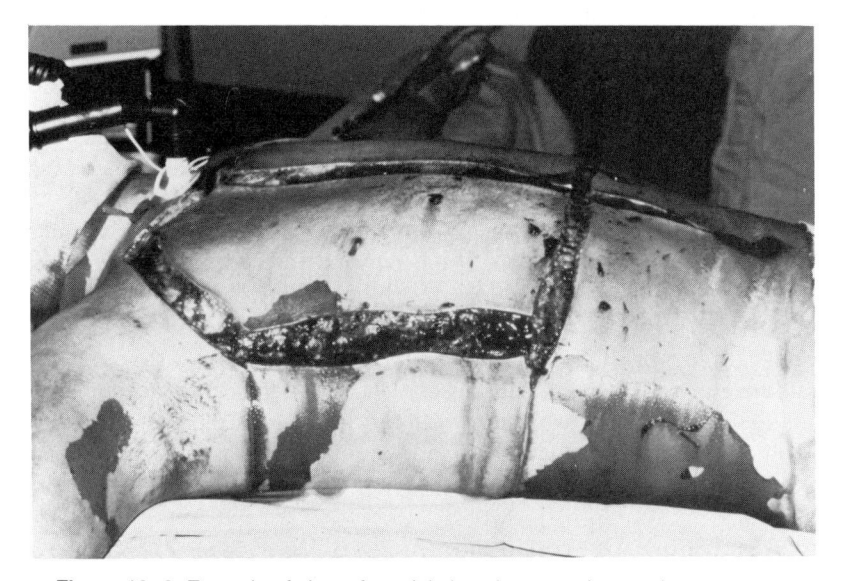

Figure 10-2. Example of circumferential chest burn causing respiratory compromise, treated with escharotomy.

cellular necrosis and a surrounding inflammatory reaction. There is usually very rapid decrease in temperature of inhaled smoke as it travels distally in the airway, so that direct heat damage is normally limited to the upper airway, especially the supraglottic area. When steam is present in inhaled gas, however, the heat-carrying capacity is greatly increased, and more severe distal airway injury may result.

Toxic chemicals are produced in fires due to incomplete combustion of burning materials. Commonly produced toxic chemicals include nitrous oxide, sulfur dioxide, hydrochloric acid, and hydrocyanic acid, among many others. Contact of these chemicals with respiratory epithelium results in membrane damage, inflammation, and possible necrosis. Unlike heat injury, which does its maximal damage in the proximal airway, chemical injury tends to occur throughout the respiratory tract with significant injury to the small airways and alveoli.

Following damage to the respiratory epithelium by heat and toxic chemicals, a number of pathologic changes in the lung result. A loss of ciliary activity results in poor clearance of bronchiotracheal secretions and predisposes to alveolar fluid accumulation and infection. Variable direct damage to the subepithelial parenchyma may occur or this damage may result, indirectly, from the loss of the epithelial barrier. In either case, parenchymal edema and hemorrhage usually result and bacterial invasion of these tissues is common. Furthermore, a more generalized injury to the pulmonary capillary bed may occur, resulting in increased permeability and a generalized increase in interstitial edema.

A number of physiological sequelae may result from these pathologic changes. Edema surrounding the airway may result in obstruction, particularly in the supraglottic area where loose connective tissue predisposes to edema formation. The generalized increase in interstitial edema of the lung parenchyma may result in decreased compliance of the lungs and may contribute to ventilatory failure. Hypoxia frequently results from inhalation injury. This appears to be the result of mismatching of ventilation and perfusion, probably the result of patchy and uneven vasoconstriction of the pulmonary microcirculation.

Finally, the injury following the inhalation of smoke is very frequently followed by pulmonary infection. Predisposition to these infections is caused by (1) damaged pulmonary epithelium with loss of its antimicrobial barrier, (2) edematous and poorly perfused parenchyma (providing a fertile bacterial environment), (3) loss of ciliary function, (4) possible increase in pathogenic organisms in the airway associated with hospital care, and (5) a generalized decrease in immunologic defenses associated with the systemic burn. The development of pneumonitis in patients with inhalation injury exacerbates all of the primary pathologic deficits.

Adult Respiratory Distress Syndrome (ARDS)

Respiratory failure can complicate the course of seriously burned patients, even if no direct inhalation injury occurs. The respiratory failure in these cases is quite similar to that occurring in other critically ill patients and has been termed ARDS. The precise etiology of ARDS has not been agreed upon. It is clear, however, that patients who are likely to develop ARDS are those who have experienced shock and multiple transfusions, and especially those who subsequently develop systemic sepsis. Seriously ill burned patients certainly meet these prerequisites and are quite prone to develop ARDS, particularly in association with septic complications.

DIAGNOSIS OF RESPIRATORY COMPLICATIONS

The diagnosis of respiratory damage is often suggested by history and physical examination of the burn patient upon presentation to the hospital. Pulmonary damage is much more likely if burns occur in a closed space fire. The patient's complaints of shortness of breath are an important indication of possible respiratory damage. Patients who sustain facial burns are more likely to have respiratory damage, though many patients without facial burns also develop pulmonary problems.[7] Tachypnea, wheezing, stridor, singed nasal hairs, and the production of carbonaceous sputum are all suggestive findings on physical examination; however, these findings are not always present when significant pulmonary damage has occurred, nor does their presence necessarily indicate severe respiratory disease. The chest x-ray is often normal initially, even if severe pulmonary damage has occurred.

The arterial blood gas analysis may also be normal initially since much of the pulmonary damage takes hours or days to develop. An early arterial blood gas sample is essential in any patient in whom respiratory disease is considered, however, since this represents a baseline against which subsequent values may be compared. Sequential arterial blood gas sampling remains as the best physiologic indicator of the progression of pulmonary damage; arterial gases should be analyzed as often as every several hours in patients at high risk.

Several more sophisticated diagnostic modalities have been suggested to increase the accuracy of early diagnosis of inhalation injury. Probably the most widely utilized of these is bedside diagnostic bronchoscopy. Early bronchoscopy may reveal soot in the bronchial tree, tracheal or laryngeal edema, and irritation, inflammation, and ulceration of the airway. These findings confirm suspected airway injury and justify early aggressive therapy. An alternative to bronchoscopy is lung scanning utilizing xenon-133 intravenous injection. Xenon is normally quickly excreted into the alveolae and results in a homogeneous pulmonary scan. When bronchial damage and edema occur, however, the xenon clearance may be delayed and uneven and this is reflected in the scan. In experienced centers, xenon scanning is a relatively sensitive and accurate indicator of pulmonary damage.[8] A third diagnostic modality which has been found useful in diagnosing pulmonary damage is bedside spirometry. Patients with significant respiratory burns have shown decreased expiratory flow rates. Spirometry can be used subsequently to both diagnose respiratory compromise and to follow its response to therapy.

TREATMENT

The treatment of burn patients with respiratory complications does not differ in principle from that of other acutely ill patients. Treatment priorities include maintenance of an airway with or without endotracheal intubation. Pulmonary toilet should be vigorous, utilizing such modalities as coughing, incentive spirometry, bronchodilators, percussion and postural drainage, tracheal suctioning, and therapeutic bronchoscopy if necessary. When infection is suspected, aggressive efforts should be utilized. Arterial oxygen tensions need to be frequently monitored and maintained by supplemental oxygen administration. Ventilation must be assured and, again, should be monitored with blood gas analysis; assisted ventilation is frequently necessary, particularly since ventilatory requirements are increased in seriously burned patients. Circulation must be maintained and shock avoided, as inadequate pulmonary perfusion will exacerbate the pathology. Consideration should be given to escharotomy in all circumferential thoracic burns.

In addition to these general principles, four situations deserve particular attention. (Recall that these four problems are those identified as the causes of death for patients following the Coconut Grove fire.)

Carbon Monoxide Poisoning

Carboxyhemoglobin is formed due to the high affinity of carbon monoxide for oxygen-binding sites of hemoglobin; this binding is, however, competitive and very high concentrations of oxygen displace carbon monoxide therefore improving tissue oxygenation. Thus, the crux of therapy is administration of supplemental oxygen. With mild carbon monoxide poisoning, i.e., minimal symptoms and a carboxyhemoglobin level less than 40 percent, utilizing a 100 percent oxygen rebreathing mask is usually effective. For more serious cases, intubation and direct endotracheal administration of 100 percent oxygen is indicated, since this results in significantly higher arterial oxygen tensions (PaO_2).

There is a direct relationship between the PaO_2 achieved and the rate of decay of carboxyhemoglobin. Breathing room air, the half-life of carboxyhemoglobin is approximately 6 hours (assuming an initial value of 50 percent). This decay can be decreased to less than 3 hours if PaO_2 values of about 400 torr are achieved.[9] Even more rapid decay occurs with higher PaO_2 values, and these are achievable by utilizing hyperbaric oxygen if available; hyperbaric oxygen of 2½ to 3 atmospheres is indicated in serious cases, as breathing 100 percent O_2 under these conditions drops the half-time of carboxyhemoglobin decay to less than 1 hour. Oxygen therapy should be continued until an end point of a 20 percent carboxyhemoglobin level is reached at which point it may be discontinued.

A frequent aftermath of serious carbon monoxide poisoning is cerebral edema secondary to brain cell ischemia. Therapy in this setting should be directed at minimizing intracranial pressure, utilizing such modalities as hyperventilation, elevation of the head of the bed, avoidance of excess fluids (especially salt and water), and possibly corticosteroid administration. A logical additional approach to carbon monoxide poisoning would be to decrease the metabolic rate and, thus, the oxidative needs while carboxyhemoglobin is decaying. Such modalities as hypothermia and barbiturate administration might be useful to decrease the metabolic rate, but only limited experience has been reported.[10]

Airway Obstruction

Airway obstruction following burns is most often due to edema in the supraglottic area. This area is most susceptible due to the high temperatures to which it may be exposed, and due to its loose mucous membrane and submucosal tissues which are prone to edema formation. This edema formation may be pronounced quite early in severe inhalation injury, but is not maximal until 12 to 24 hours following burn.

Because of this progressive nature of supraglottic edema, early signs of airway obstruction should be sought and aggressive therapy instituted early. Hoarseness and stridor are ominous signs requiring prompt evaluation. Direct evaluation of the supraglottic area, either by a laryngoscopic exam or at the time of bronchoscopy, is useful to confirm this diagnosis. If supraglottic injury, inflammation, and edema are present, particularly early after a burn, then conservative management is endotracheal intubation. Either nasotracheal or orotracheal routes may be chosen; nasotracheal intubation is more comfortable for the patient but may be more difficult to perform. These tubes may usually be removed 3 to 5 days following burn, assuming the supraglottic edema is resolving and the patient does not have parenchymal lung injury requiring airway access. If signs of supraglottic edema are sought and an early diagnosis made, orotracheal or nasotracheal intubation is usually successful. This eliminates the need for tracheostomy. Tracheostomy has several disadvantages. It provides a more direct access of bacteria to the lower airway and may be associated with a greater incidence of airway infection and pneumonitis. It may also be difficult to accomplish through an edematous, burned neck, particularly if coagulopathy has developed.

All patients with supraglottic edema will not develop airway obstruction, and there is a role for therapy short of tracheal intubation. This consists of breathing cool, humidified mist and nebulized racemic epinephrine. While this approach may be successful, it requires very close patient monitoring for signs of obstruction, and the ability to perform skillful intubation on short notice should the edema progress. If in doubt, intubate (Table 10–1).

TABLE 10-1. INDICATIONS FOR ENDOTRACHEAL INTUBATION FOLLOWING INHALATION INJURY

1. Early supraglottic inflammation and edema on endoscopy
2. Progressive hoarseness associated with supraglottic hoarseness
3. Early hypoxemia (i.e., Pao$_2$ < 60 torr on 40% O$_2$ mask) or progressive hypoxemia
4. Tachypnea (i.e., respiratory rate > 30/min)
5. Hypercarbia—Pao$_2$ > 45 torr

Early Respiratory Failure

Early respiratory failure following burns is most often associated with severe inhalation injury. Patients develop progressive tachypnea and hypoxia over the hours following burn. Bronchoscopy reveals tracheal and bronchial mucosal damage with inflammation and edema. Chest x-ray shows a progressive pulmonary edema pattern. It is extremely important to recognize such patients early as their respiratory failure is progressive and to promptly institute a therapeutic approach based on physiologic goals. In order to reasonably titrate therapy, physiologic monitoring is essential. Further, it is important to monitor hemodynamic as well as respiratory functions as these are intimately interrelated.

Monitoring pulmonary function in these patients is fundamental. Oxygenation is best assessed by frequent blood gas determination. Continuous noninvasive monitoring, such as with the heated transcutaneous oxygen monitor, is also useful though such monitoring does not always accurately reflect the adequacy of oxygenation. Accurate assessment of the physiologic deficits, however, requires calculation of the alveolar–arterial Po$_2$ difference and the pulmonary venous admixture or shunt. These calculations are extremely useful in assessing the severity of the respiratory failure and its response to therapy. Adequacy of ventilation is best assessed by the arterial CO$_2$ tension (Paco$_2$). Continuous noninvasive Pco$_2$ monitoring is now feasible using end-tidal CO$_2$ monitoring, although end-tidal CO$_2$ may not accurately reflect Paco$_2$ if physiologic dead space is great, and this is frequent in severe respiratory failure. Also of significance is the amount of lung water. This is usually assessed by chest x-ray but, unfortunately, radiologic findings often lag behind the physiologic picture by hours or days. More direct measurement of lung water is possible by utilizing double indicator dilution techniques; it remains unclear, however, whether and how measurement of lung water should affect therapy.

Essential to burn patients with respiratory failure is restoration of circulating blood volume: an inadequate blood volume results in inadequate preload, low cardiac output, and inadequate pulmonary perfusion among other organs. Excess fluid administration, on the other hand, may result in increased pulmonary interstitial water and pulmonary edema. Thus assessing ventricular preload is extremely important. Central venous pressure monitoring is frequently utilized; however, monitoring right atrial pressure may be extremely misleading in burn patients with pulmonary failure. Pulmonary artery catheterization and monitoring of wedge pressure is to be preferred. Furthermore, utilizing the pulmonary artery catheter, thermodilution cardiac output determinations can be sequentially obtained.

Using these monitoring parameters, therapy can be physiologically titrated. Several aspects of therapy for patients with respiratory failure deserve emphasis.

Restoration of Blood Volume. The need for aggressive fluid therapy in burn patients is well recognized and is emphasized throughout this book. This is no less true for those burned patients who have coexisting inhalation injury. In fact, inadequate fluid replacement in an attempt to "keep lungs dry" will result not only in inadequate system circulation, but may also intensify the respiratory failure by worsening pulmonary vasoconstriction. Thus, as in other burn patients, fluid therapy should be titrated to that point where systemic perfusion is adequate. As discussed elsewhere in this book, this may require supernormal cardiac output in the postburn period. It is desirable to maintain wedge pressures as low as possible to minimize pulmonary interstitial fluid, yet the first priority must be to provide adequate preload to support cardiac output. Wedge pressures of between 10 to 15 mm Hg are usually required to achieve this goal.

The choice of fluids to administer remains controversial. The optimal fluid for patients whose hematocrits are less than about 30 percent is whole blood or packed red blood cells. For other patients there is less agreement. Colloids, such as human albumin, dextran, or hydroxyethyl starch, have theoretical advantages in that blood volume may be restored with less salt and water administration than with crystalloid administration. However, a possible capillary membrane leak associated with inhalation injury may, to some extent, limit this advantage. Nonetheless, our approach is to utilize blood and colloid fluids as the primary resuscitation fluids for such patients and to restrict salt and water administration. Considerably less fluid is required for resuscitation and edema is minimized.

Diuretics are a useful tool in the therapy of salt and water overload patients as well as in hypervolemic overtransfused patients. However, the effects of diuretics in the acutely burned patient are not specific for reducing pulmonary edema; that is, the overzealous use of diuretics may result in hypovolemia, decreased preload, and inadequate cardiac output. Diuretics, then, in the absence of clear evidence of plasma volume overload should be used with great caution.

Restoration of Flow. When blood volume has been increased to optimal levels, cardiac output is also optimized. In patients with compromised ventricular function or very severe pulmonary failure, however, cardiac output may remain low or elevation of wedge pressure may limit fluid administration. In such patients, afterload reduction such as with sodium nitroprusside should be considered; afterload reduction may improve cardiac performance and decrease wedge pressure. Positive inotropic agents, such as dobutamine, isoproterenol, dopamine in low doses, calcium, and digitalis, are also useful if indicated. Pressor agents with alpha-adrenergic action should be avoided, if possible, however, as these may intensify pulmonary vasoconstriction and worsen pulmonary shunt.

Ventilation Therapy. A major advance in caring for patients with respiratory failure has come with an understanding of positive end-expiratory pressure (PEEP) (Table 10–2). PEEP prevents alveolar collapse and atelectasis by increasing functional residual capacity, and also improves pulmonary compliance both by recruiting additional areas of the lung for ventilation and by conserving surfactant.[11] Thus PEEP may improve both oxygenation and ventilatory mechanics. The adverse effects of PEEP include barotrauma, usually seen as pneumothorax or pneumomediastinum, but also causing damage to the lung parenchyma. Further, PEEP may depress cardiac output in the hypovolemic patient. This may be disastrous to the burn patient whose survival depends on increased peripheral oxygen delivery; in such patients, PEEP that elevates Pao_2 may be harmful if cardiac output is simultaneously depressed.

Several therapeutic maneuvers including intravascular volume loading and intermittent mandatory ventilation (IMV) may minimize the adverse effects of PEEP. Cardiac depression after PEEP is most pronounced in the hypovolemic patient, but patients whose blood volumes have been restored to optimal levels have very little depression of cardiac output even at relatively high levels (20 to 25 mm Hg) of PEEP. Furthermore, cardiac depression occurring after the onset of PEEP can be reversed with intravenous fluid infusion, thus allowing the continued benefit of PEEP on oxygenation while restoring oxygen delivery to the tissues.

IMV is often useful in patients who may not require assisted or controlled ventilation. Many of these patients, despite pulmonary shunt and hypoxia, have high minute ventilation and low $Paco_2$. Oxygenation may be aided by continuous positive airway pressure (CPAP) or by a combination of CPAP and IMV to minimize or avoid high positive airway pressures. This has several advantages. First, since peak inspiratory pressures rather than PEEP per se are largely responsible for barotrauma, the substitution of IMV for controlled

TABLE 10–2. GENERAL PRINCIPLES OF VENTILATORY SUPPORT OF PATIENTS WITH INHALATION INJURY

1. Volume-cycled ventilator
2. Monitor blood gases, systemic and pulmonary arterial pressures, and cardiac output
3. Utilize at least 5 cm PEEP, with PEEP increased to maintain Pao_2 > 70 torr at lowest possible Fio_2
4. Maintain cardiac output at optimal levels
5. Utilization of intermittent mandatory ventilation to minimize number of positive pressure breaths necessary

ventilation gives more spontaneous breaths and fewer positive pressure breaths. This decreases the peak and mean airway pressure and decreases the likelihood of barotrauma. Second, there is less cardiac depression during spontaneous respiration with CPAP than there is during controlled ventilation with PEEP because of the negative pressures generated by spontaneous breathing and decrease in peak airway pressure.

Though the complications of PEEP can be minimized, it remains crucial to choose the optimal level of PEEP to give maximum benefit and minimum damage to the lungs while simultaneously maximizing tissue oxygenation. Various approaches have been taken to choose the "best PEEP" level, including consideration of Q_s/Q_t, cardiac output, mixed venous oxygen, oxygen delivery, physiologic dead space, and pulmonary compliance. We have utilized measurement of all these to determine optimal PEEP, as well as consideration of tissue oxygenation as estimated by whole body VO_2 and by transcutaneous oxygen measurement.

Administration of systemic corticosteroids has been widely utilized for inhalation injury, the rationale being that decreasing the inflammatory response is beneficial. However, controlled studies have failed to show an advantage in steroid administration. Further, the immunosuppression associated with high dose steroid therapy could be detrimental.

Late Respiratory Failure (ARDS)

In the days and weeks following a major burn, the development of late respiratory failure looms as an ominous complication. This late respiratory failure may represent severe pneumonia complicating inhalation injury to the lung, or it may appear in patients who did not initially experience respiratory difficulties. In either case, these patients usually have systemic sepsis, either primarily pulmonary in origin, from invasive burn wound sepsis, from infected intravenous catheters, or from other infected organ systems. Gram-negative organisms are frequently the etiologic agents in this setting. When a worsening of respiratory function occurs in burned patients, a source of sepsis must be suspected and vigorously sought in addition to providing aggressive respiratory support. If a specific site of sepsis can be identified and quickly reversed, i.e., removal of an infected intravenous catheter, the respiratory failure may also rapidly improve. If, however, no obvious source of sepsis is found, the burn wound must be suspected. In such cases, very aggressive burn wound debridement is necessary. If sepsis cannot be controlled, respiratory failure is usually progressive despite supportive therapy.

REFERENCES

1. Cope O: Management of the Coconut Grove burns at the Massachusetts General Hospital. Ann Surg 17:801, 1943
2. Stone HH, Martin JD: Pulmonary injury associated with thermal burns. Surg Gynec Obstet 129:1242, 1969

3. Achauer BM, Allyn PA, et al.: Pulmonary complications of burns: The major threat to the burn patient. Ann Surg 177:311, 1973
4. Moylan JA, Alexander LH Jr: Diagnosis and treatment of inhalation injury. World J Surg 2:185, 1978
5. Pruitt BA Jr, Flemma RJ, Di Vincenti FC, et al.: Pulmonary complications in burn patients. J Thorac Cardiovasc Surg 59:7, 1970
6. Walden A, Summerlin WT, Mason AD Jr, et al.: Respiratory complications in the acutely burned patient. Mil Med 13:2379, 1967
7. Hunt JL, Agee RN, Pruitt BA: Fiberoptic endoscopy in acute inhalation injury. J Trauma 15:641, 1975
8. Agee RN, Long JM, Hunt JL, et al.: Use of 133 xenon in early diagnosis of inhalation injury. J Trauma 16:218, 1976
9. Winter RM, Miller JN: Carbon monoxide poisoning. JAMA 236:1502, 1976
10. Brach BB, Yin F, Timms R, et al.: Reduced inspiratory effort during intermittent mandatory ventilation with PEEP. Crit Care Med 4:144, 1976
11. Waxman K, Shoemaker WC: Management of postoperative and posttraumatic respiratory failure in the intensive care unit. Surg Clin North Am 60:1413, 1980

CHAPTER 11
Preventing and Treating Complications
Anthony A. Meyer and Donald D. Trunkey

The incidence and importance of systemic complications has risen steadily as improved resuscitation of burn victims has greatly reduced early mortality. Presently, systemic complications are the major cause of death in these patients.[1,2] A better understanding of the clinical manifestations and pathophysiology of these complications may help to prevent or limit the morbidity and mortality from them. The factors influencing systemic complications, a method for classifying them, and a review of the complications by organ system with attention to their prevention and treatment are discussed in this chapter.

Risk factors that affect the incidence and severity of complications after thermal injury are age, pre-existing disease, associated injury, and mechanism of burn. They are summarized in Table 11–1. Age is an important factor in burn injury with increased mortality in the very young and elderly. The elderly have more cardiovascular complications due to underlying disease and diminished reserve. Young children have greater infectious and respiratory complications due to immature organ systems. Pre-existing disease, such as diabetes, alcoholism, chronic obstructive pulmonary disease (COPD), and renal impairment are all associated with increased postburn complications.[2] Associated injuries also increase the incidence of complication and death. Such injuries are frequently blunt trauma from vehicular accidents or blast injury from explosion. Concomitant inhalation and thermal injuries have a higher incidence of death and complication than do either alone. The mechanism of burn may also affect the incidence of complications. Electrical and chemical burns may produce cardiac arrhythmias or systemic poisoning re-

TABLE 11-1. FACTORS INFLUENCING THE INCIDENCE AND SEVERITY OF SYSTEMIC COMPLICATIONS IN BURN PATIENTS

Age
Pre-existing disease
Associated injury
Mechanism of burn

spectively. All of these factors need to be considered with their regard to the incidence, severity, and treatment of systemic complications in burn patients.

One method of examining systemic complications in thermally injured patients is to divide them into groups according to their etiology. This is useful in determining how and why these complications arise and which are preventable. For this purpose, systemic complications from burn injury will be divided into four groups. They are complications due to (1) burn injury, (2) inadequate treatment, (3) sepsis, and (4) therapeutic maneuvers. These etiologies, some examples, and possible means of prevention and treatment are listed in Table 11-2.

The first group of complications are the result of the burn injury itself. Inhalation injury from noxious chemicals and extremity necrosis from burns involving muscle and bone are examples. There is no way to prevent this type of complication. Appropriate, supportive care or surgery may limit its severity and effect on the patient.

A second group of systemic complications is the result of delayed or inadequate care of the burn patient. Examples of this are renal failure from insufficient fluid resuscitation and airway obstruction from failure to intubate a patient with glottic edema and stridor. Anticipation and prevention are the answer to this group of complications. Knowledge of the management of burn patients and frequent assessment will limit their occurrence.

The third group of complications usually have no single obvious cause but are nearly always related to sepsis. They represent the organ system failure that frequently follows sepsis in burn patients. Prevention of this group of complications requires avoiding sepsis by early wound grafting or aggressively treating sepsis with debridement, systemic antibiotics, and topical antimicrobials. Treatment of these complications requires standard supportive care and elimination of the sepsis by the most direct means possible.

The fourth group of systemic complications of burns is the result of treatment given the patient. Septic thrombophlebitis after intravenous cannulation and nephrotoxicity from necessary aminoglycoside antibiotics are examples of this group of complications. These treatments are correct, indicated, and monitored, but complications from such therapeutic maneuvers are increased in burn patients because of their altered physiologic responsiveness, the protracted course of their injury, and the number and relative risk of these maneuvers. Prevention of this group of complications is not always possible. However, close monitoring of methods and means of treatment

TABLE 11–2. CLASSIFICATION OF SYSTEMIC COMPLICATIONS OF BURNS ACCORDING TO ETIOLOGY

Group	Etiology	Examples	Prevention	Therapy
I	Initial injury	Inhalation injury	None	Supportive care (e.g., ventilation, dialysis)
II	Inadequate treatment	Renal failure from inadequate resuscitation or from unmonitored nephrotoxic drugs	Correct initial treatment and frequent re-evaluation	Continued close monitoring (organ system function, cultures, drug levels)
III	Unclear, probably sepsis	ARDS, DIC	Early, aggressive treatment of sepsis	Operative treatment Debridement of dead and infected tissue Correction of surgical problems Prompt wound coverage
IV	Complications of appropriate treatment	Septic thrombophlebitis	Good technique and close monitoring	Excise vein
		Nephrotoxicity from unnecessary drugs		Fluid restiction, dialysis

should reduce the incidence and severity of these complications. If such complications do arise, they need to be treated with supportive care and appropriate surgical intervention. *Alternative* methods must be considered. This classification serves only to help identify the causes of systemic complications so that preventable ones can be avoided and others limited.

It is important to anticipate and identify any complications *early*. This can best be done by *frequent patient assessment*. One convenient method of assessment is to review the organ system function of the patient frequently. This permits a rapid but thorough evaluation of the patient and reduces omission. Furthermore, it is easier for other physicians to review information in such a format. It is important to remember that all organ systems are interrelated, and that dysfunction of one may affect others. A sound understanding of the pathophysiologic effects of burn injury and subsequent complications are necessary to appreciate these interrelationships. This is especially true of sepsis. Finally, it is imperative to maintain sight of the entire patient and not as merely an integral of many organ systems.

Each organ system will be discussed regarding the physiologic disturbances, the most common and life-threatening complications, and the prevention and treatment of these specific complications. These organ systems and some of the complications are summarized in Table 11-3.

CARDIOVASCULAR COMPLICATIONS

The most serious cardiovascular complications are acute myocardial infarction (MI), high-output failure, hypertensive crisis, and bacterial endocarditis.

TABLE 11-3. ORGAN SYSTEM APPROACH TO SYSTEMIC COMPLICATIONS IN THERMALLY INJURED PATIENTS

Organ System	Major Complications
Cardiovascular	MI, hypertension; endocarditis
Respiratory	Inhalation injury, pneumonia, ARDS, pulmonary edema
Renal	Renal failure, myoglobinuria
Gastrointestinal	Curling's ulcer, hepatic dysfunction, acalculous cholecystitis
Metabolism and nutrition	Nutritional deprivation, prolonged catabolism
Endocrine	Adrenal hemorrhage, insulin–glucagon disequilibrium
Neurologic	"Burn encephalopathy," carbon monoxide intoxication
Musculoskeletal	Extremity loss, septic thrombophlebitis
Hematologic	Anemia, coagulation disorders
Immune	Sepsis

One immediate effect of severe burn injury is to reduce cardiac output by approximately 50 percent for up to 16 hours. This may be due to a serum factor that depresses the myocardium.[3] This low-output state is present despite appropriate fluid resuscitation and normal filling pressures.[4-6]

This decreased perfusion may produce myocardial ischemia and infarction in the early postburn period. This complication may be prevented by limiting further stress on the heart from hypovolemia, hypoxia, and increased myocardial oxygen demand. Any documented MI should be treated by means similar to nonburned patients. ECG monitoring, oxygen supplementation, and maneuvers to decrease the work of the heart, such as by controlling hypertension, are important measures in the treatment of MI after burn injury.

The hyperdynamic cardiac failure seen later in the course of the burn patient is most pronounced in sepsis.[7] Treatment of this high-output, low-resistance state must concentrate on treating the source of infection. The use of vasopressors to increase peripheral vascular resistance and thus the blood pressure will increase the numerical value, but may decrease effective perfusion to vital tissues. There are some occasions when blood pressure falls too low and a β-adrenergic agent increases perfusion.[7] It is very important, however, that attention be directed to the cause of sepsis and its treatment.

There is also a syndrome of acute hypertension after burn injury, especially in children.[8-10] This occurs in up to 10 percent of serious burns. It is not associated with an increase in renin, angiotensin, or catecholamines when compared to burn victims without hypertension. The most serious sequelae of this complication are seizures and encephalopathy.[11] Early recognition and treatment with antihypertensives are important in reducing complications.

Bacterial endocarditis and septic thrombophlebitis of central veins occurs more often in severely burned patients. These are usually seen with central venous catheters and especially with pulmonary artery catheters.[12-14]

Several recent studies have documented this growing problem and its high mortality.[15] Most burn patients can be measured without central lines except in the case of significant cardiopulmonary dysfunction. If these lines are needed, they should be changed frequently; preferably every 5 days or less. They should also be removed when they are no longer necessary. Treatment of endocarditis is an extended course of antibiotics, and occasional valvular replacement is necessary; however, the mortality is greater than 90 percent. Septic peripheral vein requires prompt, complete excision.

RESPIRATORY COMPLICATIONS

Complications of the respiratory system are very common after a major burn.[6,16] The complications of this organ system, especially those involving infection, contribute to the cause of death in the majority of patients who do not survive.

The major problems are inhalation injury, airway obstruction, pneumonia, pulmonary edema, adult respiratory distress syndrome (ARDS), and those related to tracheostomy, pulmonary embolism, and methemoglobinemia.

Inhalation injury is discussed in Chapter 10. There are also many good reviews available.[17,18] However, it is important to review the basic principles of this complication. Pulmonary injury is produced either by breathing superheated air or steam in a closed space, or by inhalation of noxious chemicals.[19-22] Respiratory failure develops usually at 24 to 48 hours after injury and is associated with significant morbidity and mortality. Furthermore, inhalation injury is associated with an increased incidence of subsequent pulmonary complications such as pneumonia and ARDS.[16,23-25] Treatment requires supportive care with humidified O_2 and often ventilation. Steroids are of no proven benefit and are probably detrimental.[26,27]

Acute airway obstruction may result from laryngeal edema secondary to inhalation injury and the diffuse soft tissue edema associated with burns of greater than 25 to 30 percent body surface area. This swelling and bronchospasm may be reduced by judicious fluid replacement and treatments with racemic epinephrine, but the patient must receive adequate resuscitation. If there is a reasonable chance of airway compromise, the patient should have endotracheal intubation early. If in doubt, intubate. Delay in obtaining a protected airway may lead to the need for an emergency tracheostomy and its subsequent complications.

The later pulmonary complications, pulmonary edema, pneumonia, and ARDS are very interrelated. Pulmonary edema, as measured by extravascular lung water, does not increase during resuscitation despite net gains of over 20 liters of fluid.[28] However, lung water increases dramatically after the onset of sepsis. Pneumonia may be the cause of sepsis, but more commonly develops after sepsis from burn wounds because of the increased pulmonary fluid and compromised lung function. The inflammatory and fibrotic changes seen with ARDS may then develop. The relation of this syndrome to sepsis is well documented.[22]

Tracheostomies can produce major and sometimes untreatable complications. It is associated with an increased incidence of pneumonia, necrotizing tracheobronchitis, and erosion of major vessels.[29,30] Tracheostomy is seldom needed in burn care because burn patients develop few problems from prolonged intubation with high-volume, low-pressure cuffed endotracheal tubes.[31] Laryngeal problems of stenosis and fistula from tracheostomy or endotracheal tubes can be repaired after the patient recovers from the burn injury.[32,33] Respiratory failure may develop from the inability of O_2 to bind to hemoglobin. This is usually associated with carbon monoxide intoxication, but may also develop from methemoglobinemia associated with topical silver nitrate.[34] Use of silver nitrate concentration of 0.5 percent will limit the chance of this problem. Pulmonary embolism is another respiratory complication that has been described, but is uncommon.[35]

RENAL COMPLICATIONS

The complications of the renal system reviewed here will be renal failure and metabolic acidosis from bicarbonate loss in the kidney.

Renal failure in burn patients is less uncommon because of the careful attention to fluid resuscitation in the first 24 hours after injury. Still, it continues to occur as a result of inadequate perfusion from hypovolemia or septic shock and as a result of nephrotoxic substances. Attention must be directed to maintain adequate renal blood flow at all times. Urine output remains the best monitor of perfusion in the burn patient. Nephrotoxic agents must be eliminated or monitored closely to prevent irreversible damage. Myoglobinuria from extensive thermal or electrical injury to muscle is best treated by early debridement or amputation.[36-39] Antibiotics such as aminoglycosides and amphotericin B must be monitored for their nephrotoxic effect. Dosage adjustments or use of other antibiotics are necessary if continued renal impairment occurs.[40] If a patient develops progressive oliguria, it is advantageous to try to convert oliguric renal failure to nonoliguric renal failure. Mannitol may help to do this when used in doses up to 100 grams per day. If this fails, a slow channel calcium blocker, such as verapamil or nifedipine, may augment urine output. If severe renal failure does develop, early dialysis and adequate nutritional support are important. However, only 15 percent of patients recover sufficient renal function to stop dialysis and the mortality remains high.[36]

Metabolic acidosis may develop as a result of excess bicarbonate loss from the kidney. Sulfamylon is a carbonic anhydrase inhibitor which may produce such severe acidosis that respiratory compensation is inadequate or produces respiratory failure.[15,41] Close monitoring of ventilatory rate and acid-base balance will indicate if this complication is significant. Treatment requires bicarbonate administration and changing to another topical agent.

GASTROINTESTINAL COMPLICATIONS

Complications of the gastrointestinal tract following severe thermal injury occur relatively frequently. Gastroduodenal ulceration, acalculous cholecystitis, abnormal liver function, pseudoobstruction, and superior mesenteric artery (SMA) syndrome are some of the complications.

Gastric and duodenal erosions have been reported in 66 percent of severely burned patients, with significant ulceration in nearly 20 percent.[42] Bleeding is the major clinical problem from these lesions and its presence and severity do not correlate with gastrin and acid.[43,44] Prevention is crucial with this complication and is best done by antacids and enteral feedings.[45-47] Cimetidine, though used successfully, is probably not as efficient and is more expensive than antacids.

Acalculous cholecystitis is another gastrointestinal complication of burns and other major illnesses. It may be caused by ischemia of the gallbladder wall from distention, hypercoagulability, and decreased perfusion. Although more insidious in onset, it has a much higher mortality than calculous cholecystitis.[48-50] Enteral administration of fat to decrease distention of the gallbladder and avoidance of shock may help decrease the incidence of this complication. Ultrasound and isotope studies can help delineate these problems. Treatment is cholecystectomy or cholecystostomy; antibiotics alone are inadequate.

Hepatic dysfunction after thermal injury is well documented. Several factors probably contribute to this including pre-existing disease, shock, sepsis, and hepatocellular damage from metabolic abnormalities which will be discussed separately. Mortality with significant hepatic failure is nearly 100 percent. Unfortunately, there are no apparent means to prevent this complication other than to limit the above-mentioned factors and attempt to maintain adequate nutrition. Treatment consists only of trying to reduce the demand on hepatic function, such as reduction of parenteral carbohydrate load.[51,52]

Pancreatitis has also been noted in burn patients. The etiology is unclear, but apparently involves tissue ischemia from hypoperfusion. If pancreatitis develops, it should be treated with standard therapy of reducing pancreatic stimulation and nutritional support.

Pseudoobstruction and SMA syndrome have been described in the burn patient.[53-55] The former may be helped by decreasing opiate doses, ambulation, and increasing dietary fiber. SMA syndrome may severely limit oral alimentation. Jejunostomy or transoral jejunal feeding tubes may be necessary until adequate gastric emptying returns.

COMPLICATIONS OF METABOLISM AND NUTRITION

The increased metabolic needs of the burn patient are well documented. Difficulty in meeting these needs is increased by the altered carbohydrate, protein, fat, and mineral metabolism, the need for which is greatest in the early postburn period and when the patient is septic.[56-59] Nutritional dysfunction from incorrect amounts of protein, carbohydrate, fat, minerals, and vitamins is one of the most common and severe complications of burn injury.[60,61] Protein–calorie malnutrition will lead to poor wound healing and failure of other organ systems. Administration of too much glucose can produce nonketotic hyperosmolar coma and acute fatty liver.[6,60] Specific substrate deficiencies, such as fat, zinc, or phosphate, can produce multiple complications too numerous to elicit here.

The method of nutritional supplementation can also produce systemic complications. Gastric distention from tube feedings may lead to acute respiratory failure or aspiration. Tubes can necrose the nares or perforate the bowel. Parenteral alimentation has a much higher complication rate including pneumothorax, hemothorax, catheter sepsis, or embolization. Early enteral feedings of a balanced diet with protein supplementation are the means of preventing this complication as well as treating it. If enteral feeding is not possible or inadequate, parenteral hyperalimentation may be required. The effectiveness of nutritional support is difficult to measure in burn patients, but nitrogen balance is still useful in measuring relative change. It is essential to monitor this system at all times because inadequate nutrition will lead to the failure of all other organ systems.

ENDOCRINE COMPLICATIONS

Systemic complications of the endocrine system are not common in burn patients. However, the hormonal changes after burn injury are important and have profound effect on the rest of the body. These effects have been well documented in several studies and include the hypothalmic–pituitary axis, adrenocortical hormones, catecholamines, insulin–glucagon interrelationship, and thyroid hormone.[62-66] The endocrine perturbations are most severe immediately after the injury and with any episodes of sepsis.

The physiologic effects of burns and some of the subsequent complications are frequently manifested by alterations in the level and activity of the hormones mentioned above. They frequently act as the messengers between the other systems that are discussed in this chapter.[67] Fluid and electrolyte shifts, hypermetabolism, and glucose intolerance are several effects of the burn injury itself and the subsequent complications of sepsis.[61]

Primary systemic complications of the endocrine system are relatively uncommon. One such problem is adrenal insufficiency following hemorrhage and necrosis.[68] No apparent cause is known for this complication. Other clinical factors mask the symptoms and diagnosis is difficult. Support with steroids is indicated, but the mortality for this problem is very high.

NEUROLOGIC COMPLICATIONS

Neurologic complications from burns can be separated into direct neuronal injury from the accident itself and cerebral dysfunction of several types. These include burn encephalopathy and early and late neurologic injury from carbon monoxide.

Direct nerve injury from thermal burn is very rare, but it is common in electrical injuries because the low resistance nerve tissue preferentially conducts the current. Treatment of such an injury consists of avoiding further nerve damage from pressure and ischemia and physical therapy. Most patients have partial or full recovery of nerve function.[35,69]

Burn encephalopathy may appear as a spectrum from altered mental status to seizures and coma.[1,11,70,71] Focal symptoms can occur without an apparent focal injury. This is frequently associated with sepsis, but also occurs in nonseptic patients associated with other metabolic and hemodynamic abnormalities.[72] This is probably the most severe problem seen with the acute hypertensive crisis in pediatric burns mentioned previously.

No consistent etiology has been found for this complication and there is no apparent method for predicting or treating it other than treating coexisting complications such as sepsis. Fortunately, it is usually self-limited with total resolution, but in some cases global or focal deficits are permanent.

Acute carbon monoxide intoxication is well known to produce neurologic impairment that roughly correlates with the carboxyhemoglobin level.[22] These symptoms are frequently reversible but may lead to residual deficits. Treatment is generally restricted to increasing the inspired oxygen content to 100 percent in patients with acute carbon monoxide poisoning, and providing mechanical ventilation if necessary. There is no present means to identify those patients likely to have residual problems. There is also no acknowledged therapy to prevent or limit the problem.

An even less understood complication is delayed neurologic injury following carbon monoxide intoxication.[73] It is frequently associated with sublethal levels of carbon monoxide and does not become apparent until 1 to 2 weeks after the injury. There are demonstrable changes in the brain that correspond to the defects, often in the globus pallidus. It has not been determined if the etiology is different from defects seen in acute carbon monoxide neurologic injury. As in the neurologic complications, there is no way of predicting or treating this problem.

MUSCULOSKELETAL COMPLICATIONS

Discussion of the systemic complication of the musculoskeletal system will be limited to the extremities since such complications of axial structures are very uncommon. The major complications of the extremities involve limb loss or disability. Limb loss from thermal injury and disability from subsequent scarring are reviewed in other chapters. The problems that may lead to amputation or disability are ischemia, pressure, and infection.

Ischemia may occur early due to compromised circulation from eschar or vascular damage, particularly from electrical burns.[69,74,75] Appropriate escharotomies will limit or prevent ischemia in the former situation. Vascular grafting has been done in the situation of major arterial injury to preserve limb viability.[76] Arterial occlusion may also occur in the presence of arterial catheters because of the hypercoagulable state of these patients described in the next system. Limbs distal to such catheters must be observed frequently. Catheters must be removed if perfusion fails and anticoagulation or thrombectomy may be required.

Increased tissue pressure may produce compartment syndromes and superimposed ischemic injury.[77] Blood flow to soft tissue vascular beds does not increase in the hyperdynamic state except in the area of the burn. Therefore, these tissues have no increased protection against the increasing tissue pressure from edema.

Compartment pressures can be measured if there is concern over soft tissue injury (see Chap. 8).[78] Fasciotomies should be done if symptoms develop or if compartment pressures are elevated. Permanent nerve injury, muscle necrosis, and subsequent infection may result if this complication is not considered and evaluated in time.

Late limb complications from infection are frequently the result of the primary burn injury. However, septic thrombophlebitis and necrotizing soft tissue infection may lead to inordinate muscle and neurovascular damage or amputation.[15,79] These problems must be considered as potential complications in the musculoskeletal system. Proper intravenous catheter care and early, aggressive surgical treatment of soft tissue infections will treat these and most often prevent them from spreading further. Suppurative thrombophlebitis requires excision of the involved venous system.

HEMATOLOGIC COMPLICATIONS

Systemic complications of the hematologic system can be divided into clotting and red cell production. Anemia is a common complication that is caused by many factors including blood loss and nutritional deprivation. Many burn patients have significant hemolysis that may last for weeks. Supportive transfusion and adequate nutrition are necessary to treat this anemia.[55,80]

The disturbances in the clotting mechanisms are often underestimated in regard to their importance. Within minutes after suffering burns, patients become hypercoagulable. Platelet counts fall early after burn injury and again during septic episodes.[81] They have activation of the intrinsic clotting mechanisms, fibrinolysis, and complement pathways through factor VII activation from burn tissue and intravascular contamination.[82] This produces an early disseminated intravascular coagulopathy (DIC) syndrome associated with excessive bleeding. Thrombosis in skin and subcutaneous tissue cause partial thickness injury to progress to full thickness. Attempts at treating this with heparin have no conclusive improvement in outcome.[83] Appropriate resuscitation and support with transfusion may help to limit or reduce this early systemic complication.

Later complications of clotting are usually due to sepsis or massive transfusion. Fibrin degradation products are frequently found in septic, burned patients. The bleeding problems produced are only part of the effects of this DIC. The activation of complements and kinins significantly alters pulmonary vascular endothelium and has profound effects on the function of the immune system, to be discussed later. The treatment of this type of DIC is appropriate treatment of the sepsis.

Complications from coagulopathy due to massive transfusion are mostly confined to blood loss and hypovolemia, but some of the systemic effects seen with sepsis are also present, but limited. This complication can generally be avoided by limiting surgical treatment to a certain blood loss.[84] Treatment is essentially the same as any coagulopathy from massive transfusion. Control of identifiable bleeding vessels and administration of platelets, and occasionally fresh frozen plasma.

SEPSIS

Sepsis is the major complication of the immune system. Infection is directly or indirectly responsible for nearly 95 percent of deaths from burns that occur more than 2 days after injury.[85-88]

The increased risk of infection after burn injury is due in large part to the loss of the protective skin barrier and the subsequent immune dysfunction following thermal injury. Defects of specific and nonspecific immune function involving both cellular and humoral components have been documented. Lymphocyte populations are altered with relative increase in suppressor cells.[89] Monocyte and leukocyte mobility and bactericidal activity are depressed.[90-94] Impairment of the general reticuloendothelial system has been noted.[95] Soluble components of the immune system are also impaired or decreased after burn injury. Antibody, complement, and opsonic proteins have been found to be significantly depressed.[91,96-101]

The mechanism of this depression is unclear, but may involve some serum factor with immunosuppressive activity.[102,103] Furthermore, many of the other physiologic effects of burns—endocrine, nutritional, and hematologic—have direct effects on the immune system also. The converse is also true. Treatment methods may also affect immune function. General anesthesia has been documented to decrease immune reactivity and silver sulfadiazene has been found to produce neutropenia in a significant number of cases.[104,105] The immune mechanism is reviewed in Chapter 3.

Sources of infection are not restricted to the burn wound itself, though it is a major focus. Pulmonary, urinary, and intravascular causes of sepsis are other frequent routes of infection. All these infections may produce sepsis and the subsequent effects on other organ systems. Multiorgan system failure is a common problem in septic burn patients, and successful treatment is dependent upon control of the infection.

Infection is also not restricted to bacteria. Candida and other fungi frequently become pathogenic organisms after antibiotics eliminate or suppress the sensitive flora.[106,107] Viral infections are also relatively common, but frequently not identified until recovery or postmortem.[108]

Prevention of complications of the immune system is difficult. Some attempts have been made to enhance immune function by active immunization and passive transfer of immune globulin in serum.[86,109-112] Excellent sterile technique and wound care is important, but patients rapidly become infected with endogenous bacteria. Early nutritional support will help maintain some immune competence.[113] Conversely, sepsis will impair the effectiveness of nutritional support.[58] Excellent nursing care will provide chest physiotherapy and vascular and urinary catheter care which are important in prevention of infection and sepsis. Early wound coverage is probably the best means of prevention of infectious complications.[114]

Early diagnosis and treatment of sepsis are important steps in managing this complication.[115,116] Routine quantitative culture and biopsy of the burn wound have proved to be very useful.[117] Infection should always be the likely cause of any deterioration of a burn patient, whether or not it is heralded by fever, leukocytosis, or visual evidence of infection. Cultures of blood, sputum, urine, and the burn wound should be done. Indwelling vascular catheters should be changed. Appropriate antibiotics should be started.[40] If the burn wound appears to be the source, a different topical agent may be used, subeschar clysis may be performed, or the wound excised and preferably covered with allograft or xenograft.[118] If another source of infection, such as septic thrombophlebitis, acalculous cholecystitis, or perinephric abscess is identified, standard therapy, including surgery, must be started without delay.

Complications of other systems from sepsis should be treated appropriately. Septic shock may require treatment with pressors. These drugs generally increase peripheral vascular resistance and so the blood pressure, but do not increase effective perfusion. Renal function must be supported with adequate fluids, while also considering respiratory failure from sepsis. Glucose intolerance and the general catabolic state will not reverse until the infection is under control.

PRINCIPLES OF TREATMENT

This review of organ system function should help in early diagnosis and treatment of systemic complications from burn injury. With this method of review, however, it is crucial to integrate the information into a general assessment of patient status to plan further treatment and monitoring.

Although the causes and manifestations of systemic complications of burns are multiple, the treatments follow a few general rules. These are supportive care, close monitoring, and appropriate operative treatment. Support of the organ system that is not functioning is imperative. This is accomplished by different means depending on the complication. Respiratory failure may require ventilation, renal failure may be severe enough to require hemodialysis, and nutritional failure requires adequate protein and calorie administration. These methods do not cure the complication, but provide a state of physiologic homeostatis until the organ system and the patient can recover.

The organ system in question must be frequently re-evaluated for progression of the complication. Furthermore, the other organ systems need to be assessed for the effects on them by the one malfunctioning and for unrelated complications.

Finally, operative treatment of certain systemic complications may be necessary. Basic surgery principles apply; debridement of infected and necrotic tissue, drainage of pus under pressure, access for other therapy, and correction of surgical problems such as cholecystitis or perforated ulcer.

The best means of treatment, however, is prevention of systemic complications in burns with no exception. Early grafting closes the burn wounds and starts to return the patient to a normal physiologic state. Thus, early burn wound covering is the best means of preventing these systemic complications.

REFERENCES

1. Pruitt BA Jr: Complications of thermal injury. Clin Plast Surg 1:667, 1974
2. Sevitt S: A review of the complications from burns, their origin and importance for illness and death. J Trauma 19:358, 1979
3. Baxter RC, Cook WA, Shires GT: Serum myocardial depressant factor of burn shock. Surg Forum 17:1, 1966
4. Baxter CR: Problems and complications of burn shock resuscitation. Surg Clin North Am 58:1313, 1978
5. Dodson EL, Warner GE: Early circulatory disturbances following experimental thermal trauma. Circ Res 5:69, 1957
6. Pruitt BA Jr: Fluid and electrolyte replacement in the burned patient. Surg Clin North Am 58:1291, 1978
7. Drueck C, Welch GW, Pruitt BA Jr: Hemodynamic analysis of septic shock in thermal injury: Treatment with dopamine. Am Surg 44:424, 1978
8. Brizio-Moltei L, Molteni A, Clontier LC, et al.: Incidence of post burn hypertensive crisis in patients admitted to two burn centers and a community hospital in the United States. Scand J Plast Reconstr Surg 13:21, 1979
9. Faulkner B, Roven S, DeClement FA, et al.: Hypertension in children with burns. J Trauma 18:213, 1978
10. Popp MB, Friedberg DL, MacMillan BG: Clinical characteristics of hypertension in burned children. Ann Surg 191:473, 1980
11. McManus WF, Hunt JL, Pruitt BA Jr: Postburn convulsive disorders of children. J Trauma 14:396, 1974
12. Dudrick SJ, Long JM: Applications and hazards of intravenous hyperalimentation. Ann Rev Med 28:517, 1977
13. Ehrie M, Morgan AP, Moore FD, et al.: Endocarditis with the indwelling balloon-tipped pulmonary artery catheter in burn patients. J Trauma 18:664, 1978
14. Sasaki TM, Panke TW, Dorethy JF, et al.: The relationship of central venous and pulmonary artery catheter position to acute right-sided endocarditis in severe thermal injury. J Trauma 19:740, 1979
15. Pruitt BA Jr, McManus WF, Kim SH, et al.: Diagnosis and treatment of cannula related intravenous sepsis in burn patients. Ann Surg 191:546, 1980

16. Achauer BM, Allyn PA, Furnas DW, et al.: Pulmonary complications of burns: The major threat to the burn patient. Ann Surg 177:311, 1973
17. Fein A, Leff A, Hopewell PC: Pathophysiology and management of the complications resulting from fire and the inhaled products of combustion: A review of the literature. Crit Care Med 8:94, 1980
18. Moylan JA, Chan CK: Inhalation injury: An increasing problem. Ann Surg 188:34, 1978
19. Crapo RO: Smoke inhalation injuries. JAMA 246:1694, 1981
20. Head JM: Inhalation injury in burns. Am J Surg 139:508, 1980
21. Peters WJ: Inhalation injury caused by the products of combustion. Can Med Assoc J 125:249, 1981
22. Trunkey DD: Inhalation Injury. Surg Clin North Am 58:1133, 1978
23. Getzen LC, Pollack EW: Fatal respiratory distress in burned patients. Surg Gynecol Obstet 152:741, 1981
24. Pruitt BA Jr, Erickson DR, Morris A: Progressive pulmonary insufficiency and other pulmonary complications of thermal injury. J Trauma 15:369, 1975
25. Stone HH: Pulmonary burns in children. J Pediatr Surg 14:48, 1979
26. Moylan JA: Diagnostic techniques and steroids. Inhalation Injury. J Trauma 19:(Suppl)917, 1979
27. Welch GW, Lull RJ, Petroff PA, et al.: The use of steroids in inhalation injury. Surg Gynecol Obstet 145:539, 1977
28. Tranbaugh RF, Lewis FR, Christensen JM, et al.: Lung water changes after thermal injury. Ann Surg 192:479, 1980
29. Majeski JA, MacMillan BG: Tracheo-innominate artery erosion in a burned child. J Trauma 18:137, 1978
30. Moylan JA, West JT, Nash G, et al.: Tracheostomy in thermally injured patients: A review of five years experience. Am Surg 39:119, 1972
31. Lewis FR Jr, Schlobohm RM, Thomas AN: Prevention of complications from prolonged tracheal intubation. Am J Surg 135:452, 1978
32. Eliachar I, Moscona R, Joachims HF, et al.: The management of laryngotracheal stenosis in burned patients. Plast Reconst Surg 68:11, 1981
33. Majeski JA, Schreiber JT, Cotton R, et al.: Tracheoplasty for tracheal stenosis in the pediatric burned patient. J Trauma 20:81, 1980
34. Ternberg JL, Luce E: Methemoglobinemia: Complications of the silver nitrate treatment of burns. Surgery 63:328, 1968
35. Coleman JB, Chang FC: Pulmonary embolism: An unrecognized event in severely burned patients. Am J Surg 130:697, 1975
36. Davies DM, Pusey CD, Rainford DJ, et al.: Acute renal failure in burns. Scand J Plast Reconstr Surg 13:189, 1979
37. Hunt JL, Mason AD, Masterson TS, et al.: The pathophysiology of acute electrical injuries. J Trauma 16:335, 1976
38. Rouse R, Dimich AR: The treatment of electrical injury compared to burn injury: A review of pathophysiology and comparison of patient management protocols. J Trauma 18:43, 1978
39. Shakespeare PG, Coombes EJ, Hambleton J, et al.: Proteinuria after burn injury. Ann Clin Biochem 18:353, 1981
40. Waisbren BA: Antibiotics in the treatment of burns. Surg Clin North Am 50:1311, 1970

41. White MG, Asch MJ: Acid-base effects of topical mafenide acetate in the burned patient. N Eng J Med 284:1281, 1971
42. Pruitt BA Jr, Goodwin CW Jr: Stress ulcer disease in the burned patient. World J Surg 5:209, 1981
43. Czaja JA, McAlhany JC, Pruitt BA Jr: Gastric acid secretion and acute gastroduodenal disease after burns. Arch Surg 111:243, 1976
44. Rosenthal A, Czaja AJ, Pruitt BA Jr: Gastrin levels and gastric acidity in the pathogenesis of acute gastroduodenal disease after burns. Surg Gynecol Obstet 144:632, 1977
45. McAlhany JC Jr, Colmic L, Czaja AJ, et al.: Antacid control of complications from acute gastroduodenal disease after burns. J Trauma 16:645, 1976
46. Solem LD, Strate RG, Fischer RP: Antacid therapy and nutritional supplementation in the prevention of Curling's ulcer. Surg Gynecol Obstet 148:367, 1979
47. Watson LC, Abston S: Prevention of upper gastrointestinal hemorrhage in 582 burned children. Am J Surg 132:790, 1976
48. Alwanek I: Acute acalculous cholecystitis in burns. Br J Surg 65:243, 1978
49. Glenn R, Becker CG: Acute acalculous cholecystitis: An increasing entity. Ann Surg 195:131, 1982
50. Munster AM, Goodwin MN, Pruitt BA Jr: Acalculous cholecystitis in burned patients. Am J Surg 122:591, 1971
51. Chlumsky J, Dobias J, Vrabek R, et al.: Liver changes in burns as seen in the clinical morphologic picture. Acta Hepatogastroenterol (Stuttgart) 23:118, 1976
52. Czaja AJ, Rizzo TA, Smith WR, et al.: Acute liver disease after cutaneous thermal injury. J Trauma 15:887, 1975
53. Lescher TJ, Teegarden DK, Pruitt BA Jr: Acute pseudo-obstruction of the colon in thermally injured patients. Dis Colon Rectum 21:618, 1978
54. Lescher TJ, Sirinek KR, Pruitt BA Jr: Superior mesenteric artery syndrome in thermally injured patients. J Trauma 19:567, 1979
55. Reckler JM, Bruck HM, Munster AM, et al.: Superior mesenteric artery syndrome as a consequence of burn injury. J Trauma 12:979, 1972
56. Curreri PW: Metabolic and nutritional aspects of thermal injury. Burns 2:16, 1976
57. Gump FE, Kenney JM: Energy balance and weight loss in burned patients. Arch Surg 103:442, 1971
58. Morath MA, Miller SF, Finley RK Jr: Nutritional indicators of postburn bacteremic sepsis. JPEN 5:488, 1981
59. Wilmore DW: Nutrition and metabolism following thermal injury. Clin Plast Surg 1:603, 1974
60. Wilmore DW: Carbohydrate metabolism in trauma. Clin Endocrinol Metab 5:731, 1976
61. Wilmore DW, Aulick LH: Metabolic changes in burned patients. Surg Clin North Am 58:1173, 1978
62. Bane JW, McCae RE, McCae CS, et al.: The pattern of aldosterone and cortisol blood levels in thermal burn patients. J Trauma 14:605, 1974
63. Evans EI, Butterfield WJH: The stress response in the severely burned patient. Ann Surg 134:558, 1951
64. Shuck JM, Eaton RP, Shuck LW, et al.: Dynamics of insulin and glucagon secretions in severely burned patients. J Trauma 12:215, 1972

65. Wilmore DW, Long JM, Mason AD, et al.: Catecholamines: Mediator of the hypermetabolic response to thermal injury. Ann Surg 180:653, 1975
66. Wilmore DW, Orcutt TW, Mason AD, et al.: Alterations in hypothalmic function following thermal injury. J Trauma 15:657, 1975
67. Wilmore DW, Long JM, Mason AD, et al.: Stress in surgical patients as neurophysiologic response. Surg Gynecol Obstet 142:257, 1976
68. Foley FD, Pruitt BA Jr, Moncrief JA: Adrenal hemorrhage and necrosis in seriously burned patients. J Trauma 7:863, 1967
69. Esses SI, Peters WJ: Electrical burns: Pathophysiology and complications. Can J Surg 24:11, 1981
70. Hughes JR, Cayaffa JJ, Boswick JA Jr: Seizures following burns of the skin. III. Electroencephalographic recordings. Dis Nerv Syst 36:443, 1975
71. Mohnot D, Snead OC, Benton JW Jr: Burn encephalopathy in children. Ann Neurol 12:42, 1981
72. Haynes BW Jr, Bright R: Burn coma: A syndrome associated with severe burn wound infection. J Trauma 7:464, 1967
73. Sawa GM, Watson CPN, Terbrugge K, et al.: Delayed encephalopathy following carbon monoxide intoxication. Can J Neurol Sci 8:77, 1981
74. Aulick LH, Wilmore DW, Mason AD Jr, et al.: Muscle blood flow following thermal injury. Ann Surg 188:778, 1978
75. Salisbury RE, McKeel DW, Mason AD Jr: Ischemic necrosis of the intrinsic muscles of the hand after thermal injuries. J Bone Joint Surg 56:1701, 1974
76. Wang XW, Wu JN, Sung YH, et al.: Early vascular grafting to prevent upper extremity necrosis after electrical burns. Burns Incl Therm Inj 8:303, 1982
77. Justis DL, Law EJ, McMillan BG: Tibial compartment syndromes in burn patients. A report of four cases. Arch Surg 111:1004, 1976
78. Kingsley NW, Stein JM, Levenson SM: Measuring tissue pressure to assess the severity of burn-induced ischemia. Plast Reconstr Surg 63:404, 1979
79. Davies DM: Gas gangrene as a complication of burns. Scand J Plast Reconstr Surg 13:73, 1979
80. Loebl EC, Baxter CR, Curreri PW: The mechanism of erythrocyte destruction in the early post-burn period. Ann Surg 178:681, 1973
81. Hergt K: Blood levels of thrombocytes in burned patients: Observations on their behavior in relation to the clinical condition of the patient. J Trauma 12:599, 1972
82. Caprini JA, Lipp V, Zuckerman L, et al.: Hematologic changes following burns. J Surg Res 22:626, 1977
83. Curreri PW, Wilterdink ME, Baxter CR: Coagulation dynamics following thermal injury: Effect of heparin and protamine sulfate. Ann Surg 181:161, 1975
84. Canizaro PC, Sawer RB, Switzer WE: Blood loss during excision of third degree burns. Arch Surg 88:800, 1964
85. Alexander JW, Ogle CK, Stinnett JD, et al.: A sequential prospective analysis of immunologic abnormalities and infection following severe thermal injury. Ann Surg 188:809, 1978
86. Cason JS: Some aspects on prevention and treatment of infection in burns. Prog Pediatr Surg 14:3, 1981
87. Lowbury EJ: Wits vs. genes: The continuing battle against infection. J Trauma 19:33, 1979
88. McMillan BG: Infections following burn injury. Surg Clin North Am 60:185, 1980

89. Baker CC, Miller CL, Trunkey DD: Predicting fatal sepsis in burn patients. J Trauma 19:641, 1979
90. Alexander JW: Serum and leukocyte liposomal enzymes. Derangements following severe thermal injury. Arch Surg 95:482, 1965
91. Alexander JW, Wilson D: Neutrophil dysfunction and sepsis in burn injury. Surg Gynecol Obstet 130:431, 1970
92. Altman LC, Klebanoff SJ, Curreri PW: Abnormalities of monocyte chemotaxis following thermal injury. J Surg Res 22:616, 1977
93. Butterfield WC: Experimental stress ulcers: A review. Surg Ann 7:261, 1975
94. Deitch EA, Gelder F, McDonald JC: Prognostic significance of abnormal neutrophil chemotaxis after thermal injury. J Trauma 22:199, 1982
95. Schildt BE: The present view of RES and shock. Adv Exp Med Biol 73:375, 1976
96. Alexander JW, McClellan MA, Ogle CK, et al: Consumptive opsoninopathy: Possible pathogenesis in lethal and opportunistic infection. Ann Surg 184:672, 1976
97. Arturson G, Hogman CF, Johansson SGQ, et al.: Changes in immunoglobulin levels in severely burned patients. Lancet 1:546, 1969
98. Bjornson AB, Alexander JW: Alterations of serum opsonins in patients with severe thermal injury. J Lab Clin Med 83:372, 1974
99. Bjornson AB, Altemeier WA, Bjornson HS: The septic burned patient: A model for studying the role of complement and immunoglobulins in opsonization of opportunistic microorganisms. Ann Surg 189:515, 1979
100. Dhennin C, Pinon G, Greco JM: Alterations of the complement system following thermal injury: Use in estimation of vital prognosis. J Trauma 18:129, 1978
101. Munster AM, Hoagland HC, Pruitt BA Jr: The effect of thermal injury on serum immunoglobulins. Ann Surg 172:965, 1970
102. Constantian MB: Association of sepsis with an immunosuppressive polypeptide in the serum of burn patients. Ann Surg 188:209, 1978
103. Hakim AA: An immunodepressive factor from serum of thermally traumatized patients. J Trauma 17:980, 1977
104. Chan CK, Jarret F, Moylan JA: Acute leukopenia as an allergic reaction to silver sulfadiazene in burn patients. J Trauma 16:395, 1976
105. Kiker RG, Carvajal HF, Mecak RP, et al.: A controlled study on the effects of silver sulfadiazene on the white blood cell counts in burned children. J Trauma 17:835, 1977
106. Spebar MJ, Lindberg RB: Fungal infection of the burn wound. Am J Surg 138:879, 1979
107. Spevor MJ, Pruitt BA Jr: Candidiasis in the burned patient. J Trauma 21:237, 1981
108. Linnemann CC Jr, McMillan BG: Viral infections in pediatric burn patients. Am J Dis Child 135:750, 1981
109. Fellner PR, Metyger E: Active immunization in burns. Burns 2:54, 1976
110. Jones RJ: Passive immunization against gram-negative bacilli in burns. Br J Exp Pathol 51:53, 1970
111. Jones RJ, Roe EA, Guptei JL: Controlled trial of pseudomonas immunoglobulin and vaccine in burn patients. Lancet 2:1263, 1980
112. Wassermann D, Schlotterer M, Paul P, et al.: Systematic utilization of an antipseudomonas vaccine in a severe burn unit. Scand J Plast Reconstr Surg 13:81, 1979

113. Wunder JA, Stinett JD, Alexander JW: The effects of malnutrition on variables of host defense in the guinea pig. Surgery 84:542, 1978
114. McManus WF, Goodwin CW, Mason AD Jr, et al.: Burn wound infection. J Trauma 21:753, 1981
115. Carvajal HF, Feinstein R, Traber DL, et al.: An objective method for early diagnosis of gram-negative septicemia in burned children. J Trauma 21:221, 1981
116. Parks DH, Linares HA, Thomson PD: Surgical management of burn wound sepsis. Surg Gynecol Obstet 153:374, 1981
117. Loebl EC, Marvin JA, Heck EL, et al.: The method of quantitative burn wound biopsy cultures and its routine use in the care of the burned patient. Am J Clin Pathol 61:20, 1974
118. Baxter CR, Curreri PW, Marvin JA: The control of burn wound sepsis by the use of quantitative bacteriological studies and subeschar clysis with antibiotics. Surg Clin North Am 53:1509, 1973

PART V
Special Considerations

CHAPTER 12
Chemical and Electrical Burns
Philip A. Edelman

The discussion of nonthermally induced burns requires a definition of "burns" which will be general enough to encompass the diversity of injuries. A burn is an injury caused by an exogenous agent that produces a characteristic reaction to local tissues. The injury may vary from mild erythema to full thickness destruction of the dermis and deeper tissues.

The term nonthermally induced burns needs some explanation. The "nonthermal" agent possesses some form of energy which may be translated into thermal energy by the interaction of that force with biologic matter. However, the energy source would not generally be considered to have significant thermal energy prior to its interaction with tissue. For example, an electric current does not have any thermal properties when traveling in a material of very low resistance. The generation of heat requires the interaction with a resistance. Essentially, the current is a potential energy. Thermally induced burns may result by the interaction of biologic tissues with a material which is sufficiently energized to produce heat that will result in a cytotoxic reaction. Heat is then transferred, principally by conduction, to the tissue. In general, the heat dissipates as a function of distance from the heat source, and thus, in general, tissue injury likewise diminishes. Another mechanism of burns involves the chemical action of an agent on cellular constituents such that a cytotoxic reaction occurs. The inactivation of essential enzymes (fluoride) or cell membranes (e.g., lipid peroxidation) are examples.

The nonthermal burns share many characteristics with thermally induced injuries, however, there are notable distinctions. Nonthermal burns include those caused by radiation, both ionizing and nonionizing (e.g., radiofrequency radiation, ultraviolet, microwave); laser injuries; chemically induced injuries; electrical injuries; as well as biologic agents that may cause a clinical picture that might be described as a burn.

This chapter will describe the injuries caused by electrical and chemical agents.

Nonthermal burns have the potential for delayed effects as well as injury that is not suggested by the appearance of the overlying integument. In addition, electrical and chemical injuries may cause injuries to other organ systems with or without a burn.

An organism generally removes itself from a noxious stimulus when it can be recognized as such. Although anyone would withdraw from a hot iron that was hot enough to induce a second degree burn, people are able to develop second degree burns from ultraviolet radiation via a sunlamp or from the sun. Thus, the intensity of the exposure and the duration are important factors in the determination of the severity of the injury, its prognosis, and treatment. However simple this concept, it is surprising how often people fail to remove themselves or their patients from continued chemical exposure. Anyone burned by a hot object would certainly remove it from their skin, but frequently chemicals are left in contact with the skin for prolonged periods even after a burn is noted to exist.

ELECTRICAL BURNS

A brief review of some of the common terms used in electronics is helpful in understanding electrical burns.

Amperage is a measure of the charge present. It represents the total amount of electricity in a current. In an analogy with a garden hose, amperage is the total amount of water flowing through the hose, it is not the water pressure. The generally used unit is the amp.

Voltage is a measure of the force of the flow of the current. It is the potential difference between two points along a conductor. Again referring to the garden hose, voltage is analogous with the water pressure in the hose. House current in the United States is generally 120 volts. Heavy duty equipment, such as a clothes dryer, may require a 240-volt line. Industrial situations may require much larger voltages for different processes or equipment. Most dry cell commercial batteries range from one-and-a-half to nine volts. Automobile batteries are typically 12-volt batteries, some are six-volt.

High tension current is defined as being greater that 1000 volts. However the shock from 100 volts may be fatal, and the shock from 10,000 volts may be survived. Thus the voltage involved in an injury is not sufficient data, of itself, to determine the severity of the injury.

Alternating current (AC) describes a current whose polarity changes over a period of time. With AC, the frequency and periodicity are generally termed as cycles per second or hertz (Hz). In practice, ACs are regular in their periodicity and in the United States, AC is supplied at 60 cycles per second, and is very closely regulated. In contrast, direct current does not change polarity. This is typified by a battery-operated current.

Direct current is commonly used in industrial processes. It is more effective in electrolytic reactions and thus is used in the purification of metals (e.g., aluminum from bauxite), in electroplating operations, and in galvanoplasty. It is also utilized in the transportation industry, in particular by the railroads.

In electrical burns, the duration of contact and the intensity of the current are the primary factors governing the severity of injury. Another important factor in an electrical current is the resistance of the system.

Resistance is measured in ohms; resistance is inversely proportional to the conductance of a material. Metals such as copper conduct electricity well and therefore have a low resistance; porecelain does not conduct currents well and has a high resistance, and therefore it is often used as an insulator. Electrolyte solutions are good conductors and their conductance is proportional to the ionic strength of the solution.

With these definitions, we can see their relative importance in burn protection by examining the formula for the production of heat by a current:

$$\text{Power} = \text{Current}^2 \text{ (amps)} \times \text{Potential difference (volts)}$$

and therefore:

$$\text{Power} = (\text{Current})^2 \times \text{Resistance}$$

and,

$$\text{Heat} = (\text{Current})^2 \times \text{Resistance} \times 0.239 \times \text{Time}$$

Joule's law therefore states that heat is proportional to the square of the amperage, the duration of the contact, and the resistance of the material through which the current is flowing. Alternatively, we could say that the heat is inversely proportional to the conductance of the medium.

The resistance of the medium is a characteristic of different tissues. Biologic media conduct current as a function of their electrolyte content. In order of declining resistance, the human tissues may be listed skin > bone > fat > nerve > muscle > blood > body fluids.[1] This means that a given current flowing through fat will generate more heat in the local tissues than will the same current in blood.

Further, calloused skin is more resistant to current flow than is thin skin, and dry skin is more resistant than sweaty skin.

The above equations require that all the electrical energy is converted to heat along the course of the resistance which must be pure and independent of the applied current. Certainly many conductors vary as a function of current, and therefore deviate from this formula.

It should also be understood that the development of heat is not the same as the increase in temperature of a conductor. The temperature of a conductor will depend upon its heat capacity (heat supplied to an object compared to the actual rise in temperature), and the rate at which heat can escape from the conductor by conduction, convection, and radiation. An example of this concept is illustated by closing the circuit on an incandescent lamp. The temperature quickly rises to reach a plateau; at the same time the light and heat radiated from the source increases. Therefore, at an equilibrium condition the energy supplied equals the energy radiated away from the source (or by convection or conduction). If this were not the case, the temperature of the bulb would rise infinitely.

Electric arcs may occur when a body approaches a conductor of electricity. The arc may jump a given distance (in air) as a function of its voltage. An electric arc may generate temperatures as high as 4000°C. Table 12–1 relates voltage to distance in air that a current may arc.

Rescue of the Electrical Burn or Shock Victim

As with other types of rescue, the rescuer must always be certain that he or she will not succumb to the same agent that felled the first victim. This is an obvious point, but too frequently neglected by rescuers who react before assessing a situation properly. It is apparent that a victim must be removed from the electrical source. There are several ways of accomplishing this; if there is still a wire or other source that may be continuing to provide a current, the wire must be removed from the victim, or the victim from the wire. In either event, the rescuer must be certain that he or she will not become the next victim. Nonconducting materials should be used to remove the wire or the victim, before touching the person.

Another approach is to shut off the power to the line that is causing the problem. Remember that a person who has received a shock, particularly from a machine, may have received it from an improperly grounded casing or a faulty switch. Therefore, try to shut the power off from a point that you are certain was not involved in the accident, and presumably is safe. A good central circuit breaker is usually a safe spot.

When the offending current has been shut off or removed, check the victim for the basics: airway, ventilation, and circulatory status. Institute cardiopulmonary resuscitation (CPR) if necessary. Electric shock victims may have excellent recovery when CPR is instituted early. If awake, determine mental status. Examine the victim for major injuries.

TABLE 12–1. DISTANCE AN ELECTRIC ARC MAY TRAVEL IN AIR AS A FUNCTION OF VOLTAGE

Voltage	Distance
1×10^3	Few millimeters
5×10^3	1 centimeter
2×10^4	6 centimeters
4×10^4	13 centimeters
1×10^5	35 centimeters

This last point is important as electrical currents may cause injuries other than burns. Alternating currents ranging from 39 to 150 hertz may cause severe tetany, and currents with characteristics of greater than 150 hertz become less dangerous.[2] Therefore, the victim may not be able to release his or her grasp from a live wire, thus grossly increasing the duration of contact of the current. Severe tetany may cause rupture of muscles and tendons as well as skeletal fractures.

Evaluating the patient with an electrical injury requires the determination of all the characteristics of the current as described above. It is also essential to determine the path of the current.[3] Obviously a current passing through the heart or brain will be far more lethal than one passing through the foot. It is also known that current through a body does not follow the path of least resistance, but rather follows a direct path to the ground.[4]

Therefore, a history should determine the location of the contact with the current and an attempt to determine any potential grounding spots on the body. For example, if the victim was holding the live wire in the right hand while holding a grounded metal pipe in the left hand, the current would likely travel across the upper extremities and through the organs of the thorax. It is not uncommon for a current to exit through the nails in a victim's shoes if he or she is standing on a grounded surface. The history should obviously be corroborated with the physical findings.

In addition to the examination of the entrance area of the current, the patient must be totally stripped and a search conducted for any exit wound. The exit wound of an electric current may be far worse than the entrance wound. If a victim is exposed to a large metal surface over a large area of the forearm, and the same current exists via a very small area of contact, such as the nail head in a shoe, the current may be far more concentrated at the exit site; therefore, the exit wound could be more serious.

The path of the current may cause significant damage to underlying tissues, and the appearance of the skin may be very misleading. Further, swelling of subjacent tissues may be severe with resulting neurovascular compromise. The area should be elevated, and the patient should be closely observed for a compartment syndrome requiring fasciotomy or other intervention to decompress the tissues.

With high voltage injuries, the extremely diffuse tissue destruction is a mitigating factor in the cause of mortality or morbidity. With lower voltages, the path of the current is more important; cardiac ventricular fibrillation is a common cause of sudden death in these injuries.

Certainly morbidity and mortality may be augmented by the electric current causing hemolysis and tissue injury. Hyperkalemia may result along with hemoglobinemia and myoglobinemia. This may lead to the accumulation of heme proteins in the renal system with resulting renal failure due to the toxicity of these proteins to the kidneys. Therefore, diuresis with volume load and an osmotic diuretic (mannitol) is necessary; diuretic agents may also be utilized.

The burn typically appears as a central, charred black area, surrounded by a gray-white region of coagulation necrosis with another outer ring of bright erythema. Typically, the surrounding blood vessels are thrombosed and cause further tissue destruction. The endothelial cells and intima are often damaged. These changes may cause delayed erosion of arterial walls with ensuing late hemorrhage. This is often seen in infants who place exposed electrical cords in their mouth and develop severe coagulative burns of the corner of the mouth. It is a known complication for the superior labial artery to erode hours to days after such an injury.

Transthoracic currents have been demonstrated to cause pulmonary edema and hemorrhagic injury to the lungs. Certainly, this is not a reaction limited to the pulmonary system and may be found in tissues in the path of the current. Visceral rupture has in rare circumstances been reported.

The effects of currents on the musculoskeletal system have also been reported. The bone typically becomes whitened and avascular. The injuries to bones and joints may be due to sudden tetanic contractions and their characteristics have been described by Barber.[5]

The acute effects on the heart may vary and are dependent on the intensity of the current and the voltage. Low voltage injuries may cause chest pain and dyspnea, however a few hours later, the symptoms abate and the electrocardiogram is normal. More significant currents may cause actual injury to the heart: ventricular fibrillation or cardiac arrest may occur. In addition to the acute effects of current on the heart and its conducting system, there may be persistent symptoms of angina (angina pectoris electrica), and it may be associated with palpitations, sweating, restlessness, and labored breathing.

Neurologic sequelae from electric shock may be acute, delayed, and chronic.[2] Acutely there may be altered mental status, amnesia, headache, and convulsions. Deafness, visual disturbances, weakness, and twitching may develop. Cataracts, particularly unilateral, may develop after electrical injury, but they are rare. The victim may also develop ventilatory or generalized paralysis. A delayed and potentially long-term effect may be the development of vestibular dysfunction. Despite the absence of symptoms initially, the patient may develop significant vertigo and nausea, often with emesis, when he or she attempts to walk a day or two later. Any patient who has sustained a shock sufficient to cause a loss of consciousness should be observed in the hospital with the benefit of continuous cardiac monitoring for at least 24 hours. This may be accomplished in a speciality unit or cardiac telemetry facility.

Treatment

The assessment and treatment of electrical burns requires an understanding of the above principles of electricity and the injuries caused by such currents. As the severity of the injury is often not apparent at the time of initial examination the treating physician must suspect deeper injuries and anticipate the potential problems associated with them. The path of the current and its characteristics will help lead the clinician to determine the treatment. Most often the extent of the injury is underestimated and fluid resuscitation is therefore likewise underestimated.

In addition to the usual principles of resuscitation of any injured patient—namely, attention to airway, ventilation, and circulation—the physician must understand the systemic effects of the current. Respiratory paralysis, renal failure, musculoskeletal injuries, cardiac arrhythmias, and multiple organ injury may accompany electrical injuries to the skin and subjacent tissues.

Therefore, close observation is mandatory, and baseline studies of renal function (creatinine and blood urea nitrogen) should be obtained as well as a urinalysis. It is important to be sure that the urine is tested for blood after it has been centrifuged, as this may be helpful in identifying free heme proteins. Cardiac and hepatic enzymes should be monitored closely, as should the electrocardiogram. Isoenzymes of CK (CPK or creatine kinase) should be obtained to distinguish skeletal muscle from cardiac bands. Plasma free hemoglobin or haptoglobins may be helpful in documenting hemolysis, but a complete blood count with attention to the hematocrit is more useful especially as this study is easily obtained for serial studies.

Complete roentgenographic studies should be obtained to reveal any occult injury. Chest x-rays should also be obtained. Hyperkalemia should be suspected and can be followed by serial serum determinations as well as by electrocardiographic evidence of a tall, tent-shaped, peaked T waves, which are often symmetric with a narrow base. However, a peaked T wave is not always seen in hyperkalemia.

Repeated complete abdominal examinations are advised. A comatose patient should have skull x-rays and preferably a computerized tomographic (CT) brain scan. Appropriate central lines, central venous pressure (CVP) or flow-directed balloon-tipped pulmonary artery catheters, may be required.

Electrical burns require early debridement of devitalized tissue. Except in minor cases, this is done in the first 24 to 48 hours postinjury. Usually repeated debridements are required because of the difficulty in assessing the extent of damage at the first procedure. Technestium 99 scans have been proposed as a helpful adjunct in locating devitalized muscle.[6] Magnetic resonance scans may be helpful.

Immediate reconstruction is tempting but one must be certain that all of the devitalized tissue has been removed. One exciting development is immediate revascularization which has been proposed by Wang of China.[7] This approach seems to attack the basic underlying problem of continued tissue devitalization. Any deterioration of the patient's condition (fever, hemoglobinuria, or hypotension) is an indication for repeat debridement or amputation.

CHEMICAL BURNS

Injuries of the skin and the subjacent tissues may be classified in several ways when a chemical agent is involved.[8,9] The classification may be a pathologic one, that is describing the injury as coagulation necrosis, liquefaction, or desiccation. Alternatively, the injury may be classified on the basis of the nature of the agent, such as oxidizing agents, acids, caustics, corrosives, or agents causing an exothermic reaction.

Regardless of the method used, many of the principles of thermal and electrical burns apply to chemical injuries. Namely, the duration and strength of the chemical is important in the determination of the injury. As in the case of electrical injuries where amperage is so important, the concentration of the chemical is very important. Concentration may be expressed in many different units and may vary depending on the physical state of the chemical. Common units of concentration include percent (weight per volume), molarity, molality, normality, pH (negative log of hydrogen ion concentration), and parts per million. The precise definitions may be found in standard chemistry textbooks.[10]

Unfortunately, it is not uncommon to see a patient with a chemical contamination who has made it through the emergency room and into an intensive care unit without ever being decontaminated. This causes further injury to the patient and may expose hospital personnel to unnecessary risks. Ideally the patient should be decontaminated immediately, even before entry into the hospital. Laboratories and other facilities using potentially dangerous chemicals should have flood showers. The criteria for flow and design of such showers is suggested in many manuals of laboratory safety and is also listed in NIOSH (National Institute of Occupational Safety and Health) documents.

Very few chemicals cannot safely be washed off the skin with water, and even the reactive metals such as sodium (in small amounts) are probably best washed with a flooding stream of water such that the heat from the exothermic reaction of the metal with water will be rapidly dissipated.

Curreri et al.[11] reviewed statistics from the Brooks Army Medical Center, Institute of Surgical Research. Table 12–2 is adapted from their papers.

Both groups of patients had 10.5 percent third degree burns. The difference in the two groups suggests that chemical burns may heal more slowly, but also the extent of injury may have been underestimated more frequently in chemical burns than in thermally induced injuries, and that there may have been injuries to other organ systems causing longer hospitalization.

Several factors, as alluded to above, are involved in determining the severity of the burn. In addition, some of these factors may also determine

TABLE 12–2. EXTENT OF INJURY, MORTALITY, AND HOSPITALIZATION OF CHEMICALLY INDUCED BURNS VERSUS ALL BURNS

Patient Group	Burn (%)	Mortality (%)	No. of Days
Chemical burns	19.5	5.4	104
All burns	28.5	19.3	74

% burn is % total body burn (all degrees); No. of days is total number of hospital days.
(From Curreri PW, et al., 1970, with permission.[11])

the likelihood of injury to other organ systems. These factors include (1) the strength or concentration of the agent, (2) quantity, (3) manner and duration of the contact, (4) extent of tissue penetration, and (5) mechanism of toxicity.

It must be remembered that injury continues until the chemical is inactivated by reaction with cellular components. Chemicals which cause denaturation of essential membrane proteins, enzymes, or cause interruption of essential metabolic pathways may have effects that are substantially delayed. Some agents may require metabolism to effect their toxicity and for that reason may cause a delayed reaction. Some chemicals, including drugs, may induce a severe allergic reaction which may be delayed. This injury may be otherwise indistinguishable clinically from other burns.

Ammonia may be studied as a representative chemical causing significant injury. Ammonia is a pungent gas. It is a strong alkali and is very soluble in water. It is relatively nonpolar as a gas. Ammonia causes liquefaction necrosis of tissues. Severe ophthalmic injuries occur from ammonia.

Because ammonia is a relatively small molecule and because of the alkalinity of ammonia in solution, it is an extremely hazardous solution or vapor if introduced into the eye. It readily penetrates tissue membranes and causes deep injury. Blindness may occur after ophthalmic exposure. Ammonia "burns" of the eye should be treated with immediate irrigation of the eye which may be continued for 24 hours.

The injury due to ammonia exposure is also dependent on the concentration and duration of exposure. Close et al. demonstrated that high concentration short exposures produced injuries in the upper airways which were treated with tracheal intubation or tracheostomy without long-term sequelae.[12,13] The lower dose, longer exposure was able to produce injuries at the lower lungs which were permanent.

The duration of contact with a chemical should be minimized as much as possible, early removal of contaminated clothing, and copious irrigation before transport are essential. The morbidity of chemical burns was considerably less in patients who had early decontamination as compared to those who did not.[14]

In general, the mineral acids cause a coagulation necrosis whereas the alkalis cause a liquefaction necrosis. The effects of most acid burns are seen immediately (hydrofluoric acid is one example of an exception, however the injury is not really an "acid" injury). On the contrary, alkalis often cause delayed injury with extension of the injured area over time.

Many chemicals which cause skin injury may cause other injuries as well. *Phenol* burns are distinctive and the victim may readily absorb the phenol (or alkylated phenol) such that the victim's breath is tainted as the chemical is excreted via the lungs. The phenol compounds are central nervous system depressants. In addition, there may be injury to the kidneys and a rise in the activity of serum hepatic enzymes may be seen hours after a dermal exposure (Fig. 12-1). The injury from phenol may produce an anesthetic lesion due to the properties of the chemical. The injury due to phenol is characterized by coagulation of the tissues.

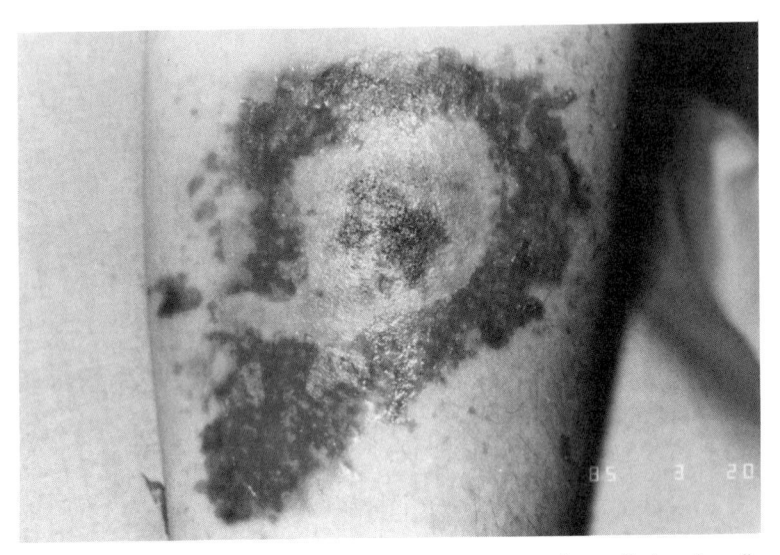

Figure 12–1. This 32-year-old concrete maintenance worker spilled a phenolic stripping compound on his calf. The ensuing phenol burn caused a beefy red appearance consistent with a second degree injury. However, he persisted in having severe muscle pain, increased calf girth and pain with walking. This persisted for several weeks and necessitated anti-inflammatory medication for resolution.

Formaldehyde can cause serious injuries to mucosal surfaces and can also cause injury to the skin. Sensitized individuals may develop severe dermatitis which can lead to the appearance of a burn.

Nitric acid causes a typical yellow appearance to the tissues. This is caused by the production of xanthoproteins by the nitric acid. *Sulfuric acid* typically produces a blackened eschar. *Picric acid* is an extremely corrosive material. *Chromic acid* is also an exceptionally corrosive chemical; the typical "chromeholes" attest to the deep penetration and total destruction of tissue caused by this acid. The chromeholes are deep diffuse ulcers with a relatively small necrotic central area on the skin (Fig. 12–2).

Acetic acid is a strong acid and has the ability to penetrate readily into tissues and cause severe injury. *Formic acid* may cause serious injuries which appear to spread even after the exposure has ceased. This may be partly due to the spreading of this materials by blister fluid. A group of children developed circumferential bullae of the fingers after an exposure to copper naphthenate 3 days earlier. The oozing blister fluid allowed new lesions to form. Certainly in this case the blister fluid was contaminating previously unexposed tissue causing a new but less severe injury.

The simple mineral acids, e.g., *hydrochloric,* cause an injury which is usually readily apparent early after the exposure. The injuries are generally

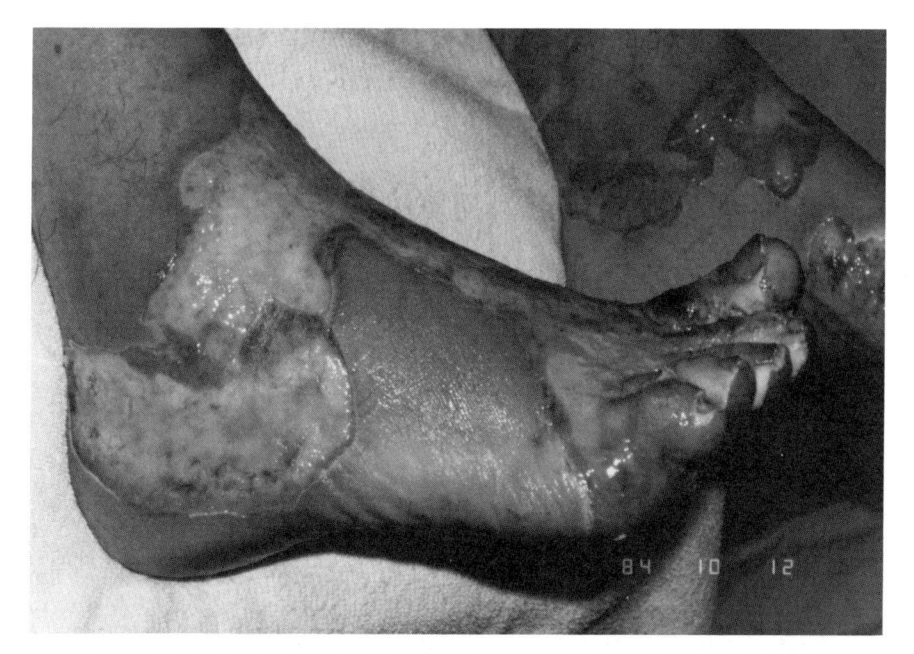

Figure 12-2. This individual spilled chromic acid on his feet (through his shoes); this injury is 48 hours postburn. Burns caused by chromic acid may cause renal failure on rare occasion.

not deep and there is no systemic injury from the chemical. This is partly because the acid is almost totally dissociated and the ions are unable to readily penetrate the tissues.

Picric acid has also been implicated as causing some mild toxicity to the kidney, however other chemicals are far more capable of systemic injury. Some of these include the hydrocarbons. *Methylene chloride* (dichloromethane) causes severe injuries to the skin and subjacent tissues. There may be liquefaction necrosis and an early black, leathery appearance to the skin as an eschar forms. Dichloromethane is unique as it is the only exogenous agent that is metabolized to carbon monoxide in vivo. Therefore, increased expired carbon monoxide and carboxyhemoglobin may be detected. Central nervous system depression can therefore result from the effect of the organic solvent as well as the metabolite, carbon monoxide. Electrocardiographic changes due to the effects of *halogenated solvents* may be combined with the ischemic effects of the decreased oxygen transport capabilities of the blood secondary to the production of carboxyhemoglobin.

Gasoline burns, due to prolonged skin contact (without ignition) are well documented.[15] The absorption of tetraethyl lead from dermal contact with leaded gasoline is well known. Unleaded gasoline contains 0.5 to 3 percent *benzene*, another absorbable, potentially toxic agent (although probably not a serious consideration with a one-time exposure to gasoline) (Fig. 12–3). The gasoline can cause central nervous system depression with the potential for further injury.

Cement is another etiologic factor in many severe burns and is often overlooked. The pH of wet cement is in the range of 12.5 to 14. Cement powder that gets onto wet skin or in the eyes must be copiously irrigated without any delay. Cement burns have been well documented.[16–20]

Many other agents may cause burns including antiseptics such as *thiomersol* and *povidone–iodine* if allowed to remain in contact with the skin for prolonged periods, with pressure and a pool of solution, as may occur in the operating room.[21] *Paraquat* has also been shown to cause burns.[22]

In addition to the systemic effects of *ethylene oxide* (nausea, vomiting, dizziness, and headache) and the potential for pulmonary injury of the inhaled gas, this material can cause dermal injury. The gas is heavier than air and can accumulate in low places, such as in shoes. Care must be taken to prevent this injury.[23]

The lacrimatory agents, such as *chloracetophenone*, can cause burns especially when there is prolonged contact in a confined space.[24] *Trichloracetic acid* is commonly used in laboratories and industry. It is utilized in the biochemical laboratory as it is an excellent agent to precipitate proteins—it is

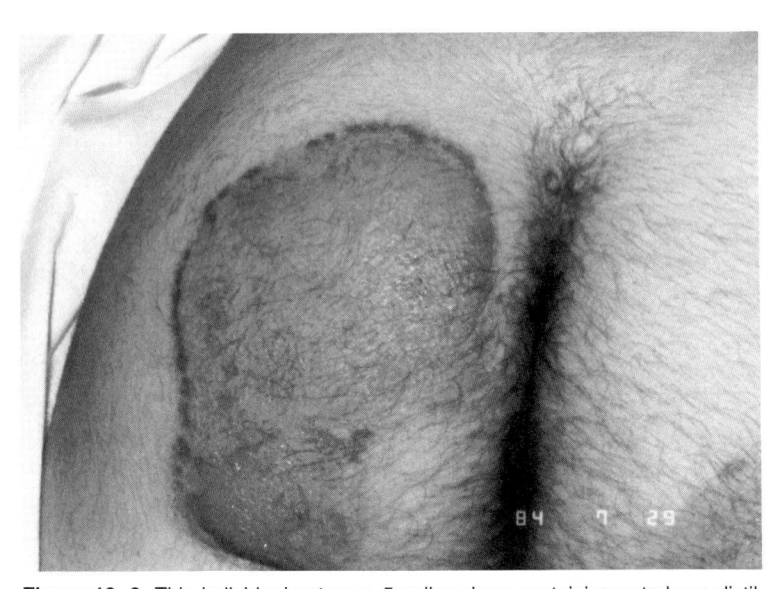

Figure 12–3. This individual sat on a 5-gallon drum containing petroleum distillates on a very hot day. There was some leakage of the petroleum distillates onto the surface of the can saturating the patient's pants. He had pain that evening and yet there was no indication of any injury when seen the next morning in an emergency room. By the following day, there was significant erythema and at 48 to 72 hours, the skin began to break down revealing a second degree burn. There was no apparent systemic toxicity resulting from this exposure.

equally effective in vivo. *Tungstic acid, phosphomolybdic,* and *tannic acids* can cause significant injury. The latter acid can also induce liver injury after dermal exposure.

As with dichloromethane, the *trichloroethanes, trichloroethylene,* and other organic solvents may cause burns. In addition to possible skin injury, *methyl (n)butyl ketone* and *n-hexane* may cause peripheral neuropathy after chronic exposure due to their common metabolites *2,5-hexanedione* and *2,5-hexanediol.*

Ointments left in contact with the skin for prolonged periods, especially when pressure is applied, may cause maceration of the skin and a burn appearance. *Hypochlorite* used in household bleach (5 percent) or a concentrate used for swimming pools may cause significant injury, however there is no pulmonary toxicity unless the material is mixed with an acid-liberating *chlorine gas.* Many household bleaches may be stabilized with *alkalis* resulting in high pH solutions. Aromatic amino and nitro compounds when absorbed may cause methemoglobinemia in addition to skin injury.

In addition to *tannic acid, phosphorus* may cause hepatic necrosis. Phosphorus and picric acid are nephrotoxic. Acid vapors, ammonia, and phosgene may cause pulmonary injury. The ability of a chemical to induce a pulmonary injury is dependent on the solubility, concentration, and form of the agent. The more water-soluble agents will be absorbed totally in the upper airways precluding alveolar injury. However, if in a respirable aerosol, the acid droplets may reach the parenchyma. Also, respirable particulate may have irritants adsorbed to their surfaces so that pulmonary injury may occur. Ammonia illustrates this point, and anyone with a history of inhalation of a significantly strong vapor or with burns on the face should be suspected of having injury to the upper airway with the potential for the development of edema which may compromise the airway.

Other typical agents that cause burns include *silver nitrate*, which is used medically for cautery, and causes a typical blackened area. *Permanganate* ions are extreme oxidizing agents and are capable of significant injury. *Oxalic acid*, if absorbed, may cause hypocalcemia and renal failure.

Nickel-containing materials may cause bullous reactions. *Metallic sodium, lithium,* or *potassium* cause severe desiccating injuries and, when they are in contact with water, cause severe exothermic reactions. (If they are to be removed with water a flood of cold water should be used.)

White phosphorus, although not available in this country in amateur pyrotechnics, is still used in several industries including combat munitions. This material must be removed rapidly with large amounts of water.

Cryogenic materials, such as *liquid nitrogen* or propane, may cause severe frostbite to the skin and subjacent tissues (Fig. 12–4).[25] Microvascular thrombosis is again an important factor in determining the extent of the injury. Most gases when escaping from a pressurized container through a narrow orifice will produce freezing of tissues (Joule–Thompson effect). Halogenated hydrocarbons, such as *freons,* can cause myocardial sensitization

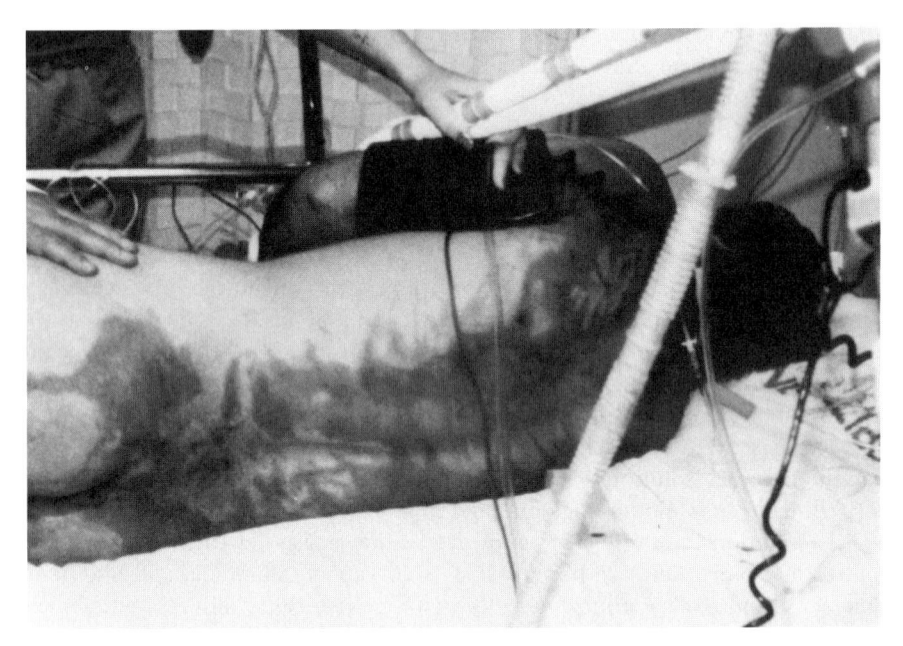

Figure 12–4. This individual was rendered unconscious due to a pure nitrogen atmosphere when he entered a confined space where there had been a substantial liquid nitrogen spill. The patient fell and was lying supine in a pool of liquid nitrogen for 5 to 10 minutes. These injuries seen several hours after the accident eventually resulted in severe frostbite injuries as deep as the spinal processes.

with subsequent ventricular arrhythmias from endogenous or exogenous sympathetic agents (epinephrine should be avoided with the intoxication by any halogenated hydrocarbon).

Hydrofluoric acid is used in many industries for cleaning fabrics (rust removal), metals, as well as glass etching, and in the manufacture of silicon chips for the electronics industry. It is also used in dental offices. The effect of hydrofluoric acid is largely corrosive. Fluoride is the most electronegative element and, as such, it is really a relatively weak acid (dissociation constant about 1000 times less than hydrochloric or hydrobromic acid). Despite this, Harris et al.,[26] and Iverson et al.,[27] state that hydrofluoric acid is "one of strongest inorganic acids known." In terms of dissociation and hydrogen ion concentration this is not true. It is, however, one of the most corrosive materials known.

Because a large percentage of hydrofluoric acid is undissociated relative to other inorganic acids, the uncharged moiety is able to penetrate through cell membranes. In each tissue, a new equilibrium is established and free fluoride ion exerts its highly cytotoxic effects by reacting with essential proteins causing alteration of cellular membranes and the poisoning of enzymes such as enolase, thus blocking glycolysis via the Embden–Myerhoff pathway.

Biologically, only magnesium and calcium ions can precipitate the fluoride ion; thus in large body surface area exposures to hydrofluoric acid, hypocalcemia may occur and can be fatal.[28] Burns of the skin, even with only slight erythema, may cause injuries to subjacent structures if there is a delay in decontamination of the area.

Interestingly, weak solutions (less than 20 percent hydrofluoric acid) may cause more significant injuries than concentrated material. This is because the strong hydrofluoric acid creates immediate pain as a result of the pH, thus acting as a warning property and alerting the victim to wash the area. Conversely, the weak solution does not provide any immediate pain and the injury goes undetected for a prolonged period of time (up to 24 to 36 hours) at which time the hydrofluoric acid has had the opportunity to penetrate deeply into the tissues. The acid also can become sequestered around the nail and beneath it. This commonly causes significant injury to this area, and ulceration of the nail bed may occur unless the nail is removed early (Figs. 12–5 and 12–6). This is usually heralded by periungual pain, erythema, and swelling. Typically, the individual has been working with a dilute solution and discovers a pinhole in the tip of a finger of a glove, creating an injury to the distal potion of the finger.

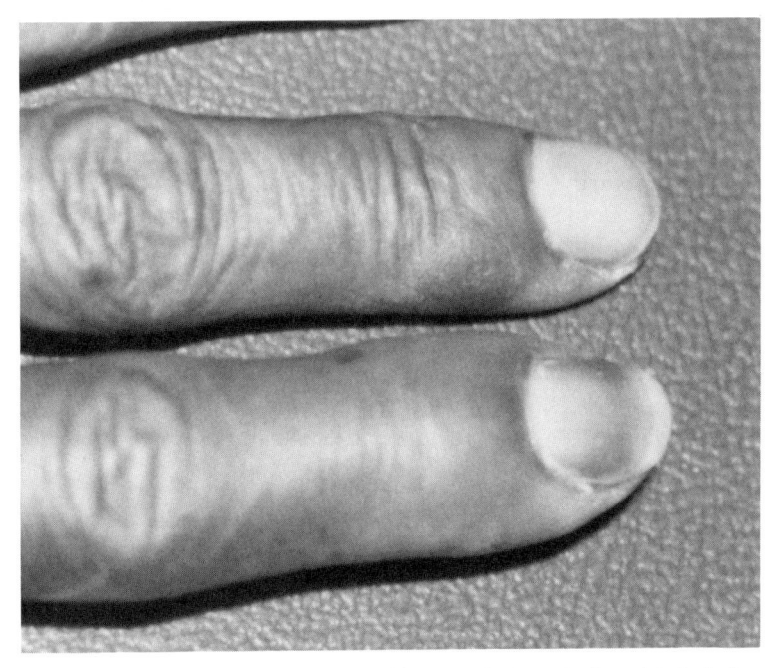

Figure 12–5. This female computer chip manufacturer had a pinhole in her protective glove allowing 2.5 percent hydrofluoric acid to come in contact with her distal index finger for a period of hours. Unfortunately the nature of the injury was not appreciated by the initial treating physicians who applied Silvadene Cream and a bandage. The patient continued to have pain and subungal discoloration.

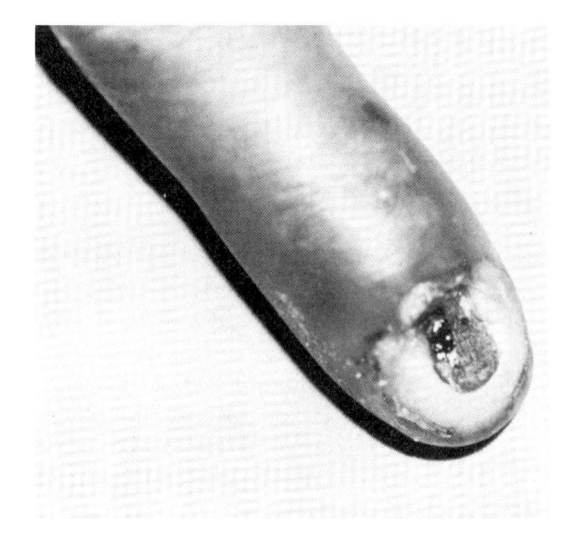

Figure 12–6. Several weeks after the injury, there was significant tissue loss and the distal phalanx is exposed and necrotic. The patient underwent amputation of the distal phalanx of the index finger.

Hydrofluoric acid injuries should be divided into categories in terms of the strength of the agent. The most concentrated acid is 70 percent or 22 molar. Strong concentration is considered 50 to 70 percent. Twenty to 50 percent is considered intermediate, and 1 to 20 percent is weak. Injuries with the weak acid, as pointed out, may be severe if there is delay in removing the material from the body surface. Intermediate acid injuries often go unnoticed for a brief time, but the pain soon alerts the patient to seek attention. These injuries are not usually severe unless the pain is unheeded. The strong acid usually produces immediate pain; however, if the material is not removed very quickly, deep injury is likely. Inhalation of hydrofluoric acid vapors may cause serious pulmonary injury. Hydrofluoric acid may be liberated from certain fluorosilicates and other fluoride-containing compounds (heating of fluorocarbons or Teflon above 350°C).

Osteolysis has occurred after exposure of skin overlying bony prominences to hydrofluoric acid. The injured area may initially appear erythematous and swollen. After several hours, there may develop a blanched area which may progress to a necrotic zone. These injuries are frequently full thickness. Certainly, weak solutions which are rapidly removed, probably will not cause significant injury.

Treatment

The treatment of chemical burns demands prompt removal of the offending agent. Therefore immediate removal of contaminated garments is mandatory. The area should be *flooded* with water. Do not delay decontamination by searching for specific neutralizing or buffering agents. With alkali burns, prolonged irrigation has been advocated. Always copiously irrigate the eyes as the obvious burns of the skin with associated pain may allow catastrophic ophthalmic injuries to be occult. Even if liquid ammonia does not get in the eyes, the vapors from a liquid injury of the body may cause eye injury.

Further general treatment includes dilution, neutralization, and debridement. All blisters are considered contaminated and are debrided. Systemically, a search for remote injury should be undertaken, preferably with the consultation of a toxicologist familiar with the effects of the chemicals or through the services of a poison control center. Enhancement of excretion of toxic materials, if absorbed, may be necessary. Antidotes in rare cases are indicated (calcium injection for oxalate or hydrofluoric acid injuries to combat hypocalcemia). A recent review article details the factors governing cutaneous absorption of chemicals.[29]

Recall that absorption will be greater through thin skin, highly vascular areas, and skin which has been damaged. Abrasions, lacerations, defatting (as occurs after exposure to many solvents such as diethyl ether), occlusive dressings, prolonged exposures (including bullae), lipid solubility, concentration, and exposed surface area all determine the degree of local injury and absorption into the bloodstream. These facts also give the clues to treatment.

Substances such as phenols, which are highly lipid soluble, are best removed from the skin using mineral oil which will absorb more phenol per milliliter than will water. Binding may be used to neutralize hydrofluoric acid by using magnesium sulfate soaks to the area. The resulting magnesium fluoride is precipitated. Recall that the hydrofluoric acid may penetrate cell membranes but that magnesium sulfate is ionized and will not penetrate through tissues.

The treatment of hydrofluoric acid burns includes soaking the affected surfaces with magnesium sulfate (Epsom salts) or calcium salts after copious water irrigation. Many facilities prepare a 2.5 percent calcium gluconate gel which is highly effective. If pain persists after 45 minutes of topical application, a subcutaneous infiltration with calcium gluconate may be indicated. This is also true with injuries due to very concentrated (greater than 50 percent) solutions. Although other substances (Zephiran, alcohol, and other substances) have been championed for topical use, I choose magnesium sulfate (if calcium gluconate gel is unavailable) because it is probably at least as effective as anything else, inexpensive, and readily available. If Epsom salts are not readily available in the hospital, an ampule (injectable—usually available on cardiac "crash" carts) of magnesium sulfate may be used.

The use of calcium salts for injection dates to the 1930s [30-34] and has been controversial ever since then. Harris and Rumack,[26] reported that magnesium ions were more effective than calcium ions when injected. However, their study was invalidated by poor experimental design leading to a seven- to eightfold greater concentration of magnesium ions than calcium ions. (They used equal volumes of 10 percent solutions of magnesium sulfate versus calcium gluconate. Specific ion molarity should have been used, not a percent weight volume solution.)

We find that those patients with exposures to weak solutions, or short exposures to intermediate strength solutions, are rendered pain free after aggressive topical treatment and do not require infiltration. Exposures to concentrated solutions, or prolonged exposures to intermediate (greater than 30 minutes) or weak (several hours) solutions probably will require injection. Other mitigating circumstances include the location of the burn; bony prominences, underlying nerves or cartilage may require early injection.

However, the injection is not without risk. Calcium infiltration may cause necrosis of tissues itself, and therefore overzealous administration is worse than no injection at all. The area to be injected should not be anesthetized, as the relief of pain, which is usually rapid and distinct, signals the termination of injection. Return of pain several hours later may require repeated injections. The digits should not receive more than 0.5 cc of solution per phalanx as the increased tissue pressure coupled with the edema from the injury may cause pressure necrosis. The area involved should be elevated. When injecting an area, the finest gauge needle available should be used (a 30 gauge is ideal, a 27 gauge is acceptable). Currently, the medical community varies in injecting these injuries; some physicians inject them all, others fail to inject any. Some moderate course should be dictated by clinical judgment.

When the injury overlies osseous structures, a baseline x-ray should be otained. If the injury involves the ungual area, the nail must be removed before any topical therapy can be employed. Failure to do this has resulted in ulceration of the nail bed and resulting nail deformity. In general, if there is a periungual erythematous halo, swelling, or pain, the nail should be removed. All blisters from hydrofluoric acid burns should be considered contaminated and should be debrided.

Another specially treated chemical injury is that of white phosphorus burns. The particles need to be excised, but are often hard to see as the white particles are embedded in whitened, avascular tissue. The area should be painted with a 1 percent solution of copper sulfate; this will cause the granules to turn a pale blue making debridement easier. Copper sulfate is not the treatment, but rather aids in the identification of the residual material. Soldiers burned with white phosphorus in Viet Nam were immersed in copper sulfate, and some died of hemolytic anemia induced by copper toxicity. Again, as with calcium infiltration, the antidote should not be more noxious than the original offending agent.

SUMMARY

This chapter has not attempted to provide an exhaustive treatise on the evaluation and treatment of nonthermal injuries. Rather, by studying the physics and pathophysiology of electrical and selected chemical burns and their treatment, the clinician can understand the principles governing the nature and severity of the injury.

Prompt removal from exposure is essential and this must be accomplished in a way that does not compromise the rescuer. The extent of injury is electrical and chemical burns may be misleading, usually underestimated.

In addition to the treatment of the local injury, the physician must be alert to associated injuries peculiar to the offending agent. With electrical injuries, insults to vital organs, as well as ruptured viscus, musculoskeletal injuries, and bleeding must be looked for. In chemical injuries, the potential for systemic poisoning must be considered and potential target organs identified depending upon the chemical and the circumstances of exposure.

Delayed local and systemic effects are common with these types of injuries. Hemorrhage, central nervous system disorders, and cataracts may occur after electrical shock. Chemical injury may induce late injuries to almost any organ system depending upon the agent involved. In addition, certain agents are carcinogens, or may cause reproductive hazards, terratologic effects, or sensitization (e.g., formaldehyde, isocyanates); however, these complications usually occur only with chronic exposures.

Therefore, it is essential that the treating physician obtain a thorough history from the patient or witnesses in order to determine the likely complications. Injuries of this type may produce disastrous results if the complications are not anticipated. Finally, hospital personnel should be trained in proper decontamination, with special attention to protection of the health care team so that they are not exposed to noxious agents secondarily.

REFERENCES

1. Somogyi E, Tedeschi CG: Injury by electrical force. In Tedeschi, Eckert, Tedeschi (eds.): Forensic Medicine. Philadelphia, Saunders, 1977
2. Silversides J: Neurological sequelae of electrical burns. Can Med Assoc J 91:195, 1964
3. Robinson NW, Masters FW, Forest WJ: Electrical burns: A review of and analysis of 33 cases. Surgery 57:385, 1965
4. Weeks AW, Alexander L: The distribution of electric current in the animal body: An experimental investigation of 60 cycle alternating current. J Ind Hyg Toxicol 21:517, 1939
5. Barber JW: Delayed bone and joint changes following electrical injury. Radiology 99:49, 1971
6. Hunt JL, Sato RM, Baxter CR: Acute electric burns. Arch Surg 115:434, 1980
7. Wang XW, Zoh W: Arterial injuries in electrically burned upper limbs and effects of early reconstruction of blood circulation to the wrist. Burns 8:379, 1982
8. Jelenko C: Chemicals that burn. J Trauma 14:65, 1974
9. Lewis GK: Chemical burns. Am J Surg 98:928, 1959
10. Dickerson RE, Gray HB, Haight GP: Chemical Principles. Menlo Park, Calif., Benjamin/Cummings, 1979
11. Curreri PW, Asch MJ, Pruitt BA: The treatment of chemical burns: Specialized diagnostic, therapeutic, and prognostic considerations. J Trauma 10:634, 1970
12. Dalton ML, Bricker DL: Anhydrous ammonia burns of the respiratory tract. Tex Med 74:51, 1978

13. Close LG, Catlin FI, Cohn AM: Acute and chronic effects of anhydrous ammonia burns on the respiratory tract. Arch Otolaryngol 106:151, 1980
14. Leonard JG: Chemical burns: Effect of prompt first aid. J Trauma 22:420, 1982
15. Simpson JB, Cruse CW: Gasoline immersion injury. Plast Reconstr Surg 67:54, 1981
16. Skiendzielewski JJ: Cement burns. Ann Emerg Med 9:316, 1980
17. Flowers FW: Burn hazard with cement. Br Med J 1(6122):1250, 1978
18. Greening NR, Tonry JR: Burn hazard with cement (letter). Br Med J 2(6148):1370, 1978
19. Fisher AA: Cement burns resulting in necrotic ulcers due to kneeling on wet cement. Cutis 23:272, 1979
20. Whiting RE: Alkali burns caused by contact with cement. Pa Med 80:48, 1977
21. Hodgkinson DJ, Irons GB, Williams TJ: Chemical burns and skin preparation solutions. Surg Gynecol Obstet 147:534, 1978
22. Withers EH, Madden JJ Jr, Lynch JB: Paraquat burns of the scrotum and perineum. J Tenn Med Assoc 72:109, 1979
23. Taylor JS: Dermatologic hazards from ethylene oxide. Cutis 19:189, 1977
24. Thorburn KM: Injuries after the use of chloracetophenone in a confined space. Arch Environ Health 37:182, 1982
25. Hicks LM, Hunt JL, Baxter CR: Liquid propane cold injury. J Trauma 19:701, 1979
26. Harris JC, Rumack BH, Bregman DJ: Comparative efficacy of injectable calcium and magnesium salts in the therapy of hydrofluoric acid burns. Clin Toxicol 18:1027, 1981
27. Iverson RE, Laub DR, Madison MS: Hydrofluoric acid burns. Plast Reconstr Surg 48:107, 1971
28. Tepperman PB: Fatality due to acute systemic fluoride poisoning following a hydrofluoric acid skin burn. J Occup Med 22:691, 1980
29. Webster RC, Maibach HI: Cutaneous pharmacokinetics. Drug Metabol Rev 14:169, 1983
30. Paley A, Seifter J: Treatment of experimental hydrofluoric acid corrosion. Soc Exper Biol Med 46:190, 1941
31. Jones AT: The treatment of hydrofluoric acid burns. J Ind Hyg Toxicol 21:205, 1939
32. Blunt CP: Treatment of hydrofluoric acid skin burns by injection of calcium gluconate. Ind Med Surg 33:869, 1964
33. Wilson GA, Sanger RG, Boswick JA: Accidental hydrofluoric acid burns of the hand. J Am Dent Assoc 99:57, 1979
34. Shewmake SW, Anderson BG: Hydrofluoric acid burns. Arch Dermatol 115:593, 1979

CHAPTER 13
Pediatric Considerations
Naomi Uchiyama and John German

Burn constitutes the second most common cause of death during childhood, ranking next to motor vehicle accidents. Of approximately 300,000 Americans hospitalized with burns each year, 20 percent are children.[1] At the University of California, Irvine Medical Center Burn Unit in 1982, children less than 12 years of age accounted for 28 percent of the burn admissions.[2] Additionally, many more children are treated as outpatients (69 percent of all burned children at our institution in 1982). Physical and psychological morbidity in these children is profound.

EPIDEMIOLOGY

Age and Sex
The majority of burns in childhood occur in children less than 5 years of age (84 percent in our series).[2] The peak incidence is in the 1- to 2-year age group.[3,4] The curious and adventurous nature of this toddler age group, coupled with unsteady motor development, makes these children accident prone in general. In all series, incidence in boys outnumber that in girls.

Types of Burn
Scalds comprise the major cause of burns in children, ranging from 42 to 70 percent[2,4-6] in comparison to 20 percent in adults.[7] Spillage of scalding liquid is the greatest hazard in toddlers (Table 13–1). At our institution, scald burns accounted for 58 percent of the burns in children who were hospitalized as

TABLE 13-1. BURN INJURY: CHILDREN

Types of Burn	Percentage
Scald	57.5
Contact	25
Flame	8
Abrasion/friction	3.5
IV infiltration	2
Chemical	2
Sunburn	1.5
Electrical	0.5

well as those treated as outpatients. Spillage of hot food or beverage such as coffee and soup caused 54 percent of the scald burns, spillage of hot water in 36 percent, and hot grease or oil in 10 percent.[2] Most of these accidents occur in the kitchen.[5,7] Tap water scald burns are associated with a greater morbidity and mortality than spillage of hot liquids.[8] This type of burn occurs when a child's foot, hand, or buttock is submerged in hot water in a bathtub or sink.

Burns from contact with hot objects such as steam irons, heaters, and ovens constitute the second most common type of burn.[2] Other causes of burn injury in children include flammable liquids, matches, house fires, and electrical cords.[7] The incidence of clothes fire has decreased in recent years due to the use of flame-retardant fabric. Electric mouth burns caused by an electric cord is, unfortunately, a burn peculiar to the toddler age group.

MANAGEMENT

One of the most important concepts in the management of children with burns is that the child is not always a little adult but has his or her own unique physiologic, psychological, and developmental characteristics that are different from those in adults. In this section, these differences will be discussed. Otherwise, the management of burn injuries is as outlined elsewhere in the book.

Estimation of Burn Wound Size
Children have a relatively larger head and smaller trunk and legs in comparison to adults. Thus, the "rule of nine" (Fig. 13–1) must be modified for different age groups: ages 1 to 4 years, 5 to 9 years, and 10 to 14 years. Berkow's formula or its modification can be used.

Admission Criteria
Children with second or third degree burns that are greater than 10 percent of their body surface area (BSA) are hospitalized. A burn involving more than 5 percent of the BSA in a child less than 2 years of age constitutes admission

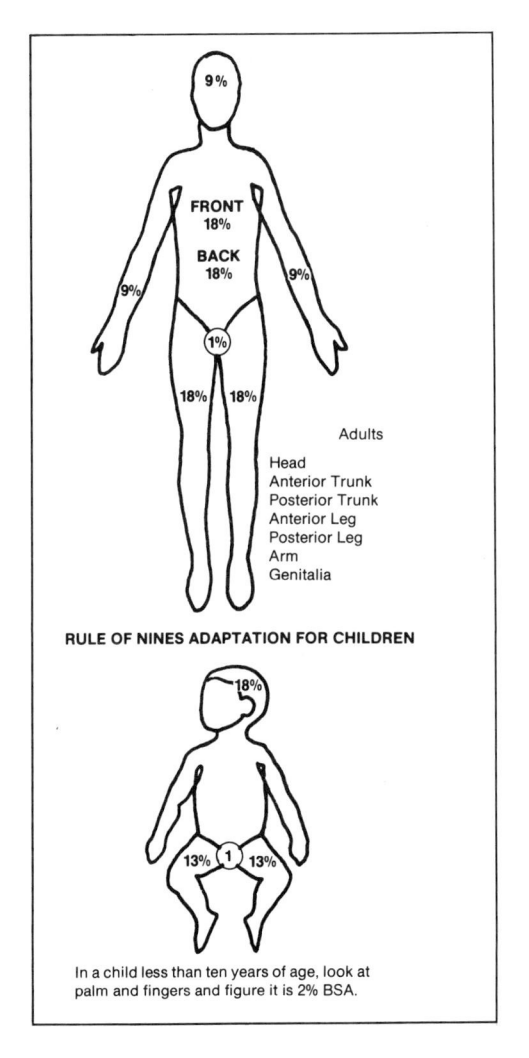

Figure 13-1. Estimation of burn wound size, Rule of Nines.

criteria at some centers.[1] Any child with burn involving the face, hands, feet, or perinium is hospitalized. Additionally, children with suspected inflicted burn, i.e., suspected battered child syndrome (BCS) may be admitted for further investigation.

Fluid Requirement

Children have a larger surface area in proportion to weight compared with adults, resulting in an increased daily fluid requirement. Between 1 and 3 years of age, this requirement may be three to four times that of an adult when calculated on a weight basis.[4] The amount of fluid is determined not only by the degree and the extent of the burn, but also the size of the child.

Daily fluid requirement consists of maintenance fluid plus replacement fluid for the losses. Various formulas have been devised to calculate the fluid deficit. One such formula is the Parkland formula:

4 ml per kg is given for each percent of BSA burn

Estimation of daily maintenance requirement may be based on the meter square, caloric, or body weight methods. In the meter square method:

1500 to 2000 ml of fluid is required for each square meter of surface area

To calculate the daily fluid on weight basis, the following formula is used:

100 ml per kg for the first 10 kg + 50 ml for each kg above 10 kg + 20 ml for each kg above 20 kg

A preferred approach by some people is to use the weight method for children less than 10 kg and the meter square one for the older child.

It must be emphasized that these formulas are approximations and should be used only as guides. It is of paramount importance to observe and constantly monitor blood pressure, pulse, urine output, and preferably central venous pressure, and adjust the fluid administration according to these parameters. Fluids should be given to maintain a urine output greater than 1 ml per kg per hour in the small child and 10 to 30 ml per hour in the older child.

Nutritional Requirement
Calorie requirements in burned children are higher with respect to size when compared to adults. Children need additional calories for growth. Various formulas have been devised, as with fluid requirements. One way is to give 60 kcal per kg plus 40 kcal for each percent of burn per day. Another method[9] is based on the meter square:

1800 kcal per M^2 + 2200 kcal per M^2 of BSA burned each day

It is rare to see a small child who is able to drink enough milk or formula orally to meet the high calorie requirement. It then will be necessary to use nasogastric tube feeding or intravenous hyperalimentation. The child should be weighed daily. The importance of daily adequate nutritional intake cannot be overemphasized. A dietitian is an essential part of the burn team.

Psychosocial Aspects
It is important to recognize in children the various developmental stages with associated behavior patterns in order to understand the child's coping mechanism in handling his or her stress such as pain and fear. For example, a 9-month-old normally has a fear of strangers and clings to the mother. When this child sustains a burn injury, this clinging behavior may be exaggerated. Fear of demons and ghosts in a normal 3-year-old may result in anxieties and nightmares in a child under stress. A previously toilet-trained 4-year-old may regress in bladder control upon hospitalization with burn.

A child with a burn injury is an integral part of the family and requires the maximal emotional support from the family. Family dynamics and its coping skills must be fully assessed. When burn injury in the child adds an extra stress on an already unstable family, decompensation may result. Family support in such circumstances is of utmost importance.

A Team Approach

Children hospitalized with a burn injury are cared for by a multidisciplinary team consisting of various professionals such as nurses, occupational and physical therapists, social workers, nutritionists, child psychologists, surgeons, and pediatricians. Additional members may include school teachers and play therapists according to the needs of the child. The nursing staff plays a key role in such a team. Everyone must remain cognizant of the needs of the child as well as the family.

Battered Child Syndrome (BCS)

Children with BCS have burn injuries that are not accidental but are inflicted upon them. The frequency of nonaccidental burn as a manifestation of child abuse has been 9 to 11 percent.[10,11] Sixteen percent of children admitted to the Children's Hospital of the Michigan Burn Center were recognized as having inflicted burns.[10] Peak age incidence is 13 to 24 months which is the same age distribution as in accidental burns.

Multiple cigarette burns and hot iron burns are considered as obvious forms of inflicted burns. However, the majority of nonaccidental burns have been due to scalds (87 to 100 percent).[11,12] Intentional scalding burns are similar in appearance to accidental burns and can easily be overlooked. A thorough initial history and physical examination become the most valuable tools in identifications of inflicted burns.[10] Criteria that can be used to confirm suspicion of child abuse by nonaccidental burns were developed by Stone et al.[10]:

1. Multiple hematoma or scars in various stages of healing
2. Concurrent injuries or evidence of neglect, such as malnutrition
3. History of prior hospitalization for "accidental" trauma
4. An unexplained delay between the time of injury and first attempt to obtain medical attention
5. Burns appearing older than the alleged day of the accident
6. An account of the accident not compatible with the age and ability of the patient
7. Responsible adults alleging that there were no witnesses to the "accident" and that the child was merely discovered to be burned
8. Relatives bringing the injured child to the hospital
9. The burn attributed to action of a sibling or other child
10. The injured child being excessively withdrawn, submissive, overly polite, or does not cry during painful procedures
11. Scalded hands or feet, often symmetrical, appearing to be full thick-

ness in depth suggesting that extremities were forcibly immersed and held in hot liquid
12. Isolated burns of the buttocks that in children could hardly be produced by accidental means

When a parent expresses inappropriate or detached emotional concern for the burned child, the suspicion of a nonaccidental burn must be considered.[11] Parents of abused children were most often abused as children themselves. Family instability and an inability to deal with stress in a crisis are important contributing factors.[11]

PREVENTION

A large proportion of burns in children is preventable. Public education coupled with legislation have been successful in some areas of preventive measures such as a ban on firecrackers and the use of flame-retardant fabrics in children's clothing. Increased public and private sector awareness is needed in the area of tap water scalds which can be avoided by lowering the thermostat temperature of household hot water tanks to less than 125°F.

Home safety in the area of burn prevention must be taught to the parents as a part of anticipatory guidance during well-child care visits as well as emergency room visits. Prevention of electrical burn by toddlers is stressed already in most of the visits to the pediatricians and family practitioners. Emphasis needs to be placed on scald burn prevention, especially in the kitchen. Young children must be kept out of the cooking area in the kitchen. Any container with hot liquids such as coffee, hot chocolate, or soup must be kept away from the reach of curious toddlers.

Every effort must be made to prevent burns in children. They suffer not only the acute pain and discomfort of the burn, but may suffer from the embarrassment of permanent disfigurement from the scars the rest of their lives that are certainly longer than the adults.

REFERENCES

1. Abston S: Burns in children. Clin Symposia 28:2, 1976
2. Uchiyama N, Madden JD, Duncan H, et al.: Epidemiology of burns in children (unpublished data)
3. Pegg SP, Gregory JJ, Hogan PG, et al.: Burns in childhood: An epidemiological survey. Aust NZ J Surg 48:365, 1978
4. Durtschi MB, Kohler TR, Finley A, et al.: Burn injury in infants and young children. Surg Gynecol Obstet 150:651, 1980
5. Joseph TP, Douglas BS: Childhood burns in South Australia A socioeconomic aetiological study. Burns 5:335, 1979
6. Smith EI: The epidemiology of burns. The cause and control of burns in children. Pediatrics 44:821, 1969

7. Jay KM, Bartlett RH, Danet R, et al: Burn epidemiology: A basis for burn prevention. J Trauma 17:943, 1977
8. Feldman KW, Schaller RT, Feldman JA, et al.: Tap water scald burns in children. Pediatrics 62:1, 1978
9. Hildreth M, Carvajal HF: Calorie requirements in burned children: A simple formula to estimate daily caloric requirements. J Burn Care Rehab 3:78, 1982
10. Stone NH, Rhinaldo L, Humphrey, CR, et al.: Child abuse by burning. Surg Clin North Am 50:1419, 1970
11. Hight DW, Bakalar HR, Lloyd JR: Inflicted burns in children. Recognition and treatment. JAMA 242:517, 1979
12. Ayoub C, Pfeifer D: Burns as a manifestation of child abuse and neglect. Am J Dis Child 133:910, 1979

PART VI
Recovery and Rehabilitation

CHAPTER 14
Nursing and the Burn Team
Suzanne E. Martinez

The specialty of burn nursing is a rewarding and challenging one. There is variety, independence, and recognition as a vital member of the burn team. The excitement of working in an area with constant, multifaceted advances in research is balanced by realization of the true value of basic nursing skills and tender loving care. Archambeault-Jones[1] points out that major burn patients require meticulous, comprehensive care if they are to survive. This care is delivered by a team of dedicated professionals. Of this group, only the nurse is with the patient 24 hours each day. The nurse's contribution to patient recovery is unquestioned.

BURN COMPLICATIONS

Children get burned as well as senior citizens and members of any other age group. Burn victims may also have been subjected to other trauma, such as fractures and chest, abdominal, or head injuries. Patients often suffer from a pre-existing or concurrent medical disease which may have caused the burn injury or may complicate treatment. Common medical problems include diabetes, seizure disorders, musculoskeletal, cardiac, pulmonary, metabolic diseases, and psychiatric disturbances. Nurses with a sound knowledge base in burn care must also be familiar with pathophysiology and current treatment methods of all these conditions.

TREATMENT

Every burn unit has a specific fluid resuscitation protocol to be followed during the initial phase of burn management. Within this protocol, parameters are established for determining effective fluid resuscitation. Nurses functioning in a critical care setting monitor the patient's physiologic status at least hourly to assure adequate fluid resuscitation. Use of pulmonary artery catheters and other hemodynamic monitoring equipment is not unusual. A clear understanding of the pathophysiology of burn injuries is essential. In order to function effectively at the bedside, a burn nurse must understand the relationship between burn injury and its effect on all body systems. The nurse must also be able to utilize the data he or she collects to maintain a stable hemodynamic state. Experienced burn nurses who function within a protocol and are able to titrate fluids based on their assessments enjoy a measure of independence when caring for the critically burned patient (Fig. 14-1).

Burn nurses have primary responsibility for the patient's daily wound care and nutritional management. Working with the dietician, nurses monitor caloric intake, temperature changes, serum electrolytes, daily weights, and the status of wound healing. Supplemental feedings are instituted early in burn management, and can be altered as necessary to prevent excessive weight loss and maintain electrolyte balance and optimum wound healing. Teaching the patient and his or her family the importance of nutrition and encouraging favorite foods brought from home is an excellent method of involving the family in patient care. Patience and persistence in helping the patient to feed him- or herself as soon as possible contributes to the return of hand and arm function.

Daily hydrotherapy and wound care are a major focus of burn management. Nurses function in this area as the team member who sees the wounds each day and is able to discern changes as they occur. The nurse must be able to identify changes and relate them to the clinical condition. Capillary damage and resultant edema can change the appearance of the wound in the early phase. The effect of inadequate nutrition on the burn is dramatic. Early signs of sepsis alter the burn surface and can be readily detected by an experienced clinician. In our burn unit, even the most critically ill patients receive hydrotherapy daily. Portable monitors and ventilators are used to provide uninterrupted observation of the patient's clinical status (Fig. 14-2).

Debridement

Debridement of the burn wound is accomplished on a daily basis by nurses using scissors and forceps to facilitate separation of eschar (Fig. 14-3). After the patient is physiologically stable and more accurate assessment of burn depth is possible, the wound may require tangential debridement. With the nurse responsible for coordination of effort, this may be accomplished in the hydrotherapy area. Ketamine is used for these sessions. Nursing responsibilities predebridement include collection of blood samples for hematocrit and platelet count, discontinuance of oral feedings early on the morning of debridement, and thorough explanation to the patient and the family regarding the debridement procedure and ketamine experience. During the procedure, nurses continue to monitor the patient's vital signs. Because of the rapid loss of heat through the burn surface, particular attention is paid to body temperature. Nurses assist in debridement using blunt debriders and the Weck knife (Fig. 14-4). Electrocautery is available. Transfusions are initiated as indicated by the amount of blood loss. Debridement is performed efficiently to maximize removal of eschar with minimal blood loss or drop in body temperature. Following debridement, the wounds are dressed and the patient returned to the burn unit for recovery. Postdebridement nursing care includes vital signs, observing the wound for unchecked bleeding, and providing a setting conducive to smooth emergence from anesthesia.

Graft and Donor Care

Graft and donor care are important aspects of wound care delivered by the burn nurse. Meticulous attention to the amount and type of exudate and graft adherence become the major focus of nursing care in the first few days postgrafting.

IMPORTANCE OF THE BURN NURSE

Pain Control

Of all members of the burn team, the nurse spends the most time with the patient. This validates the importance of her input to all aspects of burn care. One of the most valuable contributions in the nurse's work is his or her role in helping the patient with pain control. The concept of pain in burn management encompasses all areas. The pain of physical injury is compounded by the pain of therapy. Wagner[2] points out that the nurses from whom the patient seeks pain relief are also the ones who contribute to his or her pain. These varying reactions to each other establish a highly charged, but sound relationship. Emotional pain is always a part of circumstances resulting in burn injury. As with other domains, the nurse coordinates and evaluates the effort of other team members to effectively deal with the problem of pain control.

McCaffery[3] discusses the fact that although the physician orders pain medications for the patient, it is the nurse who administers them. Thus, the nurse has a considerable amount of power and responsibility in relation to the use of pain medication. Since most analgesics are ordered on a prn basis, it is the nurse who determines whether or not the medication should be given. It is the nurse who chooses which analgesic will be given when more than one is ordered.

Administration of prescribed analgesics is accompanied by careful observation of their effect on each patient. Use of agents to potentiate the effects of

UCI MEDICAL CENTER
ACUTE PHASE FLOW SHEET

Diagnosis _____
Surgery _____

Weight _____
Date _____
Time _____

PATIENT IDENTIFICATION

GLASGOW COMA SCALE

Pupil Size MM: 1 • 2 • 3 • 4 ● 5 ● 6 ● 7 ● 8 ● 9 ●

EYE OPENING
- Spontaneous — 4
- To Voice — 3
- To Pain — 2
- None — 1

VERBAL RESPONSE
- Oriented — 5
- Confused — 4
- Inappropriate — 3
- Incomprehensible — 2
- None — 1

MOTOR RESPONSE
- Obeys Command — 6
- Localizes Pain — 5
- Withdraw (Pain) — 4
- Flexion (Pain) — 3
- Extension (Pain) — 2
- None — 1

TOTAL GLASGOW COMA SCALE POINTS
- 14 - 15 = 5
- 11 - 13 = 4
- 8 - 10 = 3
- 5 - 7 = 2
- 3 - 4 = 1

TOTAL

Date _____

HEMODYNAMIC STATUS

Time: 0, 0130, 0200, 0230, 0300, 0330, 0400, 0430, 0500, 0530, 0600, 0630, 0700, 0730
Time: 0800, 0830, 0900, 0930, 1000, 1030, 1100, 1130, 1200, 1230, 1300, 1330, 140

- Temperature
- Heart Rate
- Systemic: Systolic / Diastolic
- CVP
- Pul'm Art: Systolic / Diastolic / Wedge
- Cardiac Output

SVR Formula
$SVR = \frac{(MAP - CVP) \; 80}{CO}$

$MAP = \frac{(SBP + [DBP]2)}{3}$

RESPIRATORY STATUS
- Airway
- RR
- Ventilator: Mode / Vt / Pressure Peak/End
- FiO₂
- Blood Gases: Sample Time / Source / pH / pCO₂ / pO₂ / O₂Sat / HCO₃ / B.E.

INTAKE
IV Solution Column
- Unit No.
- Blood
- Unit No.
- Blood Products
- #1
- #2

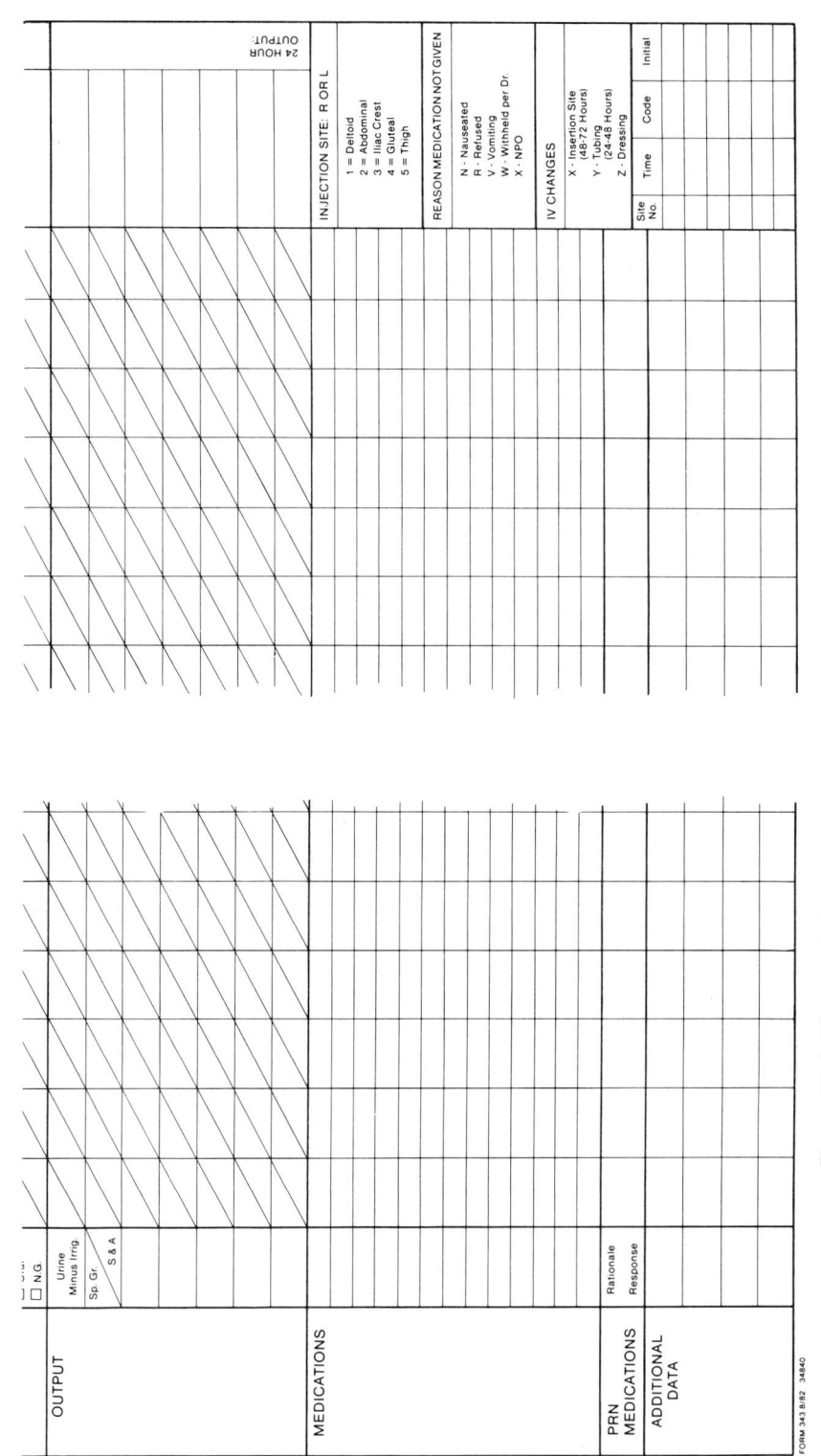

Figure 14–1. The sample flow sheet demonstrates the multiple parameters which may be assessed during the acute resuscitation of a burn injury.

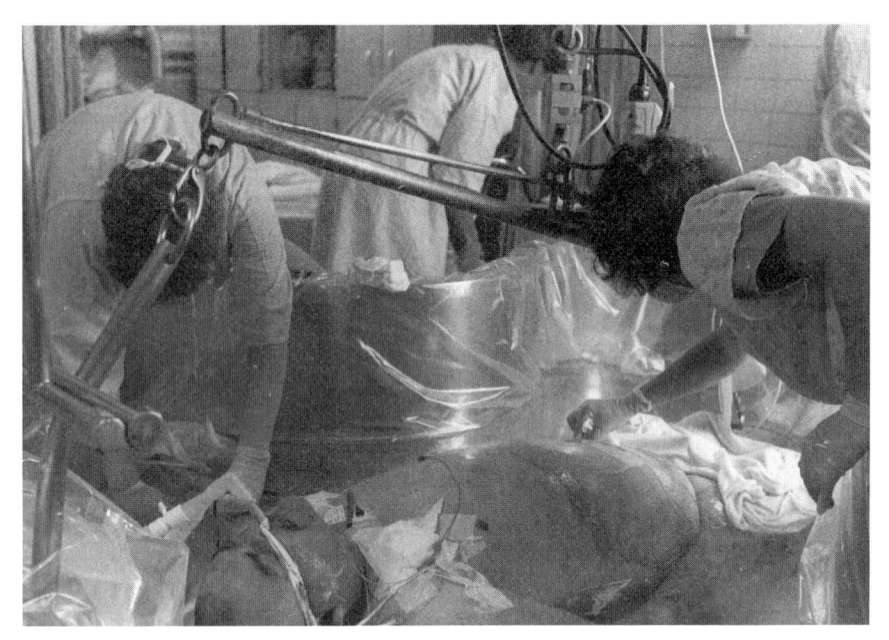

Figure 14-2. Critically ill patients may safely receive hydrotherapy under careful observation of experienced nurses and with appropriate equipment such as portable monitors and ventilators.

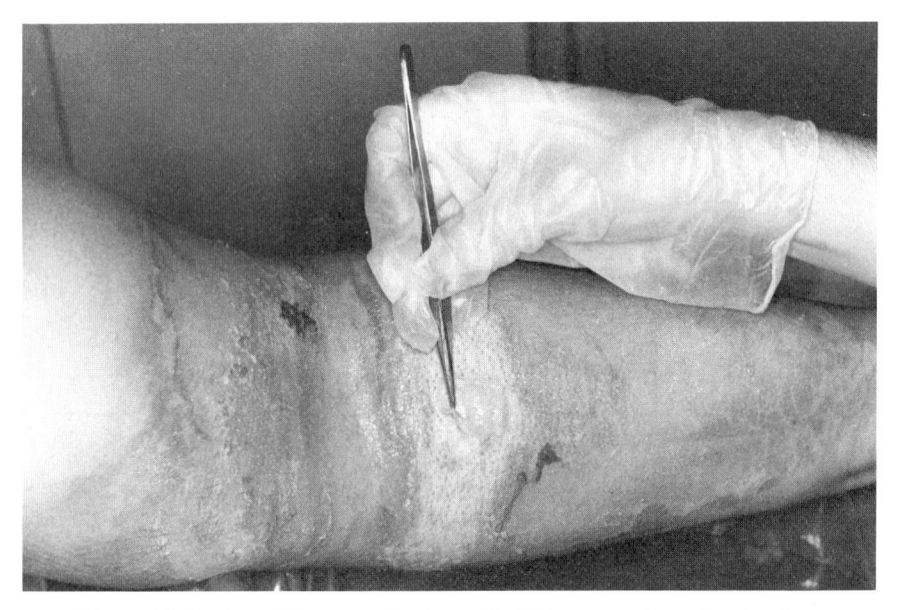

Figure 14-3. Use of forceps and scissors facilitates separation of eschar from the burn wound during the daily hydrotherapy procedure.

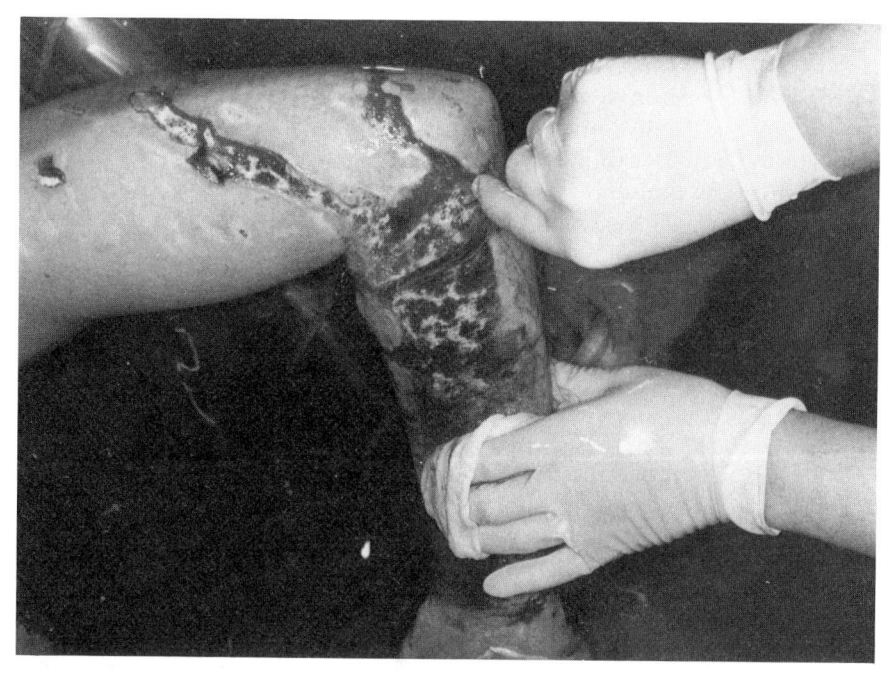

Figure 14-4. Debridement of the burn wounds with blunt instruments during ketamine anesthesia.

analgesics may be suggested. Timely administration of medications to produce optimum relief during painful therapy individualizes care.

Dealing with Discomfort

Use of tapes designed to assist the patient with relaxation technique are valuable alone or in conjunction with prescribed medications. Other forms of hypnosis, imagery, distraction, and physical comforting are utilized alone or in combination to promote a state in which the patient feels capable of dealing with discomfort.

In the area of pain management, the value of nursing expertise is demonstrated by the creative use of all methods of pain control. With experience, the nurse becomes more proficient in the use of these methods as well as providing a calm and supportive atmosphere. Advanced clinicians are adept at teaching the patient to initiate specific techniques independently. Family support can also be elicited and promotes further involvement in care.

Treatment of burns is a long-term endeavor. Burn nurses develop long and close relationships with their patients. Unlike other intensive care units where patients are transferred to less acute areas when stabilized, burn patients stay in the burn unit during their entire hospitalization, return to the same unit for outpatient care, and are readmitted to the burn unit for plastic and reconstructive procedures. Thus, staff and patients as well as their families become friends. Burn nurses are able to function as critical care practitioners, subacute and ambulatory care clinicians, as well as rehabilitation nurses. The psychosocial aspects of such long-term care are astounding. The patient and the family experience any or all of many emotions from anxiety and guilt to frustration and despair. These emotions may disappear, reappear, or change at any time throughout the course of treatment. Burn nurses must be able to effectively deal with the patients and their emotions as well as refer to the appropriate resource for psychotherapy or further emotional support. These challenges offered by the variety of nursing situations adds greatly to the continuing stimulation and interest that sustains burn nurses.

BURN CENTERS

The Burn Unit at the University of California, Irvine Medical Center is staffed mainly by registered nurses who provide all levels of care. There are more nurses assigned to the day shift to accommodate the hydrotherapy scheduled. One to two vocational nurses are also assigned to each shift. Burn technicians can be utilized to assist with practical, specialized techniques of wound and graft care.

Few hospitals employ graduate nurses in critical care areas, but require a minimum of 1 to 2 years of experience. The same is true of burn centers, although experience has shown that new graduates hired to burn units can learn, adapt, and function as effectively as nurses who have prior nursing experience. The professional requirements of licensure are equaled in importance by personal requirements of maturity, compassion, and endurance.

Nurse Orientation

Initial orientation incorporates basic critical care content as well as the specialized knowledge applicable to burn care. Orientation includes:

1. Certification in cardiopulmonary resuscitation
2. Safe use of specialized critical care and burn unit equipment such as hemodynamic monitoring equipment, Doppler, wick catheter, transcutaneous oxygen monitoring, and metabolic scale
3. Understanding of fluid resuscitation
4. Understanding of burn wound care
5. Competence in repiratory physiology and ventilator management, recognition of physiologic changes particular to the burn injury, and smoke inhalation
6. Understanding of the action, usual dosage, side effects, and toxicity of drugs used in the burn center such as morphine sulfate, meperidine hydrochloride, hydromorphine hydrochloride, acetaminophen with codeine, hydrocodone bitartrate and acetaminophen, diuretics, vasopressors, antibiotics, antihistamines, and drugs used in cardiac arrest

7. Understanding of the usual care and treatment of patients with
   a. Thermal, chemical, electrical, or abrasive injury to the skin
   b. Inhalation injuries
   c. Bacterial contamination or colonization of burn wounds
8. Understanding of and usual treatment for basic arrhythmias
9. Ability to obtain a nursing history, patient assessment, and formulate individualized care plans
10. Ability to perform venipuncture and initiate intravenous therapy
11. Develop expertise in identifying depth and percentage of burns

These goals are attained during a 4- to 6-week orientation which includes classroom learning and clinical experience on the unit with an experienced clinical partner. Critical care experience is gained by working in other intensive care units when critical patients are not available in the burn unit.

Advanced knowledge and skills which are developed and improved on a continuous basis include:

1. Competency in identification of patient condition changes and ability to take appropriate action
2. Ability to perform advanced standardized procedures such as arterial puncture, defibrillation, and cardiac output measurement
3. Ability to provide patient and family education on the hospital course and expectations following discharge
4. Increased ability to function as a member of the interdisciplinary burn team and coordinate patient care utilizing input from all members
5. Ability to troubleshoot equipment
6. Consultation on other nursing units regarding wound care
7. Education of other medical professionals on burn care
8. Public education regarding first aid for burns and fire prevention and safety

NURSE EDUCATION

Evaluation of burn nurse performance is accomplished through continued demonstration of clinical competence and maintenance of current continuing education which includes participation in burn related in-services.

Advanced degrees are not required for employment in the burn unit; however, many nurses do return to school for further education. Continuing education requirements mandated by law have some impact on the nurse's decision to return to school. However, burn nurses quickly become aware of the necessity and benefits of further education. The increased proficiency in psychosocial assessment and interactions as well as additional teaching skills are extremely helpful and can be utilized routinely in the long-term care of burn patients.

SUMMARY

Burn nursing is an exciting and challenging specialty. As in any area of the profession, there are drawbacks which make most situations less than ideal. By their nature, burn nurses are able to provide physical and emotional support to their peers as well as their patients which results in the delivery of high quality patient care and a warm, comfortable work environment.

REFERENCES

1. Archambeault-Jones C, Feller I: Burn nursing is nursing. In Wachtel T (ed): Current Topics in Burn Care. Rockville, Md., Aspen Systems Corp., 1983
2. Wagner MM (ed): Care of the Burn Injured Patient. Littleton, Mass., PSG Publishing, 1981
3. McCaffery M: Nursing Management of the Patint with Pain. Philadelphia, Lippincott, 1979

CHAPTER 15
Treatment of Joints and Scars

Robert M. Schneider and Shirley Simonton-Thorne

The burned patient's rehabilitation begins on the day of injury and may continue for several years. A therapist must be a part of the treatment team from day 1. While the physicians and nursing staff are working to stabilize the patient medically, the therapist is addressing the function of the patient by preventing stiffness and contractures.

The therapist's initial evaluation of the burned patient should include the following information which is essential for acute treatment planning: the location and depth of the burn, the presence and location of edema, hand dominance, type of employment, how the burn occurred, was it work related, and an initial active range of motion evaluation.

Therapy should begin immediately to overcome the many factors which can lead to permanent deformity. These include edema, scar formation, comfortable positioning, and the patient's fears of moving burned extremities. Therapeutic intervention initially includes positioning, splinting, active and passive exercises, and activities of daily living to prevent loss of range of motion. The therapist should encourage the patient to function independently as soon as possible. Establishing rapport between the patient and therapist is essential in accomplishing these goals.

The patient with severe burns will spend a significant amount of time in bed, therefore, proper positioning will be a major part of treatment. If the patient is permitted to position him- or herself in a comfortable, fetal, or flexed position, contractures and deformity are likely to be the result. Therefore, all body parts must be positioned in an antideformity position (Fig. 15–1).

As burn wounds heal, myofibroblasts within the skin contract is an effort

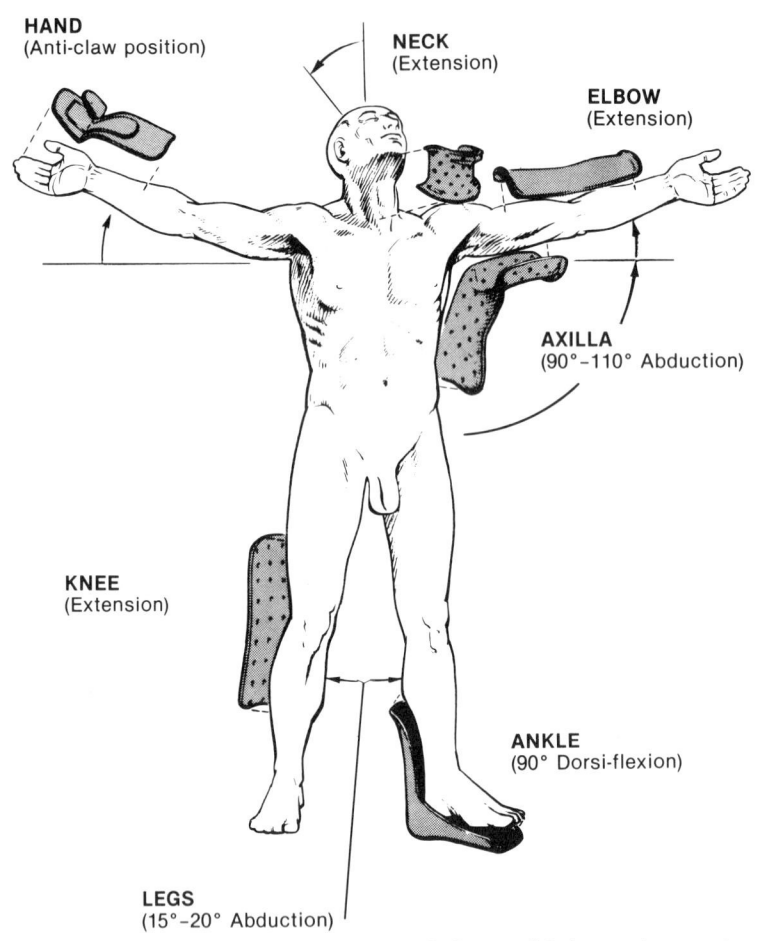

HAND (Anti-claw position)
NECK (Extension)
ELBOW (Extension)
AXILLA (90°–110° Abduction)
KNEE (Extension)
ANKLE (90° Dorsi-flexion)
LEGS (15°–20° Abduction)

Figure 15–1. Antideformity position with splinting to minimize postburn contractures.

to reduce the size of the wound and this can lead to hypertrophic scar formation.[1-3] If the burned area involves a joint flexor surface, a contracture can result in diminished range of motion. Generally, flexion and adduction are two positions to counteract. Extension and abduction will maintain skin length and prevent tightness.

Because edema often leads to loss of motion, edematous extremities should be elevated. In addition, active exercise will help reduce edema.

Splinting is indicated when positioning and active exercise are insufficient to prevent loss of range of motion.

The need for splints depends on the location of the burns. Any second or third degree burn which crosses a joint surface must be carefully evaluated for possible splinting. Splints are utilized in addition to active exercise and positioning. Complete immobilization is not recommended because it might cause joint stiffness. The occupational therapist should evaluate splints daily for proper fit and modify them as needed to accommodate increases in range of motion. Careful monitoring of all splints is necessary to identify any localized areas of redness and possible skin breakdown.

The hand is an exception to this. Hand splints are fabricated for all significant hand burns to prevent damage to the extensor mechanism of the proximal interphalangeal (PIP) joints, in addition to maintaining range of motion.

ACUTE TREATMENT

Hand–Dorsal

Potential Deformity. Burn "claw hand" deformity which consists of wrist flexion, metacarpophalangeal (MP) joint extension or hyperextension, proximal and distal interphalangeal (PIP and DIP) joint flexion, thumb adduction, and loss of hand arches.

Positioning. Wrist in 30 to 45 degree extension, MP joints in 70 to 90 degree flexion, PIP and DIP joints in full extension, and thumb in palmar abduction with interphalangeal (IP) joint extension. The entire hand should be elevated to minimize edema.

Splinting. Volar hand splints should be applied to all deep second or third degree hand burns within the first 24 hours postburn (Fig. 15–2). Burns that involve the dorsal hand, dorsal surface of PIP joints, and the edematous hand require splinting. The skin on the dorsum of the hand and PIP joints is thin and easily damaged in a burn injury. A severe dorsal hand burn can lead to destruction of the central slip of the extensor tendon resulting in boutonniere or buttonhole deformity.[4] This consists of flexion of the PIP joint with hyper-

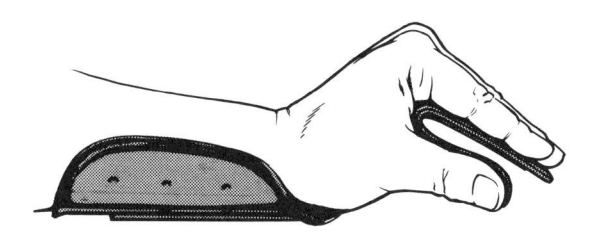

ANTI-CLAW POSITION
Wrist (30°–45° Extension)
Mp joints (70°–90° Flexion)
PIP and DIP joint (Extension)
Thumb (Opposition)

Figure 15–2. Volar hand splint in anti-claw position.

extension of the DIP joint. Because of its vulnerability, the PIP joint must be carefully maintained in extension until sufficient healing has occurred over its dorsal aspect to permit flexion.

Splinting the thumb in palmar abduction and IP joint extension will maintain the thumb-index web space, while providing a functional position.

The rationale for hand splinting postburn includes stretching the MP joint collateral ligaments, preservation of the arches of the hand, countering burn claw hand deformity, and opposing potential deformity from scarring.

With acute, deep partial and full thickness burns, hand splints should be worn at all times except during exercise and activities of daily living.[5] Alteration of the wearing schedule depends on the patient's active range of motion, patient cooperation with self-exercises, and presence of edema. Even the motivated, cooperative patient should have hand splints on at night to maintain the best position.

Proper application of hand splints is critical to prevent deformity. Improper application can *cause* deformity. In the acute phase, splints should be secured with gauze (Kerlix) wrapping (Fig. 15–3). This will provide uniform pressure over the hand as opposed to a tourniquet effect which some straps produce. The gauze is changed with each reapplication of the splint, thus keeping the wound clean. Prior to splint reapplication, splints should be cleaned with alcohol and water to prevent contamination of the burn wound.

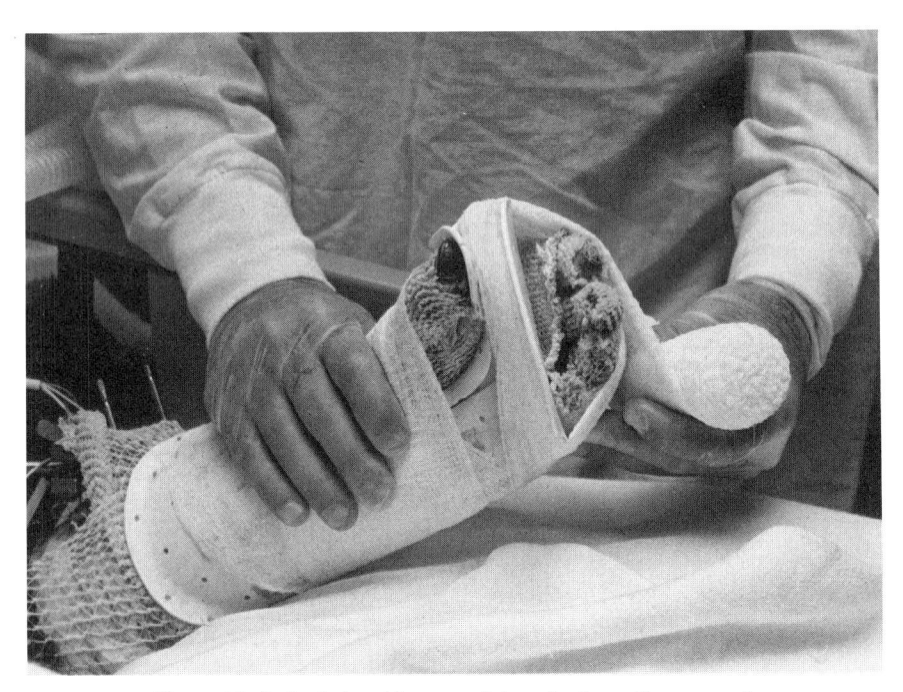

Figure 15–3. Acute hand burn—splint application with gauze roll.

Usually splints are custom fitted for each patient; however, commercially available splints can be used with modifications. As long as the splints maintain the recommended positioning, they are acceptable.

Exercises. With first and superficial second degree hand burns, all active and passive exercises can be encouraged. Deep second and third degree hand burns that include the dorsum of PIP joints should be actively and passively exercised as follows: MP joint flexion–extension with PIP and DIP joints extended, thumb opposition to all digits, thumb palmar and radial abduction, finger abduction and adduction, and wrist flexion and extension.

No fistmaking should be attempted until healing has occurred over the PIP joints. Once healing has occurred over these joints, active and passive exercises to increase full range of motion can be initiated. As much as possible, the patient should use his hands functionally in self-care activities (Fig. 15–4). This simultaneously will improve functional range of motion and increase self-esteem. By encouraging the patient to use normal utensils and devices, greater functional range of motion can be obtained. Adaptive equipment should be used only as a final alternative. Loss of strength frequently occurs following disuse in the burned hand; therefore, exercises and functional, resistive activities to increase hand strength are necessary.

Hypersensitivity often occurs following hand burns. A desensitization program to decrease hypersensitivity should be incorporated as appropriate.

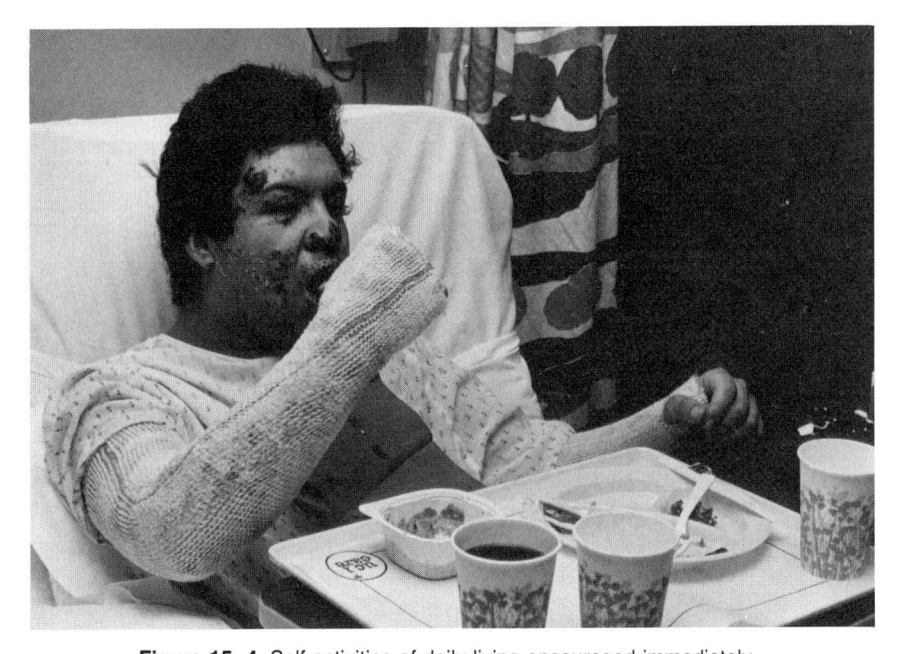

Figure 15–4. Self-activities of daily living encouraged immediately.

Hand–Palmar

Potential Deformity. Finger flexion, thumb adduction, and wrist flexion.

Positioning. Volar hand splint with wrist in 30 to 45 degrees of extension, MP, PIP, and DIP joints in extension. The thumb in midposition between palmar and radial abduction. The digits should be slightly abducted. Splints are worn at night or when not exercising.

Exercises. All active and passive range of motion exercises. Emphasis is placed on motions that counter the potential deformity such as thumb abduction, wrist extension, and finger extension and abduction.

Elbow

Potential Deformity. Elbow flexion with forearm pronation.

Positioning. Elbow extension with forearm supination.

Splinting. The elbow should be splinted in extension. A volar elbow splint (Fig. 15–5) is fabricated over the flexor surface of the elbow with the forearm supinated. This type of splint–conformer provides equal distribution of pressure. The splint is secured with a gauze wrap. The splint should be worn only at night to allow the patient use of the arm functionally to exercise during the day. If loss of range of motion continues to be a problem, the splint should be

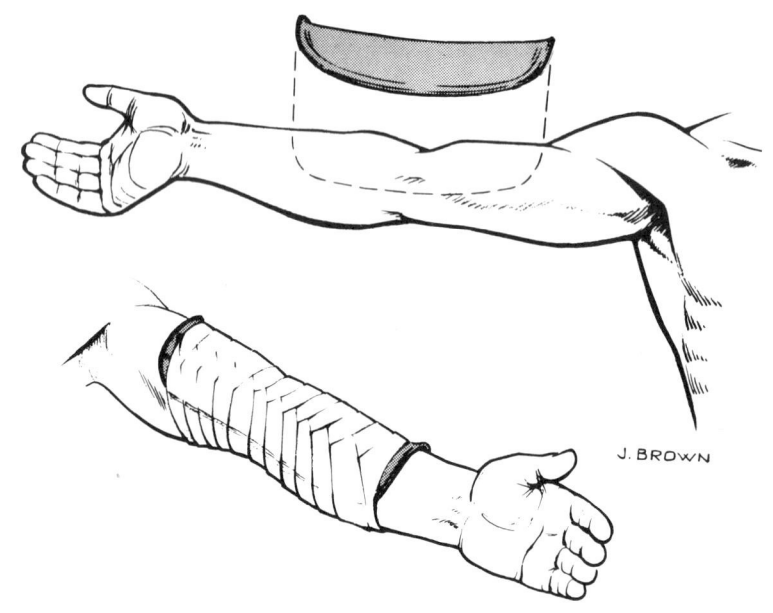

Figure 15–5. Elbow extension splint.

worn at all times except when exercising and during functional activities of daily living.

Exercises. Extension and flexion of elbow, forearm supination–pronation with elbow stabilized at side, use of pulleys, stacking cones, and functional activities of daily living (self-feeding, eating small candies, and opening door knobs).

Axilla

Potential Deformity. Adduction and internal rotation of the shoulder.

Positioning. Approximately 90- to 110-degree abduction with external rotation of the shoulder. The arm can be positioned on a bedside table, elevated on pillows to the desired angle, or in arm troughs. Troughs can be attached to an overhead traction bar in bed, intravenous (IV) poles, or attached to the bedside. Daytime positioning aids include the use of a portable IV pole with an attached arm sling to maintain the desired position of the involved axilla (Fig. 15–6).

Splinting. Axilla (airplane) splints to position the arm in 90- to 110-degree abduction.

1. Closed axilla conformer splint (Fig. 15–7): Splint makes contact along flank and includes pressure in axilla with arm support (secured with straps).
2. Open axilla splint (Fig. 15–8). Separate flank and arm cuffs with reinforcer of splint material providing stability (secured with straps).

Splints should be worn at night unless contracture with loss of range of motion indicates an increase in wearing time. If this type of splint is being used as a means of postoperative immobilization, it should be worn at all times for the appropriate length of time. Consult with the burn surgeon regarding desired immobilization time.

Exercises. Bilateral upper extremity exercises include throwing a ball, playing catch, towel dowel activities, pulleys, and stacking cones (Fig. 15–9). (Active and passive exercises are initiated to increase shoulder abduction and flexion to prevent axillary scar bands. This also reduces tightness of the skin in the axilla and flank.) Additional complications such as tendonitis and joint contractures can be prevented by the active daily exercise of each involved joint through a full range of motion. Exaggerated arm swing during ambulation and shoulder circumduction exercises are also helpful.

Neck

Potential Deformity. Anterior or lateral flexion contractures.

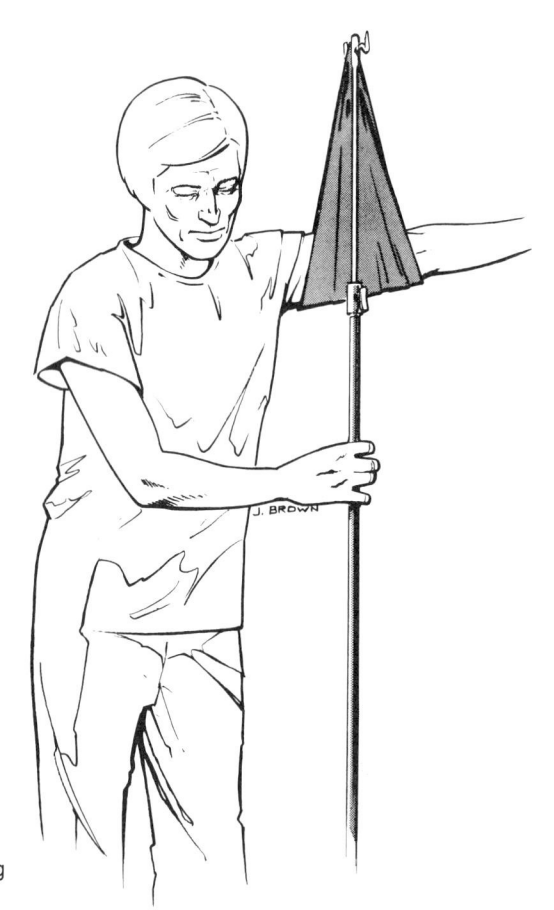

Figure 15–6. Daytime positioning aid for axilla burn.

Positioning. The patient should not have a pillow while in bed. If edema is present in the face, elevating the head of the bed rather than the patient's head alone is recommended. A smaller crib mattress can be placed on a larger mattress allowing the patient's head to be positioned in slight hyperextension. Sand bags can be placed adjacent to the burned side of the neck to prevent lateral flexion tightness.

Splinting. The splint should prevent forward or lateral flexion of the neck (Fig. 15–10). The chin and lower border of the mandible are immobilized cephalad. The splint conforms to the angle of the neck before flaring out on the anterior chest.[6] The splint is secured with a strap behind the neck. Soft neck collars are recommended by some; however, they provide pressure without maintaining the contour of the neck and they are difficult to clean. Frequently, as the skin pulls the neck into a flexed position, the lower lip will

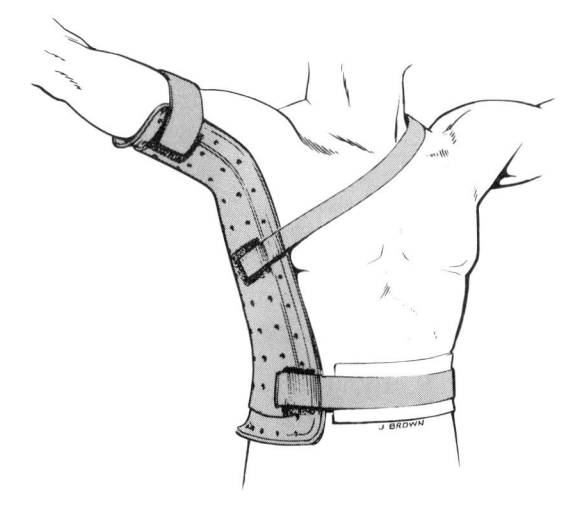

Figure 15–7. Axilla conformer (closed).

evert and pull down.[7] This will be dramatically observable when asking the patient to extend his neck, while keeping his mouth closed.

Exercises. Flexion–extension, lateral flexion, and lateral rotation of the neck. Encourage the patient to rotate his neck rather than turn the entire body. Leisure activities, such as macrame, which require the patient to look up, are helpful. The television should be positioned at an elevated height, requiring the patient to extend the neck.

Ingenuity is required if the patient has an endotracheal tube or tracheostomy. Sand bags or four poster splints are often useful.

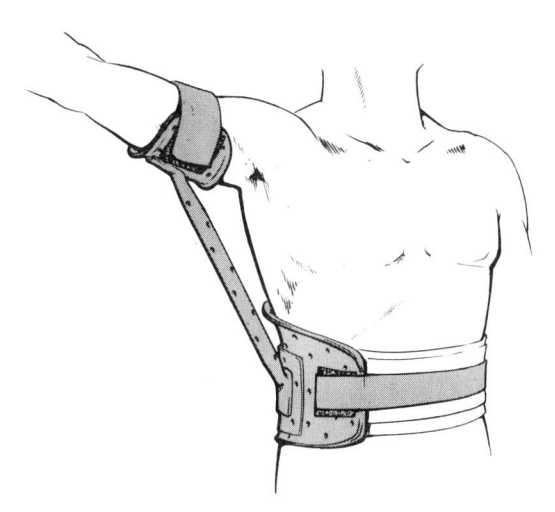

Figure 15–8. Airplane splint (open).

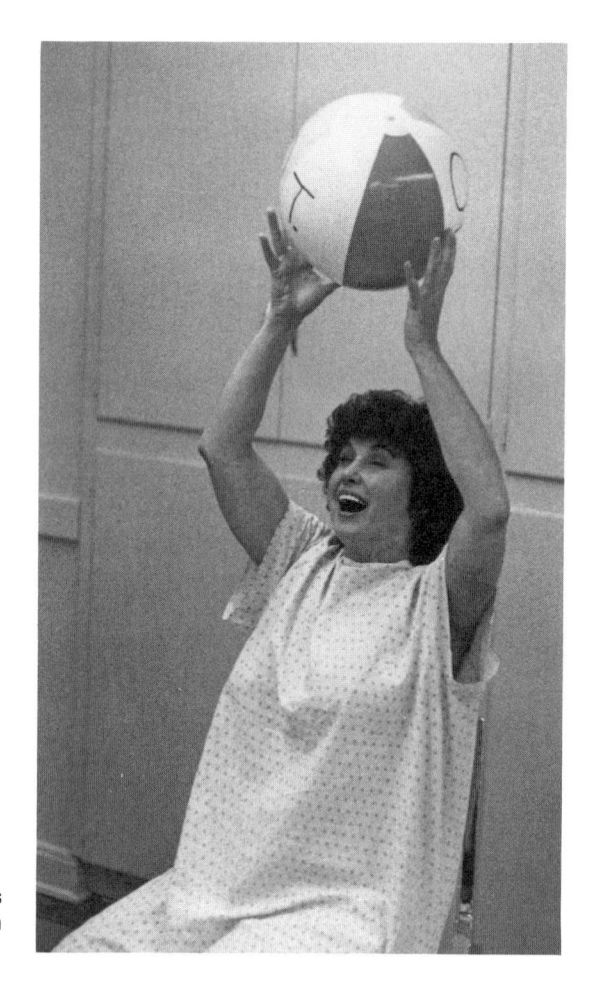

Figure 15–9. Functional activities encouraged in combination with range of motion exercises.

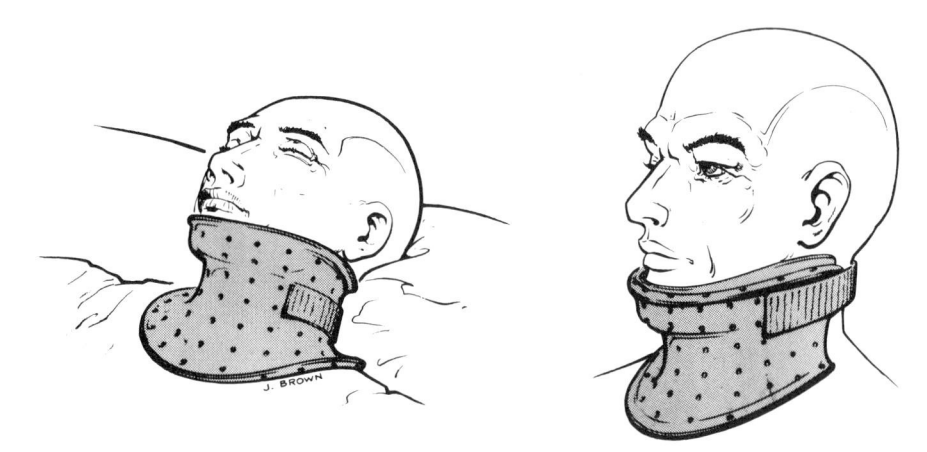

Figure 15–10. Neck splint.

Hips
Potential Deformity. Flexion, adduction.

Positioning. Extension with slight 15- to 20-degree abduction. Lying prone can be helpful if the patient continues to flex hips while supine. Pillows under the knee can help with abduction. Burns of the groin require similar positioning.

Splinting. Abdominal conformer with anterior thigh conformers, secured with straps. This device is not often indicated.

Exercises. Side-lying abduction of leg, flexing knee to chest, lying prone extending leg, and ambulation. Patients with lower extremity burns may require a tilt table exerciser to prepare for ambulation.

Knee
Potential Deformity. Flexion.

Positioning. Extension.

Splinting. Posterior knee extension shell splint (Fig. 15–11). If a deep second or third degree burn is present in the popliteal fossa, knee flexion contractures may develop. Knee extension splints are worn at night only. If loss of full extension occurs, splints should be worn at all times except during exercise. Splints are secured with gauze wrap.

Exercises. Knee flexion–extension and ambulation (both lower extremities should be wrapped with elastic bandages prior to any ambulation to increase circulation and support).

Ankle
Potential Deformity. Plantar flexion, foot inversion.

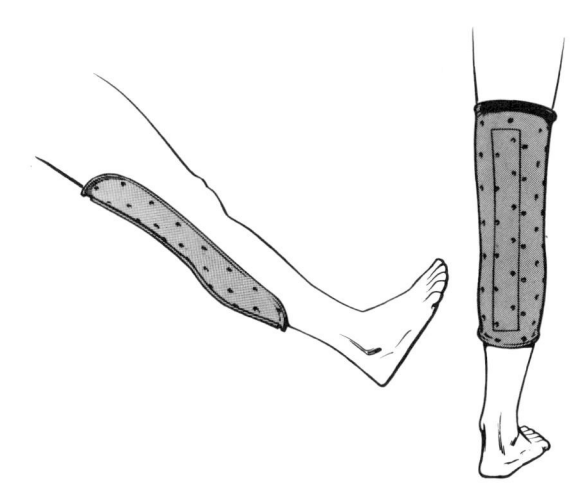

Figure 15–11. Knee extension splint.

Positioning. 90-degree dorsiflexion with foot board or splint.

Splinting. Long (including knee) and short (distal to knee) dorsiflexion splint (Fig. 15–12). Splints are secured with gauze and worn at night or during periods of daytime immobilization. The patient's heels must be carefully evaluated daily for pressure sores or ulceration. Splints are initially worn at night. Wearing time can be increased if deformity is progressive.

Exercises. Plantar flexion with dorsiflexion of the ankle, inversion–eversion and internal–external rotation, and ambulation.

Foot

Potential Deformity. Dorsal burns lead to dorsiflexion of the foot or to toe hyperextension. Volar burns produce toe flexion deformities.

Positioning. Plantar flexion of ankle, toes in extension or neutral.

Splinting. Dorsal burns can be prevented with a dorsal metatarsal conformer.[8] Volar burns are treated with individual toe extension trough splints. Splints are most commonly used after healing has occurred to correct specific deformities. Splints are worn at night or when inactive during the day (Fig. 15–12).

Exercise. Toe flexion–extension.

Face

Microstomia is a potential problem with burns surrounding the mouth. Commercially available microstomia splints can be used to stretch the oral commissures. *Exercises* include opening the mouth, eating an apple, smiling, and making facial expressions. Careful early assessment and monitoring maximum

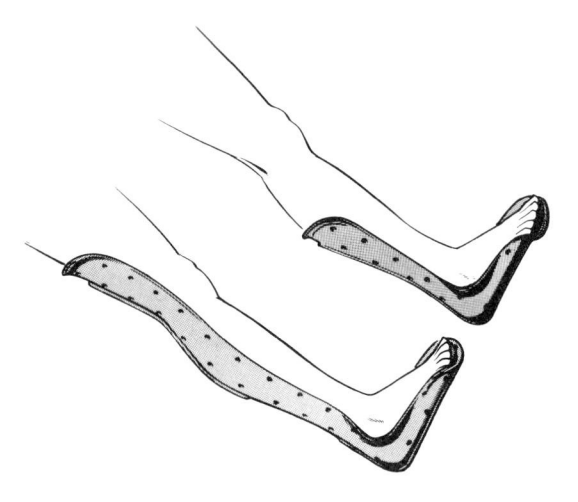

Figure 15–12. Long and short dorsiflexion splints.

length between commissures and mouth diameter are critical to reduce potential deformity.

A foam doughnut can be fabricated to prevent rubbing of the external pinna on the bed. No pillows are allowed when ear burns are present. Splints to control scar hypertrophy are illustrated in Figure 15–14.

The key to treatment of contractures and loss of functional range of motion is prevention. With appropriate assessment of the burn and careful treatment including positioning, splinting, therapeutic exercise and functional ability, limitations in range of motion and disabling contractures can be reduced.

POSTSURGICAL IMMOBILIZATION AND MOBILIZATION

The therapist can assist the surgeon with immobilizing the burn patient following grafting. Creativity in splinting is necessary. Since burns are not uniform in their locations, splinting will vary from patient to patient. Splint immobilization can immobilize the grafted area until the grafts are secure.

Grafted areas should remain immobile for approximately 5 days. Gentle, active exercise is permitted 5 to 7 days after surgery. Active assistive exercises can be initiated at 7 to 9 days. Passive stretching can be provided at 9 to 12 days and thereafter to further increase range of motion as needed. Care must be given to prevent damage to grafts. Careful assessment of the grafted area must be done daily to assure no accidental damage occurs. Close communication with the burn surgeon is essential at this critical time.

OUTPATIENT REHABILITATION

The patient is often discharged from the burn center before all burn wounds have healed. The patient will undergo daily hydrotherapy to clean and dress those wounds until they are healed or ready for grafting. The patient is seen by the therapist every other day or daily to assess healing, for continued exercises, and for scar control management.

The patient should be instructed in home exercises, home positioning, and splinting, as necessary, prior to discharge in order to maintain continuity with inpatient treatment. Periodic evaluation of active range of motion is recommended. Scar bands and contractures can be observed in their early stages, and often their deforming end results can be reduced with increased therapist-assisted exercise and splinting.

Patients with severe burns, especially to the hand, will require daily therapist-assisted treatment to increase their range of motion and function because these patients will not be able to exercise sufficiently at home to prevent contractures.

Although contractures from skin tightness and hypertrophic scarring may create increasing difficulty during the period of scar maturation, therapeutic exercise should continue in the same manner as previously outlined. While the patient is receiving passive stretching at a joint where a scar band is present, the joint should be stretched to maximum. The scar will blanch and thicken. Deep pressure massage is combined with a sustained maximum stretch. This type of treatment, in addition to splinting and positioning, should begin to increase joint range of motion. This should be done several times per therapy session, combined with active exercise and functional activities.

When not exercising, outpatients may require splinting to maintain maximum stretch on joints. This can be especially helpful at night while the patient is inactive. Dynamic splinting can be utilized in the daytime to provide passive stretching of skin and joints to further increase range of motion while not actively exercising. As long as range of motion is below normal, positioning at home should be the same as while an inpatient.

SCAR MANAGEMENT

This may represent the most challenging aspect of treating the burn patient. There are no rules, few guidelines, and frequent frustrations. Although the experience of the surgeon and therapist is important in burn scar management, no one can accurately determine how a patient will heal.

Many factors contribute to the severity of hypertrophic scarring: (1) depth of burn, (2) length of time for healing to occur, (3) grafting, (4) age, and (5) skin character. These all have to be considered when planning scar control treatment.

Scar tissue can remain immature from 12 to 18 months postburn. During this time, the skin can return to its tightened, prestretched status soon after exercise. This can lead to increased frustration by the patient who sincerely works hard. Therefore, a great deal of motivation and support is needed.

As scars mature, they will evolve through several color changes. Early on, the new skin will be pink, then red, deep red, purple, brown, and finally tan as a final mature scar. The immature scar that is between the red-brown phase will best respond to scar control treatment (usually 2 to 9 months). Then firm, vascular, red scars eventually become soft and tan colored with normal vascularity.

Causes of Scar Hypertrophy

Superficial second degree burns will usually heal with little scarring; however, hypertrophic scarring is more likely to be severe with deep second degree (dermal or partial thickness) burns. The normal parallel layers of collagen fibers located in the dermis are disrupted. Larson et al. identified a "whorl-like" nodular appearance of these collagen fibers during scar maturation.[9] Myofibroblasts have contractile components which may contribute to this whorl-like configuration of collagen. Myofibroblasts make up 50 to 75 percent of the total cellular population in the dermis of other hypertrophic scar tissues.

If partial thickness burns are allowed to heal spontaneously, hypertrophic scarring is more likely. Grafting can prevent this problem.

Third degree burns involve full thickness tissue loss and, therefore, require skin grafting. Scarring is likely to occur at the borders of sheet grafts and possibly through the holes and borders of meshed grafts.[8] The most active stages of scar formation appear to be from 1 to 6 months postburn, but this can extend beyond a year in certain individuals. During this time, the healed grafted skin is maturing and undergoing tremendous structural change. Immature scars, those which best respond to treatment, are typically firm to touch, red, and highly vascular. How this maturation process affects each person (in the form of scar tissue formation) varies.

TREATMENT

As soon as healing begins, so should scar control evaluation. Treatment will be an ongoing process for 12 to 18 months postburn, until the scarring has fully matured.

The method of choice to counteract hypertropic scarring is continuous topical pressure, which should be applied 22 to 24 hours per day until the scarring is mature.[10] Topical pressure can be maintained by using one of several devices and methods.

1. *Elastic bandages:* These can be wrapped distally to proximally over the burned extremity. It is difficult to attain consistent, even pressure. Therefore, elastic bandages are used until custom-fitted garments arrive.
2. *Tubular elastic sleeves (e.g., Tubigrip):* These are purchased in varying diameters and can provide a temporary, even pressure.
3. *Custom made elastic pressure gradient garments (e.g., Jobst garments):* For best results, these garments should provide over 25 mm Hg of pressure to the developing scar, flattening and controlling its growth.[7] Measurements for these garments are done as soon as the wound has healed. Even with scattered unhealed areas, the garments can be measured. It generally takes 1 to 3 weeks for the garments to arrive. They are then fitted on the patient.

    These garments provide even, consistent pressure to most areas of the body. Certain isolated areas where there is much differential in contour, such as the face and sternum, will require conformers or padding to apply the necessary pressure.[8] These conformers are fabricated from low temperature thermoplastics. They are thinned out and molded to the scarred area (Figs. 15–13 and 15–14). Specific areas for concern include eyelids, nose, chin, lower eyelids, neck, concave aspect of chest, and the palm of the hand. Individualized conformers can be made to fit under the pressure garments or secured with

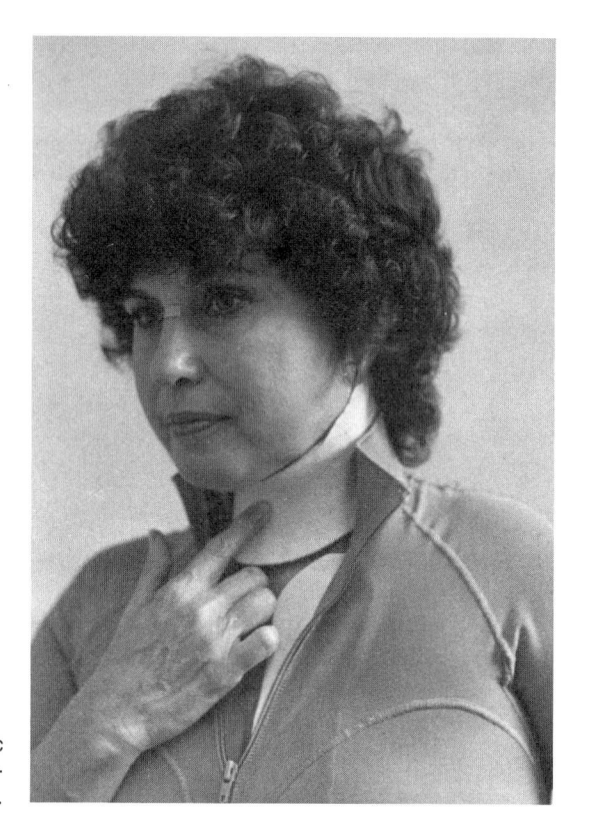

Figure 15–13. Thermoplastic neck and chest conformer to apply increased pressure on scars.

elastic bandages and modified regularly as scars change to provide the best pressure on the scars. A transparent face mask fabricated from high temperature thermoplastics can be made from a positive plaster mold. This can be worn directly on the face to decrease scarring.[11]

The foam padding under a pressure garment also can be used to apply accessory pressure to specific areas. The finger web spaces can

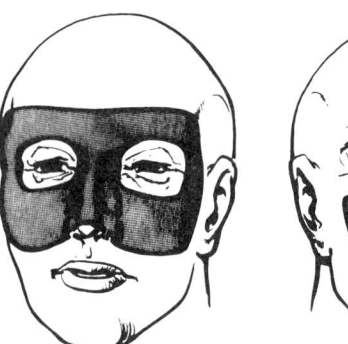

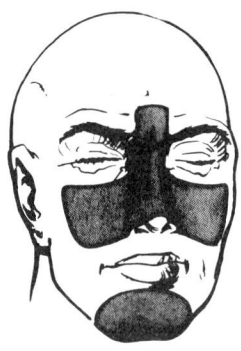

Figure 15–14. Facial, nose, and chin conformers worn under elastic pressure garments.

be maintained by applying strips of padding between the fingers under pressure gradient gloves.
4. *Flurandrenolide tape:* For scattered small areas of hypertrophic scarring, small strips of tape can be precisely cut and applied to the scar. Flurandrenolide tape contains topical steroids. The tape should remain over the scar for 24 hours and be replaced daily. (If a rash develops, the tape should be discontinued and the physician should be contacted.) A positive response occurs in most patients in 2 to 3 weeks. Treatment can be maintained for 3 or 4 months as needed.
5. *Deep pressure circular massage:* All patients should be instructed to self-massage to soften developing hypertrophic scar tissue. This massage should be done several times a day.
6. *Surgical releases:* If nonsurgical methods of scar control fail, resulting in patient frustration, joint immobility, or functional impairment, surgery should be considered. Close communication with surgeon and therapist is required.

All patients require periodic reassessment of scars. This should be done weekly or bimonthly for those patients with conformers, which may need modification, and at least every 2 to 3 months for those patients with pressure garments to monitor fit and make adjustments as needed. Early on, blisters will be a problem. Pressure therapy should continue even though modification may be necessary.

RETURNING TO WORK

The ultimate goal is to return the patients to their level of functioning prior to the burn injury. As active range of motion to hands and upper extremities increases, a work simulation or work-hardening program should be initiated. Through functional activities and simulated work tasks, which can be graded for the patient's current range of motion, strength, and dexterity, capability for return to work can be assessed, developed, and increased.

For the patient being covered by workmen's compensation, detailed reports on the following can be helpful:

1. Hand grasp and pinch strength
2. Specific sensation
3. Active range of motion and passive range of motion measurements
4. Hand dexterity
5. Standing tolerance
6. Current work capacity (level of endurance, range of motion, strength)

Judgment and understanding are necessary to return patients to work. Many jobs are compatible with wearing of pressure garments. Scars can be a devastation to the patient who works in the public eye. Patients who were injured at work may have psychological problems with returning to the same job (see Chap. 16). Many times the patient is not able to return to the same type of employment due to their contact with chemicals, fiberglass, or intense heat which causes irritation to the recently healed skin. Placement in other positions, additional schooling, or vocational counseling may be required.

Complaints of itching and pain from burn victims is common up to 6 months postburn. There can be disabling enough to delay return to work.

RETURNING TO SCHOOL

Returning to school poses problems similar to those of returning to work. Physical appearance and acceptance by peers are as important to the student as to the worker. Children returning to school with splints, conformers, and pressure garments may find adjustment difficult or impossible. Having a person who understands these problems speak to the child and parents makes this easier. A school re-entry program should incorporate the burned child's classmates and teachers. The importance of the splints, conformers, and pressure garments in the child's medical treatment must be emphasized.

BURN RECOVERY GROUP

A recovery group can be started by any interested member of the burn team. At the University of California Irvine (UCI) Medical Center, the Burn Recovery Group functions as an emotional support, self-help group composed of current and former burn victims, their families, and friends. Anyone connected with a burn injury is invited to attend the monthly meetings. The meetings are held in close proximity to the burn center to encourage current burn patients and their families to attend.

The group encourages and assists current and former patients with problems and concerns (i.e., grafting, pressure garments, what will I look like, or will my family still love me). Aid to family members enduring the trauma of a burn patient's hospitalization is another important function of the group. Mutual help between people is the goal of the group.

A monthly agenda is planned, including support for fire-related issues and offering speakers to share their expertise to the group (i.e., legal advice, make-up for burn scars, and pain control). Also, periodic social events, such as parties and picnics, are held to involve families and friends of burn patients in enjoyable, nonthreatening activities.

SUMMARY

The burned patient's rehabilitation begins on the first day of admission and continues for several years postburn for scar control management. The patient may pass through several stages of acceptance during this time. Psychological considerations must be taken into account at all times. Assisting the patient through these difficult times can be a rewarding responsibility for the burn team. The healed patient who is unable to function in society is a failure for the burn team. Emotional factors are usually responsible and must be dealt with from day 1. The successful program will treat the patient as a whole person, mind and body. The burned skin is only one aspect that requires rehabilitation.

REFERENCES

1. Baur PS, Barratt G, Linares HA, et al.: Wound contractions, scar contractures and myofibroblasts: A classical case study. J Trauma 18:8, 1978
2. Parks DH, Evans B, Larson DL: Prevention and correction of deformity after severe burns. Surg Clin North Am 58:1279, 1978
3. Willis B, Larson DL, Abston S: Positioning and splinting the burned patient. Heart and Lung J Crit Care 2:696, 1973
4. Moncreif JA: Complications of burns. Ann Surg 147:443, 1958
5. Tanijawa M, O'Donnell O, Graham P: The burned hand: A physical therapy protocol. Phys Ther 54:953, 1974
6. Willis B: The use of orthoplast isoprene splints in the treatment of the acutely burned child. Am J Occup Ther 24:187, 1970
7. Larson DL, Abston S, Willis B, et al.: Contracture and scar formation in the burn patient. Clin Plast Surg 1:653, 1974
8. Helm PA, Head MD, Pellium G, et al.: Burn rehabilitation: A team approach. Surg Clin North Am 58:1263, 1978
9. Larson DL, Abston S, Dobrkovsky M: The prevention and correction of burn scar contracture and hypertrophy. Shriners Burn Inst Pamphlet, University of Texas Med Branch, Galveston, Texas
10. Larson DL, Abston S, Evans EB, et al.: Technique for decreasing scar formation and contracture in the burned patient. J Trauma 11:807, 1971
11. Rivers E, Strate R, Solem L: The transparent face mask. Am J Occup Ther 33:108, 1979

CHAPTER 16
Psychosocial Treatment and Pain Control

Joyce K. Friedmann, Johanna Shapiro, and Lawrence Plon

Recent strides in the physical reconstruction and rehabilitation of the severely burned patient have resulted in greatly improved survivial rates and a decreased length of hospitalization. In addition, the aged, the very young, and those with complicating medical conditions are also surviving burns. It is admirable to be able to reconstruct quickly and efficiently a damaged body; however, it is imperative that medicine now consider the quality of life effecting these people who are being restored. Rehabilitation success has been defined as the degree to which the individual's ultimate functioning compares to his or her functioning prior to the injury.[1] Researchers in the area of rehabilitation outcome are beginning to use multidimensional measures of outcome which are modified to profile each individual prior to the injury.[1] The rehabilitation process itself begins in the hospital at the time of admission and must include an early and aggressive team approach if the patient is to fully utilize the technologic advances provided by the burn team. A cooperative, motivated, and socially supported patient is essential if maximum rehabilitation is to be achieved. It is becoming more apparent to those dealing with burned people that early psychological intervention is a sine qua non for rehabilitation. "The correct approach by trained people from the *beginning* of the illness and their patient continuation of contact as long as necessary will enormously reduce the suffering of both patients and their families and will avoid many tragedies."[2]

    Chang[3] studied 51 burn patients and found that 79 percent were able to return to work or school, though 45 percent required a change in work and 25 percent were not able to continue with their peer groups in school; the average time of disability was 6 months; there was significant psychological morbidity as demonstrated by self-confessed depression, juvenile delinquency, and divorce. With more than two million persons burned in the United States each year, and of these at least 100,000 requiring hospitalization, it is estimated that there are nearly nine million disability days secondary to burns.[4] Long-term follow-up of burn patients has been difficult, as many individuals seem to withdraw from society and become lost to the researcher. It is difficult to assess with certainty the meaning of this. However, it is probable that many of these patients are psychologically, emotionally, socially, and occupationally withdrawn.[5] A potential rehabilitation failure can be recognized early as the recalcitrant patient who refuses to cooperate with occupational and physical therapists; one who will not tolerate splints, conformers, and pressure garments; and one who has high pain levels, and is irritable and impatient with family members.

MacGregor[5] notes in her studies of the facially disfigured (a serious subset of burned patients) that everyone coped with the stress in some fashion. All experienced periods of marked depression and there were several suicide attempts. Defense mechanisms, such as denial and withdrawal, may be a strategem which literally holds people together. She noted in her follow-up study 20 years later that these facially disfigured people were still extremely vulnerable about their appearances. They still had feelings of impotence and anger lying close to the surface. Anger was directed at parents, surgeons, psychiatrists, society for being rigid and prejudicial, and also at society for obliging them to spend so much psychic energy devising methods to counter threats and social deprivation. It is no small wonder that these feelings of anger and helplessness interfere with successful rehabilitation.

It is important to understand the emotional experience of victims of traumatic injury and burning, in order to treat them more effectively. The psychological syndrome frequently exhibited is termed post-traumatic stress disorder (PTSD).

HISTORY OF POST-TRAUMATIC STRESS DISORDER

For many centuries man failed to recognize that fear surrounding an accident and the subsequent emotional reaction could cause a person to be physically ill. One of the earliest realizations came with the condition called "railway spine" in the 1880s which developed when a fast train, traveling at a "frightening" speed, stopped suddenly. It was first thought that vascular changes in the spinal cord caused the physical symptoms, then it was realized that emotional factors such as fright and surprise were causal. The syndrome, which was later variously termed war neurosis, combat fatigue, or traumatic neurosis, was observed and described during the Civil War as "nostalgia" or "brain weariness"; during World War I, it was generally thought that PTSD was due to physical brain damage from the nearby exploding shells, i.e., shell shock.[6]

In World War I, "physical" traumatic disorder was distinguished from psychological, and when mental breakdown could not be linked to exploding shells, the soldiers were considered to "lack moral fiber" and were accused of cowardice and threatened with the firing squad. Faced with the alternative of returning to combat or shock treatment, some committed suicide.

It was found with World War II that the underlying condition was the same; 50,000 individuals were discharged for psychological reasons. At one point, more soldiers were leaving as psychological casualties than were being drafted. Many of these became permanently disabled. There is now little doubt this could have been averted with more immediate psychological intervention.

By the Viet Nam confrontation, psychological casualties were greatly decreased from World War I levels of 101 per 1000 to 12 per 1000 due to the cardinal principles of immediacy: (1) proximity of treatment, (2) immediacy of treatment, and (3) expectancy of return to normalcy or combat. Another factor was the use of drugs, which reduced length of hospitalization. It was recognized that the severity of the physical injury was not related to the severity of the psychological injury. Probably more is known about PTSD than any other psychological entity, since the wars have provided an unparalleled opportunity to diagnosis and treatment. It is generally agreed the war and peacetime PTSD are the same syndrome.

The psychological effects of a burn injury and its treatment are multivaried and critical, not only to the patient's mental functioning, but also to his or her physical functioning. That the mind and body are related becomes patently obvious and directly affects pain levels, healing rates, surgical success, and social and occupational rehabilitation.[7,8] During the acute phase, patients face a variety of psychological problems that may include disorientation, discomfort, pain, and fear.[4] Disorientation involves a combination of physiologic, psychological, and circumstantial factors. Burn shock, sepsis, fluid and electrolyte imbalance, alcohol addiction, secondary injury, hypoxia, lack of sleep, preburn psychosis, anxiety, and many other elements elicit disorientation. Inability to recall time, place, and events is frightening for patients, and can perpetuate intense anxiety, fear of loss of control, and fear of imminent death. Pain is a central issue throughout the acute and subacute periods and is enhanced by factors such as anxiety, sensory deprivation, environmental stress, and hypermetabolism found with burns. Fears during the period immediately after injury also center around the issue of survival. When survival is no longer in question, fears often center on appearance, ability to function and work, sexual functioning, and family and social acceptance. During the convalescent phase, feelings of anxiety, guilt, and depression occur.[4]

When overwhelming anxiety develops, such as when being confronted by possible death with little possibility of escape, as in being burned, defenses against the anxiety are called into play. These defense mechanisms are useful and nonpathologic initially. Psychic numbing is a classic manifestation of Freud's repression–suppression–denial defense. If the victim is unable to handle the anxiety adequately through the various nonpathologic defenses, then long-term pathologic responses arise. PTSD casualties have been followed medically for as long as 30 years; although reduced in severity, their symptoms can be retained to a disabling degree. Seven years after World War II, fresh cases of combat fatigue were still presenting themselves at veterans' hospitals. It appears, then, that delayed onset of symptoms is possible. The symptoms can develop into conditions such as hysterias, obsessions, and compulsions, or conversion reactions such as blindness and paralysis. Burn victims often experience this PTSD which has been described by the American Psychiatric Association. The symptoms of PTSD can be[9]:

1. *Re-experiencing the event:* Dreams, nightmares, flashbacks, appearing to relive event (an attempt to retrospectively master the anxiety of the event)
2. *Psychic numbing or emotional anesthesia:* Numbing of responsiveness to, or decreased involvement with, external world (lost ability to be interested in previously significant enjoyed activities; inability to feel emotions of any type, especially intimacy, tenderness, sexuality markedly decreased)
3. *Variety of possible psychophysiologic symptoms:* Autonomic nervous system lability, impotence, headache, gastric upset, sweating, palpitation, dizziness, fatigue, decreased appetite, insomnia, hyperalertness, exaggerated startle response, depression, anxiety, emotional lability, blackouts, menstrual changes, muscle spasms, hair loss, teeth grinding, fear, impaired memory, difficulty concentrating on or completing tasks, survival guilt, avoidance of activities that may arouse recollections of event, irritability, sporadic or unpredictable explosions of aggressive behavior

Case 1:
A 39-year-old male, with a severe electrical burn to his leg, continues to have insomnia, nightmares, almost total withdrawal into his home and family nearly 4 years postburn. He is agitated, finds himself unable to control his spontaneous tearfulness, is unable to work, unable to return for further reconstructive surgery, has emotional outbursts with his wife and children, is sexually impotent, has hypertension, gastritis, a weight gain of 40 pounds, impaired memory, and is generally despondent about his loss of control of his life.

It is important to recognize that the severity of psychological disorder is not correlated with the severity, or extent, of the physical injury. In fact, a PTSD can develop as a result of merely witnessing a trauma, or its aftermath. It is not uncommon for family members to suffer PTSD as a result of participating in routine burn care.

Case 2:
A 50-year-old female patient with a small second-degree burn to the dorsal aspect of her foot developed a PTSD with symptoms of sleep disturbance, flashbacks, emotional lability, and a phobic response to her foot. She exhibited fear of looking

at, touching, or treating her wound, which seemed greatly out of proportion to the extent of her injury. Clinical interview indicated that the disfigurement triggered repressed feelings about her husband's internment in the Auschwitz concentration camp.

PROGNOSIS

PTSD is described as "acute" if less than 6 months in duration and "chronic" or "delayed" if it occurs after 6 months. It has been found that the traumatic syndrome is more severe and longer lasting when the stressor is of human design, as opposed to natural disasters, such as floods.

There may be phobic avoidances which impair functioning. The emotional anesthesia frequently interferes with interpersonal relationships. The emotional lability, depression, and guilt may produce self-defeating behavior, suicide, or substance abuse. One patient exhibited a period of shoplifting during her recovery. It should be noted that symptoms often recur, or are intensified, when the victim is exposed to situations, or activities, or news reports, resembling or symbolizing the original event. Hot, humid weather often precipitates flashbacks in Viet Nam veteran casualties. News reports of fires involving human casualties often cause anxiety attacks in burn victims. Symptoms may be intensified, of there may be a short-term relapse on the anniversary date of the injury.

PAIN

The pain of a serious burn is further compounded by the invasive and often painful procedures perpetrated by the treatment team on the victim. Healing of burns involves a number of direct physically painful contacts: (1) when the injured surface is washed; (2) pain caused while the patient is being moved, both in bed and in transport to hydrotherapy; (3) pain caused by range of motion exercise; (4) the causing of more skin damage to the patient in taking grafts. Next, the patients must endure severe itching for months after the wounds mature, along with more physical therapy and possibly more reconstructive surgery.[10] In addition to the obvious pain, there is the attendant discomfort of the pressure garments and splints, which may have to be worn 24 hours a day for 12 months. To the patient, those therapies often seem barbaric; one patient reported dreaming he was a resident in a medieval torture chamber.

PHARMACOLOGIC TREATMENT OF PAIN

Each individual responds to the sensation of pain with a unique degree of intensity. This subjective response makes the evaluation of pain medications for both acute and chronic pain difficult. Acute pain, with its usually abrupt onset and finite period of time to resolution, is the pain form most successfully treated with analgesics. Chronic, indefinite, or prolonged pain is a condition in which analgesics play a minor role. It is important to recognize that most of the studies of analgesics have been conducted in the acute pain patient.

Strong Narcotic Analgesics

These are the agents which are the first line of defense against severe pain. Of the various medications in this group, morphine is considered to be the standard narcotic analgesic against which all other narcotics are compared. These compounds seem to act centrally.[11] They do not abolish pain stimulus, but they do reduce a patient's perception of the pain and his or her affective response to it. The central effects include the desired analgesic and euphoria, as well as drowsiness, decreased respiration, and decreased cough reflex. Nausea and vomiting occur as a result of direct stimulation of the chemoreceptor trigger zone. Other affects are miosis, decreased gastrointestinal motility, and decreased vascular peripheral resistance.

There are many morphine derivatives, but no other narcotic analgesic, neither synthetic nor nonsynthetic, has been found to have any significantly greater analgesic effect or any significant differences in side effects when given in equal potent doses. Table 16–1 illustrates the differences among the various narcotic analgesics. The major differences are in duration of action and oral potency when compared to parenteral administration.

Parenteral morphine is probably the drug of choice for acute, moderate to severe pain. Meperidine, which is extremely popular, has a shorter duration of action of about 3 hours. In patients with renal impairment, normeperidine, a metabolite of meperidine, can build up in the body. Normeperidine has about one-half the analgesic properties of meperidine and has twice the consulvant properties of the parent compound.

Hydromorphone has a high degree of oral activity and is very useful when an oral narcotic analgesic is indicated, but its short duration of action, about 3 hours, limits its use in chronic pain.

For severe chronic pain, methadone and levorphanol are probably the drugs of choice. Both have a high degree of oral activity and long durations of action, about 6 to 8 hours.

If oral medication cannot be tolerated and a parenteral agent is not desired, hydromorphone and oxymorphone can be used as rectal suppositories.

The side effects of the strong narcotics can be very troublesome. The nausea and vomiting can be helped somewhat by hydroxyzine or promethazine which are frequently added to a patient's medications. Hydroxyzine has been shown to enhance pain relief when given with narcotics.[12] These agents will also potentiate the sedative properties of the narcotics. Constipation can be minimized by the use of a stool softener such as dioctyl sodium sulfosuccinate.

One method of attempting to minimize the depressive effects of narcotic agents has been the use of Brompton's solution. This mixture of morphine and cocaine has been widely used. The cocaine is intended to combat the central nervous system depression following the use of a narcotic. Cocaine apparently has no systemic pain-relieving properties, and it has a variable result in reducing the central nervous system effects.[13] It has been reported that results using just morphine are as good as that of a combination of agents. Morphine solutions containing perhaps 10 mg per 5 ml can be used for pain relief and easily titrated to meet a patient's needs. An antiemetic or stimulant, such as an amphetamine, can be then added to the drug regimen if the narcotic side effects become intolerable.

Weak Narcotic Analgesics

These drugs, such as codeine and propoxyphene, are useful mainly in the treatment of mild pain. A dose of 60 mg of codeine which is equivalent to 65 mg of propoxyphene approximates 650 mg of aspirin for the relief of pain. When given in higher doses, both of these drugs cause a significant increase in side effects without a corresponding increase in pain relief. When given with aspirin (Empirin, Ascodeen) or acetaminophen (Tylenol with Codeine, Phenaphen), it may provide slightly better pain relief than with either drug alone.[14]

Other Medications for Burn Patients

Antidepressants have been demonstrated to have intrinsic analgesic effects independent of their antidepressant qualities.[15] Agents such as amitriptyline, imipamine, or doxepin may be useful, especially in the chronic pain patient. We have found that doxepin, in addition to having strong sedative properties for outpatients, seems to decrease the incidence of nightmares our outpatients experience. Further research is needed to document this drug effect.

Basic Rules for Analgesia for Burn Patients

1. A relaxed, nonanxious patient seems to respond better to analgesics than a tense one. The use of diazepam and its pharmacologic cousins should be avoided unless anxiety is a severe problem. These drugs are depressants and can intensify the depression which a burn patient, already on depressing drugs, may experience. Alprazolam, a newer antianxiety drug, may also have antidepressant properties. Lorazepam may be useful in minimizing the memory of painful procedures and thereby decrease anxiety.
2. Analgesics should be used to prevent pain from recurring after it is initially decreased. It apparently takes less medication to prevent pain than it takes to abolish it.
3. The oral route of administration is preferable for prolonged periods of treatment.
4. Pain medication should not be administered on a prn basis for patients in severe pain. It should be used routinely. If prn is required, the patient is probably undermedicated. Routine use of the medications avoids patient–nurse issues as to who controls and evaluates the effectiveness of the medication. It also minimizes the patient from associating an injection with the specific relief of pain.

TABLE 16-1. RELATIVE POTENCIES OF NARCOTIC ANALGESICS

Drug	Parenteral Equianalgesic Dose (mg) im/sc	Duration (hr)	Bioavailability po:im	Comments
Morphine	10	3–6	1:6	IV dose 5–8 mg
Meperidine (Demerol)	75–100	2–4	1:3	Short action
Methadone (Dolophine)	7.5–10	4–8	1:2	Good po activity long t-1/2 relative to duration of analgesia
Hydromorphone (Dilaudid)	1.5	3–4	1:2–3	Available as suppository good po activity
Oxymorphone (Numorphan)	1	4–5	1:6	Available as suppository
Levorphanol (Levodromoran)	2	6–8	1:2	Good po activity long duration

Pentazocine (Talwin)	45–60	2–3	1:3	Psychiatric side effects/antagonist activity
Codeine	130	3–6	1:2	Over 60 mg greater toxicity

Oral

Drug	Oral Dose (mg)	Rectal Dose (mg)	Duration (hr)
Hydromorphone	2–4	3–6	3–4
Levorphanol	2–3	—	6–8
Meperidine	150–300	—	3
Methadone	20	—	6–8
Morphine	20–40	—	3–4
Oxymorphone	1	5–10	4
Oxycodone	20–40	—	3–4

5. Use longer acting analgesics. Meperidine's short half-life may require too frequent injections for the severely pained patient.
6. Give medications on a routine basis based on the patient's response, not on a dosing schedule which has been established by hospital tradition.

It is important to remember that most patients are undermedicated for severe burn pain, perhaps from a fear that they will become addicted to the narcotic analgesics. If one adheres to the above guidelines, adjusts doses of medications to the individual needs of each patient, and remembers that the hospital burn unit is not the type of environment in which addiction is likely, both the patient and the staff will feel more comfortable.

NONPHARMACOLOGIC PAIN CONTROL

There can be no doubt that high levels of anxiety lead to increased levels of pain perception.[16] The nonpharmacologic approach to pain control is based on the concept that a relaxed patient is more comfortable. Simple relaxation procedures such as abdominal breathing, autogenics, and hypnosis can potentiate analgesics. It is recognized that an agitated patient experiences a lowered pain threshold; most patients recognize that tension and emotional upset increase pain levels. It is helpful to have a motivated patient in order to successfully use self-control pain techniques as an adjunct to pharmacotherapy. Conceptually, it is sometimes useful for a patient to grasp that the brain controls what happens in the body and that a person's mental state modulates brain activity and, therefore, physical systems. The mind and body are interrelated. Relaxing the mind can make the body more comfortable. A mechanism for this control may be that relaxation increases endorphin output.

Hynosis can be conceived of as a relaxed state in which the patient focuses his or her mind on controlling such things as pain. Burned patients are a particularly motivated and therefore successful group of hypnotic subjects. Some specific pain control procedures, in order of usefulness are:

- Relaxation
- Dissociation
- Autonomic nervous system control
- Time distortion and amnesia
- Glove anesthesia

Case 3:
A 45-year-old male, several weeks postburn, reported difficulty sleeping. A three-deep breath hypnotic induction was used and then it was suggested that he imagine himself on a hillside, under a tree, resting comfortably (dissociation). Tears began to seep from his closed eyelids. After a few moments more under the tree, the patient was requested to return to his ordinary state of consciousness.

He did not respond. He was then told that when he returned he could bring all the comfort back he required. Upon questioning, the patient responded that he experienced the only comfort he had known since the burn and had been reluctant to leave it.

Subsequently, the patient returned to the hospital for surgical intervention for contractures. Hypnosis was again used for pain control immediately after surgery, during initial splinting. At this time it was suggested that as each spasm ended it was like it had never existed, "it was over, done with and through," he could close the door and turn his back on it (amnesia); and further that he could stretch out the time between the spasms and compress the time during the pains, "just like you are adjusting the speed control on a record player" (time distortion). This approach proved very successful with the patient. It is important to bear in mind, especially with acute pain, that it is not possible to know what a patient is internally experiencing. This patient looked and sounded like he was experiencing great pain. In fact, he reported total amnesia for the discomfort.

Group hypnotic training for burned outpatients can be expedient for symptoms such as insomnia, anxiety, occupational therapy (OT) and physical therapy (PT) discomfort, and pruritis. For itching, imagery such as cool mountain streams with pools of soothing anesthetic can be useful. Such groups when attended by spouses have proved valuable for enhancing marital harmony.

PSYCHOSOCIAL TREATMENT

Initial patient assessment should ascertain, through a necessarily abbreviated clinical interview, any premorbid psychopathology which might affect the course of treatment, i.e., alcoholism, drug abuse, suicidality, senility, and psychosis.

The immediate crisis intervention therapy should provide emotion ventilation opportunities with trained psychosocial staff. The first day treatment should include the provision of information to the patient that he or she is, in fact, a cotherapist and that his or her attitude affects important healing variables, such as comfort and sleep. Part of the information provided to the patient is that tension can affect circulation, impede the healing process, and reduce comfort levels. The direct relationship between high stress levels, increased pain, and decreased healing rates is pointed out.

Patients begin at once with simple relaxation, self-control techniques, primarily breathing, and dissociative techniques to help remove the patient from his or her uncomfortable situation to a familiar, comfortable haven such as a favorite vacation spot.[16] Brief, crisis-oriented family therapy commences during the family's first contact with the burn center, which enables them to deal with their initital feelings of shock, disbelief, guilt, and loss.

When the patient is medically stabilized, the social support system of the patient should be assessed, since it is apparent[17] that the single most important determinant in rehabilitation of a patient is the social support which is available to the patient. It is a better predictor of rehabilitation success than severity of injury. Three independent measures of social support—family support, peer support, and friend support—can be assessed by questions such as the following five[17]:

1. Do they make you feel loved?
2. Do they do things to make you feel happy?
3. Can you rely on them no matter what?
4. Would they see that you are taken care of no matter what?
5. Do they accept you just as you are?

During this phase of treatment, frequent brief psychotherapy should be provided to the patient by the psychologist, social worker, psychiatrist, or, in the case of young children, the child life specialist, for the duration of the hospital stay. Nurses, as primary front line caretakers with the most contact with the burn patients, assess the emotional and psychological status of the patient and coordinate referrals to appropriate team members. It is important that the psychotherapy be provided by a psychotherapist who is not involved in inflicting pain on the patient, so that the patient feels free to express feelings of anger and helplessness without fear of "retaliation."

In general, the focus for this period of intensive psychotherapy should be as follows: (1) Post-traumatic stress response must be recognized and treated early, to prevent withdrawal from important social, interpersonal, occupational, and educational contacts. (2) Hypnosis and abreactive techniques should be used early to obviate these effects. (3) The patient must be helped to come to terms with disfigurement and disability. Delaying truth delays rehabilitation. In studies of psychological adjustment to physiologic handicaps, mature individuals are capable and desirous of knowing facts.[18] Therapists must not project and assume people will not be able to cope. They must not overestimate patient weaknesses and underestimate their possible strengths. It is critical not to view patients' emotional disturbances necessarily as manifestations of underlying pathology.

Therapists should be more vigilant with patients who are at greater risk, i.e., patients who live alone; patients who had prior psychopathology such as depression, anxiety, or personality disorders; patients between the ages of 35 and 45; those with three or more children; those with longer hospital stays; those with more severe burns, including hands and face; children; and the aged. White[19] found that two-thirds of burned patients suffered psychological sequelae and that they were correlated with the prior categories.

Daily relaxation training–hypnosis should continue to be made available to the patient for pain control, anxiety reduction, sleep, appetite increase, and general comfort. This can be provided by a standardized tape with a diaphragmatic breathing induction, as well as individualized dissociative experience. A personal haven can be described to the patient, such as the mountains, beach, or other favorite, comfortable spot. Such training has been found to be effective with burn patients.[16,20,21] The stress inoculation procedures of Wernick[21] are useful, including education concerning the cyclic model of stress and pain, coping strategies such as relaxation training and hypnosis, and frequent coaching by team members. At least once before being discharged from the hospital, the patient and family should have the opportunity to meet with a member of the burn recovery group, i.e., someone who has been successfully rehabilitated.

During the weeks when the patient does not return for rounds, the patient should be monitored by the hydrotherapy nurses, and the occupational and physical therapists for psychosocial difficulties. The patient who does not return for medical follow-up care should be considered at psychologic risk.

Any long-term psychotherapy must take into account possible distortions projected by the various therapists. There is a tendency to assume people must be sicker than they are because they have a severe handicap. It is critical to view the patient's emotional disturbances not as a manifestation of pathology, but instead focus on the patient's interpersonal relationships, problems of interaction, and his or her functioning in a world in which his or her disfigurement is a social reality. The major factors determining whether a patient will be able to cope are not so much the premorbid personality, but perhaps previously untapped courage and resiliency of the human spirit.[5] One goal of therapy is teaching the patient to define his or her position and shift attention to him-or herself as a person behind the disfigurement. Bernstein[22] has noted that manifestations of positive self-regard and self-assurance elicit positive responses and can put at ease the nondisfigured.

CHILDREN AND THE FAMILY OF THE BURN PATIENT

One child is badly burned every 4 minutes in this country—150,000 per year. Nothing in pediatrics is more physiologically or psychologically devastating than a severe burn.[23] It is well documented that the family of the burn patient is tremendously adversely affected functionally and psychologically.[24,25] It has been pointed out that emotional adjustment in the patient is associated with more positive results from reconstructive procedures.[26] It has also been observed[27] that withdrawal in burned children is not associated with severity or location or burns, but rather with age at time of burn and the presence or absence of psychological intervention.

The initial family response to burn is often complete helplessness.[28] Other parental reactions often include difficulties in eating and sleeping. Normal family function is disrupted, and emotional lability is frequently observed.[29] Adverse effects in terms of stress on the marital relationship are also reported.[25] Negative parental coping includes blaming and denial, excessive and unresolved guilt.[25,28] Another common family problem is lack of realistic planning[30] and magical thinking about the possibilities of complete recovery.[31]

The family environment can positively or negatively influence the child's recovery. It has been pointed out that the family environment is often instrumental in reinforcing the child's regression.[32] There is also a very real danger of parents infantilizing their children and overprotecting them.[17] Further, disturbances in mothering behavior, and especially maternal guilt, are associated with behavior problems in burned children.[33] On the other hand, parents who have resolved their own guilt issues are associated with a quicker return to normalcy in the child.[34] Positive child adjustment in one study[31] was associated with the following family variables: (1) frequent and regular visits by both parents, (2) a supportive, nonblaming marital relationship, (3) parental acceptance of the outcome of the event and implications for the burned child, (4) parental ability to encourage the child to engage in normal activities, and (5) establishing a sense of mastery and control over the situation.

It has been pointed out that the family faces different adaptive tasks at different phases of treatment.[4,29,35-40] During the acute phase, the primary concern of the family is the survival of the patient, and their own feelings of guilt, helplessness, and loss of control. The family must also deal with issues of loss and grief. During this subacute phase, the family's focus is on worries about the future, the patient's appearance, ability to function, work, and resume normal familial and societal roles. Several authors have pointed out the importance of attention to the transition from hospital to home, and dealing at this point with the family's delayed grief reactions, anxiety, and dependence on hospital staff.

Play therapy is useful in the total care of the severely burned child between 1 and 14 years of age. The child's work is play and, as such, play therapy can be used by the child as a primary method for problem solving, understanding, and tolerating life. Play is a natural outlet and safety valve for explosive feelings. By providing the child with this opportunity to express him- or herself, one gains the child's trust, appeals to his natural sense of curiosity about hospital equipment and procedures, gains insight, locates problem areas, and provides interaction at the child's current developmental level.[25,40] It is during such interaction with the child, as well as family interviews, that the possibility of child abuse is assessed. It is estimated that 16 to 20 percent of pediatric burn admissions are documented child abuse cases. Data further indicate that if abused children are returned to their home environment, the likelihood of repeated injury ranges from 30 to 70 percent with a long-term mortality as high as 40 percent.[41] The first step in preventing repeat abuse is early detection, and psychosocial intervention to deal with obvious family instability, and family inability to deal with stress.[42]

DEVELOPMENTAL ASPECTS OF COPING WITH PAIN AND DEATH

There is evidence that children's responses to burns are developmentally mediated. It has been observed that the nature of the child's responses to burns vary with age—younger burn patients characteristically respond with anxiety, and older children (over 5 years) more typically engage in aggressive responses.[43] It has also been observed that adjustment is related to developmental factors. One study concludes that children burned at an earlier age make a better adjustment than those injured in middle childhood.[31] However, another study[27] came to the opposite conclusion, noting *greater*, withdrawal in children burned at an early age (under 10 years).

Several authors have identified specific issues of psychological adjustment to pain associated with particular periods of childhood.[4,24,29,44] In infancy, common reactions to pain from a burn are withdrawal, a sad facial expression, eating and sleep disturbances, and failure to positively respond to a caretaker. The primary problem is one of separation anxiety. Interventions emphasize the importance of physical contact, the maintenance of a one-to-one relationship with a caretaker, and the success of visual and auditory distraction.

In the preschool years, children react to pain by crying, and becoming immobile, clinging, and anxious. They often suffer nightmares, confusion, panic, and lose verbal and motor skills and sphincter control. Treatment approaches include the presence of a competent parent, play preparation, simple, accessible explanations, and opportunities to express feelings.

During the school years, the response to pain is characterized by hyperactivity, extreme passivity, shame, nightmares, panic attacks, encopresis, somatization, impulsivity, and depression. These children often become agitated, angry, and manipulative. The school age child needs to feel in control, which can be accomplished by behavioral contracting, self-help, participation in treatment, and relaxation techniques.

The adolescent's response to pain represents the full range of repressive possibilities (anxiety, depression, aggressiveness, manipulation); indeed, adolescent burn patients are notable for their extreme regression, probably as a result of their complete helplessness and loss of a sense of control. Self-esteem and body image are affected and the adolescent tasks of identity formation are immensely complicated by the presence of scarring. Self-hypnosis and relaxation techniques are recommended.

Burn Recovery Group, School Re-Entry Program
The burn recovery group is a vital rehabilitation tool in which patients are encouraged to maintain continued contact with each other. The group provides a supportive and educational milieu in which to ventilate frustration that occurs as rehabilitation proceeds.

The school re-entry program model has been designed by a burn patient, Barbara Kammerer, who is herself a secondary school teacher. Her program is in part based on the difficulties she experienced with re-entry, and has the unique vantage point of patient and teacher. The major goal of the program is to ease the transition of the severely burned child in returning to the classroom in order to increase the potential for recovering his or her former social and academic skills. The mechanics of the program are as follows: The school re-entry counselor should meet with the child and the family early in the recovery period to make them aware of the program. The administration and classroom teachers should be informed of the student's condition, and communication encouraged between the teachers, classmates, and the burned child to maintain the link between the burned student and the school.

Teachers should make personal contact with the child, as well as conduct classroom projects that can be taken to the child. Letters, cards, collages, and drawings are typical projects.

Approximately 1 week before the student returns to school, 1-hour long presentations are made to the entire staff and faculty, the classmates and, in some cases, the entire student body. The presentations consist of a slide program, lecture, and discussion period. From 35 to 40 slides are used in the presentation which is altered to fit the maturity level of the students. The slides demonstrate what happens to skin anatomically when it is burned by showing the three types of burns and the affects of each on the skin. Slides of patients being treated in the hydrotherapy room, the critical care unit, and occupational therapy are included. An explanation of the pressure garments and their importance in the student's recovery are shown through the use of slides of school age patients. The school re-entry program is designed to promote understanding of the burned student, the burn center, burn care, the rehabilitation process, and burn prevention. After the student has returned to school, follow-up contacts are made with the parents and classroom teachers to assess and continue to assist in the student's adjustment.[45]

The subjectively observed results of the program are positive. Other students make fewer unkind remarks, demonstrate greater concern for the burned student, accept him or her more readily, and are more supportive when the student must return to the hospital for future surgeries. When others show that they accept the burned child, he or she often feels more accepting and confident of him- or herself and his or her situation.

Excessive staring and taunting remarks seem to be the result of a lack of understanding and knowledge among the general public. The harm done psychologically and emotionally can have lasting effects which prohibit normal development. By providing a program to ease the transition of students returning to school, burn centers not only assist the burned child to return to a more humane school atmosphere, but can also impact a wider community population with an understanding of burns, burn centers, and the care provided.

The staff should also remain cognizant of the relationship between physical attractiveness and perceived functional ability. Even in nursery school, a child's popularity correlates with physical attractiveness. A nonattractive child is thought to be "scary." There is evidence that attractiveness affects nursing care as well as mothering time. Attractive children are given more attention by their teachers, more information, better evaluations, more opportunity to perform, and more support for the child's endeavors. The evidence is that the physically attractive child lives in a different social world than his or her disfigured counterparts. Attractiveness affects recommendations by experienced personnel consultants, and treatment received from authorities.[46] Studies show that appearance affects rating of work and influences salaries offered. Positive personality characteristics are ascribed to attractive people and vice versa. Even 3-year-olds ascribe to the belief that "beautiful is good."[47]

VOCATIONAL REHABILITATION

Patients are recovering faster, leaving the hospital sooner, having fewer functional disabilities and less disfigurement. However, with longer patient follow-up, it is evident that vocational and psychological rehabilitation has not been adequate. It is evident from workmen's compensation evaluations that a patient's mental status can ameliorate physical capabilities. PTSDs are more common than suspected and not easily detected.[48] The following type of patient has often been thought to be malingering.

> Case 4:
> As the result of an aircraft crash, a female patient suffered second- and third-degree flame burns to 40 percent of her body. She had reconstuctive surgery, progressed well, and was discharged to return to work. To the outside world she admitted no physical or psychological disability, until she attempted to return to work. Under the stress of constant reminders from well-wishers, she broke down and admitted having symptoms of insomnia, nightmares, nervousness, withdrawal from friends and previously enjoyed recreational activity. The precipitating event which made her seek psychotherapy was a news report of an aircraft crash which caused her to emotionally decompensate; she also noted phobic responses to aircraft-related phenomena in general and was unable to return to her former level of competence at work.

The basic psychotherapy regimen (1) encourages the open expression of anxiety and depression, (2) encourages the direct, rather than indirect, expression of anger, (3) replaces feelings of helplessness with competence, and (4) stimulates awareness of social supports.[49] There are ample data that psychological reactions to illness or injury mediate rehabilitation outcomes. The patients who later recover well from these physical stresses are those who earlier have openly expressed anxiety about them.[50]

DESENSITIZATION AND RETURN TO WORK

Hypnosis, relaxation training, and visual imagery are indispensable tools in allowing the patient to control the fear and anxiety concomitant with phobic reactions to trauma. These techniques can be used by professionals trained in their use as (1) rehearsals of return to stressful work–school situations; (2) desensitization procedures for return to the actual site of accident; and (3) techniques for dealing with anticipated stressful situations. It is, of course, essential when attempting to extinguish excessive emotional responses, to repeat the procedure until the patient feels *completely* relaxed while contemplating the stressor.

Case: 5
Louise, mentioned earlier, was taught to relax in the psychologist's office and in this relaxed state rehearsed successfully and calmly returning to work. She then repeatedly imagined herself seated in an airplane, remaining calm and in control, feeling satisfaction at being able to fly again, without having her knees knock together. Finally, she was taught self-hypnosis to be practiced at home in her den, in her recliner chair. She learned to recreate this most relaxing state, while on the airplane itself, she had only to touch her wrist. Her wrist became a talisman, a reminder, a cue that she could be just as relaxed and as in control as she was at home in her easy chair.

REFERENCES

1. Perry RR, et al.: A research model for the study of rehabilitation among adult burn patients. Rehab Lit 43:77, 1982
2. Clark AM: Thermal injuries: The care of the whole child. J Trauma 20:823, 1980
3. Chang F: Burn morbidity. A follow-up study of physical and psychological disability. Ann Surg 183:34, 1976
4. Helm PA, Kevorkian CG, Lushbaugh M, et al.: Burn injury: Rehabilitation management in 1982. Arch Phys Med Rehab 63:6, 1982
5. MacGregor F: After Plastic Surgery. New York, J.F. Bergin, 1979
6. Kardiner A: The Traumatic Neuroses of War. New York, Harper and Brothers, 1941
7. Gruen W: Effects of brief psychotheraphy during the hospitalization period on the recovery process in heart attacks. J Consult Clin Psychol 43:223, 1975
8. Capone M, Westie K, Chitwood J, et al.: A functional model for hospitalized cancer patients. Am J Orth Psych 49:598, 1979
9. Diagnostic and Statistical Manual of Mental Disorders, 3rd ed. (DMS-III). Washington, D.C., Am Psych Assoc, 1980
10. Martinez S: Behavioral manifestations of the patient requirements in pain. Graduate paper prepared for MA in Nursing, California State University, Long Beach, Calif., 1979
11. Stoelting RK: Opiate receptors and endorphins. Anesth Analg 59:874, 1980
12. Bonica JJ, Albe-Fessard D (eds): Advances in Pain Research, Vol. I. New York, Raven Press, 1976
13. Melzach R, Ofiesch JG, Mount BM: The Brampton mixture: Effects on pain in cancer patients. Can Med Assoc J 115:125, 1976
14. Mdertel CG, Ahmann DL, Taylor WF, Schwartau N: Relief of pain by oral medications. JAMA 229:55, 1974
15. Moore D: Treatment of chronic pain with tricyclic antidepressants. South Med J 73:1585, 1980
16. Crasilneck HB, Stirman JA, Wilson BJ, et al.: Use of hypnosis in the management of patients with burns. JAMA 158:103, 1955
17. Davidson TN, Bowden ML, Tholen D, et al.: Social supports and post-burn adjustment. Arch Phys Med Rehab 62:274, 1981
18. Davis F: Passage through crisis. Polio victims and their families. Indianapolis, Bobbs-Merrill, 1963

19. White A: Psychological sequellae more likely in burn patients living alone. Br Med J 284:465, 1982
20. Schafer DW: Hypnosis use on a burn unit. Int J Clin Exper Hypnosis 23:1, 1975
21. Wernick RL, et al.: Pain management in severely burned adults: A test of stress inoculation. J Behav Med 41:104, 1981
22. Bernstein NR: Medical tragedies in facial disfigurement. Pysch Ann 6:33, 1975
23. Trunkey D, Parks S: Burns in children. Cur Probl Pediatr 6:3, 1976
24. Stoddard FJ: Coping with pain: A developmental approach to the treatment of burned children. Am J Psych 139:736, 1982
25. Cahners SS: A strong hospital-school liaison: A necessity for good rehabilitation planning for disfigured children. Scand J Plast Reconstr Surg 13:167, 1979
26. Feller I, Tholen D, Cornell, RG: Improvements in burn care, 1965–1979. JAMA 244:2074, 1980
27. Molinaro JR: The social fate of children disfigured by burns. Am J Psych 135:979, 1978
28. Cook T: Psychosocial assessments of families on a pediatric burn center. J Burn Care Rehab 3:105, 1982
29. Knudson-Cooper MS: Emotional care of the hospitalized burn child. J Burn Care Rehab 3:109, 1982
30. Bartlett RH, et al.: Rehabilitation following burn injury. Surg Clin North Am 58:1249, 1978
31. Giljohann A: Adolescents burned as children. Burns 7:95, 1979
32. Bowden ML, et al.: Progress in rehabilitation. A review of three studies." Nat Inst Burns, 1982
33. Martin HL: Antecedents of burns and scalds in children. Br J Med Psych 43:39, 1970
34. Solomon JR: Care and needs in a children's burn unit. Prog Ped Surg 14:19, 1980
35. Bowden ML: Rehabilitation of the burned child. J Burn Care Res 3:109, 1982
36. Luther SL, Price J: Burns and their psychological effects on children. J School Health 51:419, 1981
37. MacGregor F: Social and psychological studies of plastic surgery. Clin Plast Surg 9:283, 1982
38. Talabere L, et al.: A tool for assessing families of burned children. Am J Nurs 76:225, 1976
39. Hill MP: Supportive followup and discharge. Am J Nurs 76:228, 1976
40. Levinson P: Art and play therapy with pediatric burn patients. J Burn Care Rehab 3:42, 1977
41. Deitch EA, Staats M: Child abuse through burning. J Burn Care Res 3:89, 1982
42. Hight D, Bakalar HR, Lloyd JR: Inflicted burns in children: Recognition and treatment. JAMA 242:517, 1979
43. Miller WC, Gardner N, Mlott, SR: Psychosocial support in the treatment of severely burned patients. J Trauma 16:722, 1976
44. Theimer V: Individual approaches. J Burn Care Res 3:101, 1982
45. Kammerer B: School re-entry program for the burned child. Paper read at the Sixth International Congress on Burns, San Francisco, August 31, 1982
46. Bercheid E, et al.: Medical tragedies in facial disfigurement. Psych Ann 6:33, 1975
47. Pertschuk M, et al.: Social and psychological effects of craniofacial deformity and surgical reconstruction. Clin Plast Surg 9:297, 1982

48. Putten T, et al.: Vietnam Returnees: A forgotten diagnosis? Arch Gen Psych 29, 1973
49. Viney LL: Patterns of anxiety in the chronically ill. Br J Med Psych 55:87, 1982
50. Viney LL: Use of a model of reaction to illness-related stress to develop a hospital-based counseling program. Paper read at the Australian Psychological Conference, Melbourne, August 7, 1982

Index

Italicized *t* and *f* indicate tables and figures respectively.

ABC's, 9, 10
Acetic acid, 192
Acetylsalicyclic acid, 39–40*f*
Acid-base status, 88
Acid burns, 191–193, 196–198*f*
Acidosis, 88, 167
Adenosine diphosphate (ADP), 28
Adenylcyclase activators, 60
Adrenocorticotropin hormone (ACTH), 43–44
Adult respiratory distress syndrome (ARDS)
　pathophysiology, 152–153, 166
　treatment, 159
Age
　incidence and severity of burn injury complications, 161
　pediatric burns and, 203
Airplane splints, 229, 231*f*
Airway obstruction, 155, 166
Albumin, serum, 137
Alkalosis, 88–89
Allograft, 103
Aloe vera plant, 35
Alpha$_2$ macroglobulin, 53
American Burn Association, classification of burn injuries, 18*t*, 109
Amitriptyline, 249
Ammonia, 191, 195
Amperage, 184
Analgesics
　administration of, 215, 219
　　basic rules, 249, 252
　narcotic, 248–249, 250*t*–251*t*
　for outpatient management, 113

Anatomical regions, frequency of burn injury, 6*f*
Ankle burns, 233–234*f*
Anorexia, 143, 146
Anthropometric measurements, in assessment of nutritional status, 136–138*t*
Antibiotics. *See also* specific antibiotics, nephrotoxicity, 167
Antibodies, role in host defense, 53
Antibody-mediated immunity, 50–51*f*
Anticlaw position, 225*f*
Antideformity position, 223–224*f*
Antidepressants, 249
Antigens, skin test, 137, 138*t*
Antimicrobials, topical, 93, 94*t*
Arachidonic acid, inhibition of metabolism, 40*f*
Arm circumference, 136, 138*t*
Autografting, 97–104*f*
Automobiles, crash-worthy fuel systems in, 8–9
Axilla burns, 229, 230*f*, 231*f*, 232*f*

Basal metabolism expenditure, 135
Battered child syndrome, 207–208
Beta-lysin, 50
Biobrane, 103–104*f*, 116–118*f*
Bleach, household, 195
Blood flow restoration, 157–158
Blood gas analysis
　for early respiratory failure, 156

Blood gas analysis (cont.)
 monitoring and, 87–88t
 respiratory failure and, 153
Blood-lymph barrier, permeability, 29–30f
Blood pressure, arterial, 80–81
Blood volume
 assessment of, 87
 deficits, 80
 restoration in respiratory failure, 156–157
B lymphocytes, antibody-mediated immunity and, 50–51f
Body surface area, injured, 11f, 14
Bone marrow-derived system (B cell), 50–51f
Brain cell ischemia, 155
Brigham Burn Budget, 71–73t, 76
Brompton's solution, 248
Bronchoscopy, 156
Brooke formula, 69, 72f, 76
Burn centers. *See also* Hospitalization
 admitting factors, 15
 distribution in United States, 17
 nurse orientation, 220–221
Burn nurses
 burn complications and, 213
 education of, 221
 graft and donor care, 215
 importance of, 215, 219–220, 222
 orientation for burn center, 220–221
 responsibilities, graft and donor care, 215
 treatment role, 214
  debridement, 214–215
Burn recovery groups, 240, 257–259
Burn transfer checklist, 15, 16f
Burn unit. *See* Burn centers

Calcium, serum, 75
Calcium salts, 199–200
Calmette–Guerin bacillus, 60
Caloric requirements, 139–141t
Capillary filtration coefficient, 28–29f
Capillary plexuses, 27f
Carbohydrate requirements, 140–141

Carbon dioxide tension, arterial ($Paco_2$), 156
Carbon monoxide poisoning
 neurologic impairment, 170
 pathophysiology, 150–151f
 patient transport, 13
 treatment, 154–155
Cardiac output, 80, 84
Cardiovascular system complications, 164–165
Case studies
 of nonpharmacologic pain control, 252–253
 of vocational rehabilitation, 259
 of work re-entry and desensitization, 260
Catecholamines, 80
Catheter placement, indwelling, 86
Cement, 194
Central venous pressure, 82–83
Cerebral edema, 155
Chemical burns
 classification of injury, 189–198f
 evaluation of, 9
 extent of injury, mortality and hospitalization, 190t
 treatment, 198–201
 treatment at scene of injury, 11–12
Chemicals, toxic, 152
Chemotactic factors, 55
Chemotaxis, leukocyte, 55–56f
Chest wall burns, circumferential, 151f
Chest x-ray, 89, 156
Child abuse, 207–208, 256
Children
 burns of. *See* Pediatric burns
 developmental aspects of coping with pain and death, 256–259
Chloracetophenone, 194
Cholecystitis, acalculous, 168
Chromic acid, 192
Chronic obstructive pulmonary disease (COPD), 13
Cigarettes
 burns from, 207
 "fire safe", 8
Cimetidine, prevention of edema, 40, 41f

INDEX **265**

Classification of burns, 23–26t
  by American Burn Association, 18t, 109
  history of, 3
Claw hand deformity, 123, 225
Clorox-Betadine solution, 110
Coagulation, zone of, 26f, 27
Coagulation system, activation in acute phase of burn injury, 31f
Coagulopathy, 171–172
Cocaine, 248–249
Codeine, 249, 251t
Collagen-chondroitin sulfate-silicone skin substitute, 104
Colloid resuscitation, 76, 157. *See also* Resuscitation
Complement, 50
Complement system, immune response and, 54f
Complications
  cardiovascular, 164–165
  endocrine, 169
  gastrointestinal, 167–168
  metabolic, 168–169
  musculoskeletal, 170–171
  neurologic, 169–170, 188
  nurses and, 213
  nutritional, 168–169
  principles of treatment, 173–174
  renal, 167
  risk factors, 161–162t
  systemic
    classification by etiology, 162, 163t
    organ system approach to, 164t
Conduction, of heat, 22–23
Contractures, 235–236
Cooling, modification depth of burn wound, 34–35, 36f, 37f
Copper sulfate, 200
Corticosteroids, systemic, 159
Cortisol, plasma, 44
Corynebacterium parvum, 60
Cryogenic materials, 195–196f
Crystalloid resuscitation, 76, 157. *See also* Resuscitation
Current
  alternating, 184–185
  direct, 185
  high tension, 184
Cyclosporine, 103

Death
  coping with, developmental aspects of, 256–259
  pediatric, 203
  rates
    of adults, 7f
    by state, 5f
Debridement
  nursing responsibilities, 214–215, 218f, 219f
  in outpatient management, 114–115
Defense mechanisms, 244
Deformities, potential. *See also* specific deformities
  of ankle burns, 233
  of axilla burns, 229
  of dorsal hand burn, 225
  of elbow burn, 228
  of foot burns, 234
  of hip burns, 233
  of knee burns, 233
  of neck burns, 229
  of palmar hand burn, 228
Dehydration, 35, 38f, 146
Delayed hypersensitivity skin testing, 137, 138t
Demerol (meperidine), 248, 250t, 251t
Depth of burn assessment in emergency department, 15
  classification by, 3
  estimation, 4f
  evaporative water loss and, 32
  modification
    by cooling, 34–35, 36f, 37f
    by pharmacologic manipulation, 35, 39–40
    by prevention of dehydration, 35, 38f
Dermal plexus, 27f
Dermatomes
  drum, 97–99f
  hand, 96f
  power, 97, 99–101f

Diagnostics, 13
Diarrhea, secondary to enteral nutrition, 146
Dicloromethane, 193
Dilaudid (hydromorphone), 248, 250t, 251t
Discomfort of patient, dealing with, 219–220
Disposition of burn patients, 12f, 15–16f
Disseminated intravascular coagulopathy syndrome, 171–172
Diuretic phase of resuscitation, 74
Diuretics, 157
Dolophine (methadone), 248, 250t, 251t
Donor care, 215
Doppler pulse, 121
Doxepin, 249
Drugs. *See also* specific drugs
  for modification of burn wound depth, 35, 39–40
  stimulation of immunologic activity, 60

Edema
  cerebral, 155
  formation following burn injury, 28–31f
  laryngeal, 166
  pulmonary, 166
  shock and, 80
  supraglottic, 155
Education
  of nurses, 221
  of patient and family, 115
Elastic pressure garments, 237–239f
Elbow burns, 228–229f
Electrical burns
  electric arc travel vs. voltage, 186t
  rescue of victim, 186–188
  severity of, 185
  terminology, 184–186
  treatment, 188–189, 200–201
  treatment at scene of injury, 12
Emergency department
  assessment of burn injury, 14–15
  treatment in, 15–19f

Encephalopathy, 165, 169–170
Endocarditis, bacterial, 165
Endocrine system
  changes following thermal injury, 42–44f
  complications, 169
Endoperoxidases, 33
Endoperoxides, 28
Endotracheal intubation, 155, 156t
Enteral nutrition
  commercially available formulas, 142–145t
  complications of, 145–147
  infusion pump, 145
  tubes, 145f
Epidemiology
  age and sex of pediatric burns, 203
  size of burn problem, 4–5f
  types of burns in children, 203–204t
Epinephrine, 95, 96
Erythrocytes, destruction and lysis, 42
Escharectomy, 95
Escharotomy
  of extremities, 121–123f
  of lower extremity burns, 128, 130
  sites, 123f
Ethylene oxide, 194
Evaluation
  of electrical burn patient, 187–188
  of extent of injury, 11f
  of patient, 10
  of scene of accident, 9–10
Evans formula, 68, 72t, 76
Exchange transfusion, 61, 95
Excision
  primary, 96–97, 125–126f
  sequential, 94–95
  tangential, 95–96, 96f, 125f
Exercises
  for ankle burns, 234
  for axilla burns, 229, 232f
  for dorsal hand burn, 227f
  for elbow burn, 228–229f
  for facial burns, 234
  for foot burns, 234
  for hip burns, 233
  for knee burns, 233
  for neck burns, 231
  for palmar hand burn, 228

Exposure, duration of, 21–22f
Extent of burn injury
  assessment in emergency department, 14–15
  chemical burns vs. all burns, 190t
  evaluation of, 11f
Extremities. *See also* specific extremity
  escharotomy, 121–123f
  intermediate care, 126, 128
  lower, burns of, 127f, 128–130f
Eye burns, 12, 191

Fabrics, flammable, 8
Facial burns
  admission to burn unit, 109–110
  exercises for, 234
  treatment, 234–235, 238f
Facial disfigurement, 244
Factor B, 54
Factor V, 42
Factor VIII, 42
Family
  assessment of support, 254
  of burn patient, 255–256
  education of, 115
  initial response to injury, 255
  support of, 116
Fats, requirements for, 141
Fibrin degradation products, 171
Fibrinogen, 42
Fibronectin, 58
Fick equation, 85t
Fire prevention, 6–9
Fire suppression systems, automatic, 7–8
First degree injury, 23
Flaps, myocutaneous
  dorsi, 129f, 130f
  gastrocnemius, 127f, 128f
Fluid requirements, pediatric, 205–206
Fluid resuscitation. *See* Resuscitation
Flurandrenolide tape, 239
Foam padding, under pressure garments, 238–239f
Follicle stimulating hormone (FSH), 43
Foot burns, 128, 234f
Formaldehyde, 192

Formulas
  burn resuscitation, 68–73t, 76, 206
  enteral nutrition, 142–145t
Fourth degree burns, 23, 25–26
Friends, support assessment, 254
Full thickness burns
  characteristics of, 15, 23, 25t
  estimation of depth, 3, 4f

Gasoline burns, 193–194f
Gastric aspiration, avoidance in enteral nutrition, 145–146
Gastrointestinal system, complications, 167–168
Glucagon, 43, 44f
Glucocorticoids, 43, 44f
Glucosuria, 146
Grafts. *See* Skin grafts

HALFD formula, 70–71, 72t
Hand burns
  antideformity position for, 124
  dorsal, 95–96, 225–227f
  initial management, 124f
  palmar, 228
  positioning and, 123–125f
  primary excision, 125–126f
Heart rate, 80–81
Heat
  conductance, 22–23
  intensity, 21–22f
  loss, following thermal injury, 42–43
  production by current, 185
  transferral, 183
Hematocrit, 42
Hematology, changes following burn injury, 42, 171–172
Hemoglobinemia, 187
Hips, burns of, 233
Histamine, 50
Histamine antagonists, 40, 41f
Histamines, 80
History
  of burn classification, 3
  of fluid resuscitation, 67–68

History (cont.)
  of post-traumatic stress disorder, 244–247
Hormones, response to thermal injury, 43–44f
Hospitalization. See also Burn centers
  admission criteria, pediatric, 204–205
  chemical burns vs. all burns, 190t
Host deficiency, 59
Humoral immunity, 52–53f
Hybridoma, 61
Hydrochloric acid, 152, 192–193
Hydrocyanic acid, 152
Hydrofluoric acid burns
  characteristics of injury, 191, 196–198f
  treatment of, 199
Hydromorphone (Dilaudid), 248, 250t, 251t
Hydrotherapy, 114–115, 214, 218f
5-Hydroxytryptamine, 31
Hydroxyzine, 248
Hyperalimentation, central venous, 147
Hypermia, zone of, 26f
Hyperkalemia, 75t, 187
Hypernatremia, 74–75t
Hyperosmolar syndromes, 146
Hypersensitivity, 227
Hypertension, acute, 165
Hypertonic formulas, 70, 72t, 76
Hypnosis, 252–255, 259
Hypochlorite, 195
Hypokalemia, 75t
Hypomagnesium, 75–76
Hyponatremia, 75t
Hypoproteinemia, 137
Hypothermia, 81

Immobilization, post-surgical, 235
Immune response
  complement system and, 54f
  components of, 49–57
  defects following thermal injury, 58–59f, 60–61, 172–173
  interactions of, 58–59f
  phagocytic cells and, 55–57f
  specific, 50–51f
  interaction with nonspecific immunity following thermal injury, 57–58
Immunity
  cell-mediated, 51–52f
  humoral, 52–53f
  nonspecific, 49–50
Immunoglobulins, 53
Immunomodulation, 60–61
Immunomodulators, ideal, 60
Immunosuppressive drugs, 103
Impramine, 249
Incidence of burn injury
  in adults, 7f
  in children, 7f
  geographic, 5
  related to anatomical regions, 6f
Indomethacin, 39–40f
Infection. See Sepsis
Inflammatory mediators, 30–31f
Inhalation injury
  diagnosis of, 153
  pathophysiology, 151–152, 166
  ventilatory support, 158–159t
Insulin, 43
Interleukin 1, 60
Interleukin 2, 60
Intermittent mandatory ventilation (IMV), 158–159
Internal fixation, for hand burn grafting, 125–126f
Intravenous infusion, 10, 12–13

Joints. See also specific joints
  acute treatment, 225–235f
  post-surgical immobilization and mobilization, 235
Joule's law, 185
Joule-Thompson effect, 195–196

Kallikrein-kinin system, 50
Ketamine, 95, 114
Kidney complications, 167
Kinins, 31, 50, 80

Knee burns, 233f
Kupffer cells, 57

Lacrimatory agents, 194–195
Laryngeal problems, 166
Lavage, 11–12
Leg burns, 127f, 128–130f
Leukopenia, 93
Levamisole, 60
Levels of burn care, 15
Levorphanol (Levodromoran), 248, 250t, 251t
Liver dysfunction, 168
Lund and Browder chart, 11f, 14
Lungs. *See* Respiratory system
Lung sounds, 13
Lung water, 166
Luteinizing hormone (LH), 43
Lymphocytes, total count, 137
Lymphokines, 60

Macrophage phagocytosis, 57
Mafenide, 93
Mannitol, 167
Massage, deep pressure circular, 239
MAST, 12
Memory cells, 51–52
Meperidine (Demerol), 248, 250t, 251t
Meshing, 101–102f
Metabolic complications from burns, 42–44f, 168–169
Methadone (Dolophine), 248, 250t, 251t
Methylene chloride (dichloromethane), 193
Methylprednisolone acetate, 35
Military Anti-Shock Trousers (MAST), 12
Mineral requirements, 141
Mobilization, post-surgical, 235
Monitoring
  approaches, summary of, 89
  of blood volume, 87
  of cardiac output, 84
  of central venous pressure, 82–83
  invasive, complications of, 86
  of nutritional status, 147–148
  of oxygen delivery and consumption, 84–85t
  physiologic variables, 85t
  principles of, 79–80
  of pulmonary artery, 83t
  of respiratory function, 87–89t
  of resuscitation, 73, 74f
  transcutaneous oxygen, 86–87
  of urine output, 81–82
  of vital signs, 80–81
Monitors, 214, 218f
Morphine, 248, 250t, 251t
Mortality, chemical burns vs. all burns, 190t
Multiple disaster burn victims, 13–14
Muramyl dipeptide, 60
Musculoskeletal system complications, 170–171
Myofibroblasts, 236
Myoglobinemia, 187
Myoglobinuria, 167

NADPH-oxidases, 32, 34f
Neck burns, acute treatment, 229–232f
Necrosis, zone of, 26f
NeoSynephrine, 95–96
Neurological system, complications, 169–170, 188
Neutrophils
  function of chemotaxis and phagocytosis, 55–57f, 58
  functions of intracellular killing, 58, 59
  oxygen burst, 32–33, 34f
Nitric acid, 192
Nitrogen loss, 140
Nitrous oxide, 152
Nonthermal burns, 183–184. *See also* Chemical burns; Electrical burns
Normeperidine, 248
Numorphan (oxymorphone), 250t, 251t
Nurses. *See* Burn nurses
Nutrition
  assessment of status, 136–138t
  complications of, 168–169

Nutrition (cont.)
  delivery of nutrients, 141–147f
  initial support of burn patient and, 135–136
  inpatient vs. outpatient, 115
  monitoring status, 147–148
  pediatric requirements, 206
  specific requirements, 139–141t

Opsonization, 58
Osteolysis, from hydrofluoric acid, 198
Outpatient management
  applications for nonburn center facility, 119
  biobrane dressing technique, 116–118f
  criteria, 109–110
  debridement, 114–115
  education of patient and family, 115
  healing and follow-up, 118–119f
  medications, 111, 113
  rehabilitation of joints, 235–236
  team concept, 113–114
  transition from inpatient status, 115–116
  wound care, 110–111f, 112f
Oxycodone, 251t
Oxygen
  consumption, monitoring of, 84–85t
  delivery, monitoring of, 84–85t
  gradient, alveolar-arterial difference, 88
  hyperbaric, 13
  transcutaneous monitoring, 86–87
Oxygen burst, 32–33, 34f
Oxygen free radicals, 32–33, 34f
Oxymorphone (Numorphan), 250t, 251t

Pain
  control
    burn nurse and, 215, 219
    nonpharmacologic, 252–253
    outpatient, 111, 113
    coping with, developmental aspects of, 256–259

  pharmacologic treatment of, 247–252t
  types of, 247
Pancreatitis, 168
Paraquat, 194
Parents, of burn patient, 256
Parkland formula, 69–70, 72t, 76, 206
Partial thickness burns
  characteristics of, 15, 23, 24–25t
  conversion to full thickness wounds, 32
  estimation of depth, 3, 4f
  hypertrophic scarring and, 237
Pathophysiology of burn wounds
  local effects of thermal injury
    classification of burns, 23–26t
    conductance, 22–23
    edema formation, 28–31f
    evaporative water loss, 32, 33f
    intensity and duration, 21–22f
    modifying depth of burn wound, 34–40f, 41f
    overview of wound physiology, 33–34
    oxygen free radicals, 32–33, 34f
    tissue response, 26–27f
    vascular response, 27–28f
  systemic effects of thermal injury, 40, 42–44f
Pediatric burns
  epidemiology, 203–204t
  management, 204–208
  prevention, 208
  response of family to, 255–256
PEEP, 158–159
Peer support, 254
Pentazocine (Talwin), 251t
Peripheral vascular resistance, 80
Permanganate ions, 195
Peroxidases, 32, 34f
Phagocytic cells, immune response and, 55–57f
Phagocytosis, 56f, 58
Pharmacologic treatment, of pain, 247–252t
Phenol burns, 191, 192f, 199
Phosphorus, 195, 200
Physician–nurse relationship, 113–114
Picric acid, 192, 193, 195

Pig skin, 103
"Pinprick sensation", 15
Plasmapheresis, 61
Platelet
 adhesiveness, 42
 aggregation, 28
 count, following burn injury, 171
 survival, 42
Play therapy, 256
Poly (AC), 60
Poly (IC), 60
Polymorphonuclear neutrophils. *See* Neutrophils
Positioning
 of ankle burns, 234
 of elbow burn, 228
 of foot burns, 234
 of hand, 225*f*
 of hip burns, 233
 of knee burns, 233
 of neck burns, 230
 of palmar hand burn, 228
Positive end-expiratory pressure (PEEP), 158–159
Postage stamp technique, 101
Post-traumatic stress disorder (PTSD)
 case studies, 246–247
 history of, 244–247
 prognosis, 247
 symptoms, 246
Povidone-iodine, 194
Prehospital care. *See* Scene of burn injury
Prevention
 of burns, 9
 of dehydration, 35, 38*f*
 of fires, 6–9
 of pediatric burns, 208
Prognosis, 17, 19*f*
Properdin, 54
Propoxyphene, 249
Prostaglandins
 in acute phase of burn injury, 31*f*, 80
 inhibition of metabolism, 40*f*
 regeneration of, 33
Prostaglandin synthetase inhibitors, 39–40*f*
Protein
 loss, extravascular, 30
 plasma levels, 136–138*t*
 requirements, 140
Pseudomonas vaccines, 61
Psychological effects, of burn injury, 244–247
Psychosocial aspects
 of long-term care, 220
 of pediatric burns, 206–207
 of treatment, 253–255
Psychotherapy, 254, 255, 259
Pulmonary artery catheterization, 83*t*, 86
Pulmonary edema, 166
Pulmonary wedge pressure, 83, 157

Rehabilitation
 burn recovery group, 240
 exercises for. *See* Exercises
 initial evaluation, 223
 outpatient, 235–236
 return to school, 240
 return to work, 239–240
 success, 243
 summary of, 240–241
 vocational, 259
Relaxation techniques, 252–255, 259
"Respiratory burst", 58
Respiratory rate, 81
Respiratory system
 complications, 149–150, 165–166
  treatment of, 154–159*t*
 diagnosis of complications, 153–154
 failure, 166
  early, 156–159
  late, 159
 pathophysiology of, 150–153*f*
 monitoring of, 87–89*t*
Resuscitation
 burn formulas, 68–71
 colloid, 76
 diuretic phase, 74
 for early respiratory failure, 157
 electrolyte disturbances, 74–76*t*
 flow sheet, 216*f*–217*f*
 history, 67–68
 monitoring, 73, 74*f*
 protocol, 214

Reticuloendothelial system
　depression after burn injury, 57–58
　phagocytic cells, 55–57f
Ringer's solution, lactated, 10
Rule of 50, 68, 72f
Rule of Nines, 10, 11f, 14

Scalds
　intentional, 207
　pediatric, 203–204t
　prevention, 8
Scars
　hypertrophic
　　causes of, 236–237
　　severity of, 236
　　splints to control, 235, 238f
　management of, 236–237
　treatment of, 237–239f
Scene of injury
　evaluation of, 9–10
　incidence and, 5–6
　treatment at, 10–12
School, return to, 240, 243–244, 257–259
Second degree burns, 23, 24
Sedation, for escharotomy, 122–123
Sepsis
　burn shock and, 80
　complications of, 162
　diagnosis and treatment, 172–173
　from invasive monitoring, 86
　signs of, 105
Serotonin, 50
Severity of burn injury, 18t
Sex, pediatric burns and, 203
Shock, burn, 79–80
Shock victim, electrical, rescue of, 186–188
Silvadene. See Silver sulfadiazine
Silver nitrate, 94t, 195
Silver sulfadiazine (Silvadene)
　advantages and limitations, 93, 94t
　for outpatient management, 111f, 112f
Skin expansion techniques, 101–102f
Skin grafts
　care of, 215
　donor sites, 105

　for hand burn, internal fixation of, 125–126f
　xenografts, 103
Skin substitutes, ideal properties of, 103t
Smoke detectors, 6–7
Smoke inhalation injury. See Inhalation injury
Social factors, in burn injury recovery, 116
Spirometry, 154
Splinting
　of ankle burns, 234f
　of axilla burns, 229, 230f, 231f
　of dorsal hand burn, 225–227f
　dynamic, 236
　of elbow burn, 228–229f
　of foot burns, 234f
　of hip burns, 233
　of knee burns, 233f
　of neck burns, 230–231, 232
Splints, 224–225
Stasis, zone of, 26–27f, 34
Steroids, 39, 159
Stress, neurohormonal response to, 135
Subdermal plexus, 27f
Subpapillary plexus, 27f
Sulfur dioxide, 152
Superficial burn wound, characteristics of, 23–24
Superior mesenteric artery syndrome (SMA), 167, 168
Superoxide dimutase, 32–33, 34f
Superoxide radical, 32–33, 34f
Surgical management, of burn wound, 94–105f, 239
Survival of burn patient, 17, 19
Swan–Ganz catheter, 83, 86

Talwin (pentazocine), 251t
Tannic acid, 195
Team approach
　in outpatient management, 113–114
　for pediatric burns, 207
Temperature
　body, monitoring of, 81
　of conductor, 185–186
Testosterone, 43

Therapists, 254
Thiomersol, 194
Third degree burns, hypertrophic scarring and, 237
Third degree injury, 23
Thrombin, 95
Thrombocytopenia, 42
Thrombocytosis, secondary, 42
Thrombophlebitis, septic, 162, 165
Thrombosis, venous, 28
Thromboxanes, 28, 40f
Thumb splinting, 226
Thymopoietin, 61
Thymosin, 61
Thymus-derived system (T cell), 50–51f
Thyroid function, postburn, 44
Tissue response to burn injury, local, 26–27
T lymphocytes
  acceleration of maturation, 60–61
  alterations following thermal injury, 59
  cell-mediated immunity and, 50, 51–52f
Toxins, bacterial, 28
Tracheostomy, 155, 166
Transferrin, serum, 137
Transfusion, exchange, 61, 95
Transport of patient, 12–13f, 15–16
Treatment. *See also* under specific type of burn
  complications from, 162, 164
  in emergency department, 15–19f
  of multiple disaster burn victims, 13–14
  with respiratory complications, 154–159t
  on scene, 10–12
Triceps skinfold thickness, 136, 138t
Trichloracetic acid, 194–195
Trichloroethanes, 195
Tube feeding. *See* Enteral nutrition
Types of burns, in children, 203–204t

University of California, Irvine, Burn Center formula, 71, 73f
Urine output, monitoring of, 81–82

Vaccines, 61
Vascular resistance, 29f
Vascular response to burn injury, local, 27–28f
Vasopressin, 95
Ventilators, 214, 219f
Ventilatory support, for inhalation injury, 158–159t
Visual imagery, 259
Vital signs, monitoring of, 80–81
Vitamin requirements, 141
Vocational rehabilitation, 259
Voltage, 184, 186t

Water
  evaporative loss, 32, 33f
  loss, following thermal injury, 42–43
  lung, 166
Weight-height index, 136, 138t
Whirlpool agitation, 110f
White phosphorus, 195, 200
Wick catheter, 121–122f
Work, return to
  desensitization and, 259–260
  disability time and, 243–244
  rehabilitation and, 239–240
Workmen's compensation, 239
Wound
  depth. *See* Depth of burn
  excision. *See* Excision
  size, estimation in children, 204, 205f
  superficial, 23–24

Xenografts, 103
Xenon scanning, 153
X-ray, chest, 89, 156

Zone of coagulation, 26f, 27
Zone of hyperemia, 26f
Zone of necrosis, 26f
Zone of stasis, 26–27f, 34, 95